Ten Lessons in Clinical Acupuncture

Ten Lessons in Clinical Acupuncture

By

Changzhen Gong and Wei Liu

Cambridge
Scholars
Publishing

Ten Lessons in Clinical Acupuncture

By Changzhen Gong and Wei Liu

This book first published 2023

Cambridge Scholars Publishing

Lady Stephenson Library, Newcastle upon Tyne, NE6 2PA, UK

British Library Cataloguing in Publication Data
A catalogue record for this book is available from the British Library

ISBN (10): 1-5275-4266-1
ISBN (13): 978-1-5275-4266-2

TABLE OF CONTENTS

PREFACE

The ancient art of acupuncture, involving the precise insertion of slender needles into the body to address ailments, has endured for millennia as a revered healing practice. Although many in the Western world have been skeptical or even dismissive, scientific scrutiny has substantiated the efficacy of acupuncture as a healing modality. Today, none but the most resistant would deny that acupuncture can be effective – sometimes stunningly effective – in its clinical applications.

It is often said that Western science is reductive in its search for the specific enzyme, molecule, chemical reaction, or neural pathway that produces the observed phenomenon or desired result. This is frequently contrasted with the "holistic" approach of traditional Eastern medicine, based in a philosophical worldview which sees all life as part of an interconnected web: to remove anything from this web and isolate it for analysis is to destroy the delicate balance of elements which sustain it.

Is there any ground on which these two approaches to science and medicine can meet? Can two worldviews not only meet, but blend, and demonstrate the best qualities of both?

Ten Lessons in Clinical Acupuncture is an attempt to merge these medical worldviews. The cases presented in this book document the therapeutic success of acupuncture in a context of validated scientific research. Acupuncturists are empowered by the knowledge that there is a solid scientific basis for their traditional practice, while Western medical practitioners are given a perspective into the depth and complexity of acupuncture's theoretical basis and its coherence as a medical system. Ideally, *Ten Lessons in Clinical Acupuncture* can inspire a synergy between ancient wisdom and modern science, opening doors to mutual respect, appreciation, and cross-pollination of ideas, transcending cultural boundaries.

The health conditions covered in this book are very commonly seen in acupuncture clinics and hospitals: low back pain; knee osteoarthritis; dysmenorrhea; stroke; nausea and vomiting; IVF for infertility; hypertension; Parkinson's disease; schizophrenia; and breech presentation. The selection of these specific ten conditions for inclusion is based on the authors' experience giving presentations and lectures to the acupuncture and medical community in the United States and around the world. Lectures dealing with these conditions were the most frequently requested – our "top ten."

Ten Lessons in Clinical Acupuncture details the classical treatment protocols for each health condition, substantiated by modern scientific studies including basic mechanism research and clinical observations, clinical trials, systematic reviews, and meta-analysis. The integration of classical tradition with evidence-based research reflects the evolution of acupuncture in the modern world. Scientific investigations breathe new life into ancient principles, revealing their efficacy and mechanisms of action. This synthesis honors acupuncture's rich heritage while acknowledging its adaptability and relevance in contemporary healthcare systems.

Since acupuncture was introduced to mainstream society in the United States in the 1970's, scientific studies of acupuncture have increased exponentially in every decade. Acupuncture has become an agenda item for internationally-recognized institutions including the World Health Organization (WHO), National Institutes of Health (NIH), National Cancer Institute (NCI), German Federal Committee of Physicians and Health Insurers (G-BA), and the National Institute for Health and Care Excellence (NICE). Numerous well-established research institutes in China, Japan and Korea have dedicated themselves to unraveling acupuncture's mysteries, shedding light on its mechanisms, efficacy, and clinical applications. The influential Acupuncture Consensus Statement issued by the National Institutes of Health (NIH) [1] stands as a groundbreaking endorsement, acknowledging acupuncture's effectiveness in treating a range of conditions. Such recognition solidifies its position as a valuable therapeutic tool. The British Medical Journal further bolstered acupuncture's scientific credibility through a comprehensive assessment of 14000 clinical trials [2], 2400 systematic reviews and meta-analyses [3], and 139 clinical guidelines [4]. This monumental effort consolidates a vast body of evidence supporting acupuncture's efficacy and safety.

In the dynamic healthcare landscape, acupuncturists must continuously expand their knowledge and skills to stay competitive. *Ten Lessons in Clinical Acupuncture* is an invaluable reference, providing practical guidance for effective treatment while enhancing acupuncturists' professional acceptance and credibility in the eyes of the public. As the chapters unfold, readers explore the complexities of the human body and are challenged to harness the full potential of acupuncture as a therapeutic modality. Marrying classical tradition with evidence-based scientific research, this work embodies progress, propelling acupuncture into an arena of acceptance and recognition, and paving the way for a future where the medical worldviews of Eastern and Western medicine coexist harmoniously.

ACKNOWLEDGEMENTS

Many people have made this book possible, including the practitioners, patients, students, and staff members who have been part of TCM Health Center and the American Academy of Traditional Chinese Medicine over the past twenty-eight years. I want to thank them all.

I am most heavily indebted to my wife, Wei Liu, and my executive secretary, Leila Nielsen: they have been fundamental to the accomplishment of this book. Wei Liu is my life companion and a remarkable acupuncture practitioner. For her, every patient is not only a respected individual, but an opportunity to expand her clinical and academic experience. All of the patient cases in this book, excluding those provided through the courtesy of other doctors, are derived from her practice. Leila Nielsen has worked as my executive secretary and chief operating officer, and has also functioned as my editor for twenty-five years. Her ability to render my prose into clear, concise English (and her frequent requests for clarification) have been instrumental in achieving my goal of presenting the theory and practice of acupuncture and Chinese medicine to healthcare professionals and the general public in a straightforward, understandable form.

I am grateful to Allerton Press for giving me permission to include some of my published articles from the *International Journal of Clinical Acupuncture*. In the capacities of associate editor and Editor-in-Chief, I have served the *International Journal of Clinical Acupuncture* for twenty years.

Of course, any errors, or incorrectly-attributed sources are solely my responsibility.

CHAPTER ONE

ACUPUNCTURE FOR LOW BACK PAIN

Introduction

Acupuncturists treat a lot of patients with back pain; so many in fact, that many acupuncture clinics in the United States rate back pain as the number one condition treated. Acupuncture and Chinese medical textbooks are full of protocols and case studies, presenting a host of treatment approaches. Treatments for back pain as well as other conditions are provided according to Chinese medicine pattern differentiation in most contemporary texts. This trend of delineating protocols based on Chinese internal medicine began in the 1950s. One unfortunate consequence of adherence to pattern differentiation is the loss of flexibility in applying acupuncture's unique meridian theory. Historically, Chinese herbal medicine focused more on internal disharmony, while acupuncturists often drew on their knowledge of meridian theory and qi-flow. These attempts to form a unified field of medicine and educational standards evoke concern among scholars and practitioners, as the medicine is dynamic and diverse, and is regarded as a constantly evolving medicinal-art in addition to being a science. This chapter presents acupuncture cases and treatment protocols derived from classical and contemporary approaches to low back pain. Chapter forty-one from one of the most respected Chinese medical sources, the *Yellow Emperor's Classic of Medicine,* is referenced for perspective. This entire chapter discusses a classical approach to the treatment of back pain. For contrast, treatment approaches within the *Yellow Emperor's Classic of Medicine* are presented along-side a more contemporary style as exhibited by Yang Jiasan. Case histories are woven through this chapter from China's leading acupuncture scholars and practitioners, these personal accounts bringing theories to life. To further substantiate theoretical expositions, historical accounts, and recent subjective experience; recent clinical trials, systematic reviews and meta-analysis follow. Hopefully, this compilation of varied information will provide what is necessary to validate the wide-spread use of acupuncture in the treatment of back pain for those who may benefit.

Many have experienced low back pain. From dull pain with subtle onset and slow progression to sudden, sharp or persistent pain emanating from below the waist to the tailbone; pain in the low back can range from bothersome to debilitating. Pain may even extend down the back or sides of the legs all the way to the feet, as is common in sciatic pain. Muscle strain, often related to excessive physical labor, heavy lifting, forceful movement, bending or twisting in awkward positions, or prolonged periods of standing still is a leading precipitating factor in the initial onset of many cases of low back pain.

Low back pain is not considered a "disease" but exists on its own as a chief complaint in otherwise healthy individuals; however, it may also co-occur along with many other conditions and disease states. From both eastern and western perspectives, a multitude of underlying problems, ranging in seriousness, may be at the root of the issue. Most LBP cases do not arise from what could be defined as a single cause but are understood to manifest after a series or combination of less-noticeable muscle or skeletal sprains, strains or tendency toward holding the body in sub-optimal alignment patterns. Habits and tendencies that affect overall health and well-being such as obesity, smoking, weight gain during pregnancy, stress, poor diet, lack of physical conditioning, poor posture and maladaptive sleeping position may contribute to low-back discomfort and pain. A larger list of potential contributing factors include osteoarthritis, degeneration of the discs between the vertebrae or spinal disc herniation, vertebral fractures, and occasionally, an infection or tumor in or near the spine.

It is not uncommon for women or men to have acute low back pain related to medical conditions of the reproductive system: endometriosis, ovarian cysts, cancer of the reproductive organs, uterine fibroids, enlarged prostate or kidney issues may all coincide with low back pain. It has been reported that almost half of all pregnant women experience low back or sacral pain as muscles and ligaments are stretched by the changes in posture and shifting center of gravity that naturally occurs during pregnancy.

Low back pain is frequently associated with musculoskeletal issues, inflammation, spinal tumors, and infections. In cases of low back pain related to musculoskeletal etiology, the problem can be purely mechanical, categorized as strain, muscle spasm, or vertebral arthritis. Herniations of the disks, stenosis or fractures may all arise spontaneously or be due to compression over time. Low back pain often coincides with inflammatory conditions such as HLA-B27 derived arthritis and related conditions such as ankylosing spondylitis, reactive arthritis or psoriatic arthritis. Inflammatory bowel disease may also present with low back pain. When tumors exist within the spine (often metastasizing from other cancers such as breast, prostate and lung), the pressure and infringement may cause discomfort, pain or debility. Sometimes, when no mechanical or other cause can be identified, an infection along the spine is found to be the source of acute or persistent low back pain.

Of the varied etiologies from which back pain may arise, nerve compression is a common element. Trauma, degeneration and declining health due to age may cause bulging or herniated discs in which the softer interior protrudes through a crack or fissure in the protective outer coating of the disk. The vertebrae then lose their cushion and the friction causes pain due to nerve compression or inflammation. Spinal stenosis, or the narrowing of the spinal canal, arthritis (spinal osteoarthritis), or spondylosis may also cause irritation due to changes in the facets and resultant bone spurs. Spondylolisthesis, or slipping of one lumbar vertebra over another, fractures due to chronic stress or trauma and osteomyelitis, a common bacterial infection of the bone, may produce low back pain. In addition to painful malignant tumors, benign masses or tumors may also arise in the spine causing undue pressure on the spine.

Medications, surgery and physical therapy are common conventional interventions, with acupuncture also gaining global recognition as an effective remedy. A discussion on the classical and contemporary acupuncture approaches to low back pain follows.

The Yellow Emperor's Approach

This section was inspired by chapter forty-one of the *Yellow Emperor's Classic of Medicine,* in which back pain is categorized by meridian differentiation. Patterns have been grouped into three sections: differentiation according to the six stages; differentiation by the extraordinary channels; and differentiation by accompanying symptoms [1].

1. Low Back Pain according to the Six Stages

Differentiation by the six stages (twelve channels) is a fundamental concept described in the *Yellow Emperor's Classic of Medicine*. The six stages belonging to taiyang, yangming, shaoyang, taiyin, shaoyin and jueyin. This categorization method is used to pair the twelve meridians (channels) according to depth. A full understanding of disease pathogenesis via the stages is illustrated in the *Treatise of Cold Febrile Disease* (or *On Cold*

Damage) written by Zhang Zhongjing (150-219 AD). Low back pain and any other condition can be viewed from the perspective of which of the six stages each individual case fits into.

Starting with the most exterior of the stages, low back pain due to a disorder of the foot taiyang, or urinary bladder meridian meets specific criteria. This type of back pain will be characterized by pain that radiates from the neck down to the lower back and to the sacrum. The patient feels heaviness and downward pressure as if carrying a heavy load on his back. In taiyang back pain, needling or bloodletting may be applied to Weizhong (BL40). During the spring season, the wood element is growing along with the supply of water. The taiyang meridian consists mainly of cold water, therefore needling Weizhong (UB40) will not draw blood.

In cases where lower back pain is due to disharmony of the foot shaoyang or gallbladder channel, symptoms will manifest more prominently on the sides of the body along the gallbladder meridian. The low back pain often feels like a needle is pricking the skin at the waist. Gradually, the pain progresses to the back and up the neck to the base of the skull. Pain prevents the patient from looking either up or downward or to either side. Needling and bloodletting the Yanglingquan (GB34), which is in the depression inferior to the head of the fibula, releases stagnation from the channel and tendons. During the summer season, fire burns intensely hot. The shaoyang channel belongs to the element of fire, therefore needle the Yanglingquan (GB34) will have no bleeding.

If lower back pain originates from a disharmony within the foot yangming, or stomach channel, pain maybe so severe that the patient cannot move his head at all. In addition to pain, any movement may cause dizziness and blurry vision. Melancholy may overwhelm the patient. Needling with bloodletting at Zusanli (ST36) three consecutive times, until blood is produced, will remove the stagnation between the upper and lower body. Since metal dominates the autumn season, and the yangming channel belongs to metal, needling Zusanli (ST36) in autumn will not produce blood.

Lower back pain manifesting from foot shaoyin, or the kidney channel often produces deeper symptoms. The pain often radiates along the spine and down the kidney channel along the inner side of the leg. Needling and bloodletting Taixi (KI3), in the depression posterior to the medial malleolus, twice removes blockage causing shaoyin low back pain. Shaoyin qi is stored during the winter. Needling Taixi (KI3) at the beginning of spring, should not produce blood. If this point does bleed in the spring, it will be difficult to treat low back pain the following winter.

When lower back pain results from imbalance in the foot jueyin, or liver channel, stiff low back predominates, as if a bow is pulled at maximum tension, ready to shoot. The pain is characterized as being both tense and taut. Palpation from the heel along the posterior side of the lower leg to the calf will reveal tension with multiple knots. Low back pain of this type will be relieved by needling these knots. If the patient also shows signs of liver yang rising, such as agitation, short-temper, speaking loudly or yelling; or seems abnormally quiet due to liver qi deficiency, needle these knots three times along with Ligou (LR5).

2. Low Back Pain Differentiated according to the Extraordinary Channels

In addition to the twelve primary channels, low back pain may manifest due to disorders of one or more of the eight extraordinary meridians. Symptoms associated with these extraordinary channels may direct the differential pattern diagnosis and treatment prescription to focus on the indicated extraordinary vessel.

When lower back pain is associated with a disorder of the jie channel, which connects with the horizontal collaterals, signs and symptoms may be noticed along the underneath the skin where these collaterals are scattered, starting from the foot taiyang bladder channel. Since jie channel circulation does not reach the head, disharmony in this vessel may be detected by pain radiating to the shoulder and causing blurry vision. Concurrently, blockage of bladder qi may cause urinary incontinence. Needling and bloodletting the lateral side of Weizhong (BL40) where it connects to the horizontal collateral channel of the knee relieves blockage along this vessel. Bleed until all the dark red blood has escaped and bright red blood appears.

Because the jie channel, which is scattered underneath the skin, runs up and down the length of the body and circulates around the entire body, lower back pain arising from a problem in the jie channel may have symptoms anywhere along the pathway. One manifestation is pain at the waist so severe that the bone feels as if it's cracked and broken. An underlying kidney qi deficiency is at the root of this manifestation, and the patient may be extremely terrified and frightened. Needling and bloodletting at Weizhong (BL40), in the center of the knot (which will be about the size of a rice grain) will unbind the qi. As above, the point is bled until the dark red blood is expelled and bright red blood begins to flow.

When lower back pain is related to the tongyin channel, which is yangqiao channel (3), the patient feels as if a small hammer is pounding at the waist; the patient's face will also be swollen. Needling Jinmen (BL63), at the end of the fibula, lateral to the malleolus, three times, relieves this kind of back pain.

Lower back pain due to a disorder of the yangwei channel manifests as facial swelling and pain. Needling the channel at Chengshan (BL57) which is the crossing-point of the yangwei meridian and the foot taiyang urinary bladder channel, located in the depression at the lower juncture of the calf muscles.

When lower back pain results from disorder of the dai mai, or belt channel, that encircles the waist, pain stops the patient from looking up or down. If the patient does look up, he tends to stumble and fall. This condition most often arises when heavy lifting has injured the lower back. Blood stagnation at the transverse fossa, is the source of the severe pain. Needling Fuxi (BL38) and Weiyang (BL39) twice until bleeding occurs will remove the blockage and pain.

When there is a disharmony of the huiyin, or Ren channel, low back pain results from both yin and yang deficiency. Spontaneous sweating, thirst, and the desire to drink due to yin deficiency, combined with increased urination due to yang deficiency are the telltale signs. Needling Chengjin (BL56), five cun below the popliteal crease, or Chengshan (BL57) three times to provoke bleeding. From the text, it seems that BL56 is intended, although Chengshan (BL57) is the point named in Su Wen's interpretation. The text also more generally mentions the horizontal collaterals, which include both points.

Lower back pain of the feiyang, or yinwei channel presents with swelling of the face that makes one look very angry; however, lack of sufficient heart qi combined with kidney yin deficiency more often correlate to feelings of extreme sadness and terror. Needling Zhubin (KI9), located five cun above the medial malleolus relieves pain and related symptoms; it is the crossing-point of the feiyang and yinwei channels.

When lower back pain is due to a disorder in the cangyang, or yinqiao meridian, in which the circulation does not reach the head, pain radiates to the chest, and the vision is blurry. In severe cases, the patient cannot unfurl, bending backward is impossible and the patient is not able to talk. Needling Jiaoxin (KI8), located two cun above the medial malleolus, twice will relieve the back pain and related symptoms. Jiaoxin (KI8) is a coalescent point on the yinqiao channel and a powerful point for movement and mobility issues.

In patients with lower back pain manifesting from blood deficiency within the scattered, or chong, channel (which is said to be scattered underneath the skin), itchy skin and surface heat sensations will manifest. The combined symptoms tend to create irritability and restlessness, and if the bladder is overly warm, urinary incontinence ensues. With low back pain due to blood deficiency in the chong meridian, the patient may feel a sense that there is a piece of wood stuck horizontally to the lower back. Needling Dubi (ST35) three times (and ST36, according to Wu's translation) will resolve this condition.

Low back pain accompanied by a cough so fiercely painful that the body spasms indicates that the rouli channel, which is a sinew channel, is imbalanced. Needling shallow sinew points along the shaoyang gallbladder meridian between points Yangfu (GB38) and Xuanzhong (GB39), bilaterally, twice will alleviate the condition.

When low back pain radiating along the spine and up to the head manifests with a very heavy head, blurred vision, stiffness and instability to the point of falling down easily, needling and bleeding Weizhong (BL40) will rectify the patient. If the patient is simultaneously suffering from low back pain and the common cold, needling the foot taiyang channel to reinforce the yang qi will be beneficial. If the patient's low back pain coincides with a fever, needling the foot jueyin meridian will reduce symptoms. If the patient is stricken with back pain that restricts the ability to look up or down, needling the foot shaoyang meridian will relieve the pain. When the patient has a cough with a moderate fever, needling the foot shaoyin meridian until bleeding occurs will expel the fever and reduce pain.

3. Acupuncture for Low Back Pain according to Accompanying Symptoms

Different kinds of back pain are can be differentiated into patterns according to accompanying symptoms. Specific groups of symptoms lead to identification of meridian involvement and precise treatment strategies. Some basic guidelines are as follows:

If external cold invasion has rendered a patient unable to turn his head, needling the foot yangming meridian is indicated.

If the patient exhibits a high fever, needling the foot taiyin meridian is likely to resolve the exterior.

If the patient is coughing and has a moderate fever, needling the foot shaoyin meridian will alleviate the condition.

If the patient is constipated, needling the foot shaoyin meridian will unblock the channel.

If the patient's abdomen is distended, needling the foot jueyin meridian will reduce the pressure.

If the patient's body movements are restricted and he is unable to bend, can neither look up nor down needling the foot taiyang meridian clears the channel.

If pain radiates along the spine and down the inner leg, needling the foot shaoyin meridian restores the kidneys to relieve pain.

When lower back pain is associated with constriction in the lower abdomen, and the patient cannot stand upright or look up, needle the eight lower baliao points in the sacral foramen, which belong to the foot taiyang meridian. Treatments for this condition are best when correlated with the wax and wane of the moon. On the first day, needle once; on the second day, needle twice. Following in this pattern allows a gradual increase in frequency while the moon is gaining, until a maximum of fifteen needle insertions are given on the fifteenth day of the month. Decrease number of needles per day in the same fashion starting with fourteen needles on the sixteenth day. The left side is needled in cases of right-sided pain, whereas the right side is needled with left-sided pain.

TCM Approach

Traditional Chinese medicine (TCM) diagnostics and treatment approaches for acute and chronic backaches vary according to the specific channels involved and the selected needling technique. Selecting which channels to treat and which needling technique to apply often take precedence over pattern identification in cases of back pain, unless herbal formulas are prescribed. In discussions on back pain, modern textbooks commonly focus on just four patterns: invasion of cold and dampness, qi and blood stagnation, kidney deficiency and liver qi stagnation. In clinical practice, combined patterns are frequently seen. For example, patients may have backache from cold-damp invasion against a background of kidney yang deficiency; or qi and blood stagnation with an underlying kidney deficiency. Methods of tonifying deficiencies are combined with practices that eliminate pathogenic factors. When a patient is suffering from chronic recurring backache from cold-damp invasion, while at the same time has an underlying persistent kidney yang deficiency pattern, herbal formula Shen Zhao Tang (*Kidney Warming Decoction)* may be administered, modified with additional kidney-yang tonics.

As a leading acupuncture scholar and practitioner in the twentieth century, Yang Jiasan [2] illustrates eight potential TCM patterns for back pain: cold dampness, damp heat, blood stasis, kidney deficiency, wind cold, phlegm dampness and strain or sprain. Out of the many possible Chinese medical approaches to take in treating back pain, some of Yang Jiasan's have been shared.

1. Back Pain due to Cold Dampness

A patient presenting with back pain arising from cold dampness may manifest with a sense of heaviness, stiffness and difficulty turning or rotating. Symptoms will tend to be worse on rainy, snowy or cloudy days, and will improve in warm, dry weather. Low back will feel cold, and the patient may carry extra water weight. Abdominal distention may arise due to undue stress on the spleen, along with clear urine which may be excessive or hindered due to cold and dampness affecting the kidney and urinary bladder. The tongue coating may be white and greasy, while the tongue body may be swollen, tooth-marked and pale or bluish. The pulse may be slow, soggy and full. Yang Jiasan states there are no fixed ashi or trigger points for this pattern.

In back pain due to an invasion of cold dampness, pain is due to damp cold obstructing the meridians and collaterals impairing the free flow of qi and blood. Both yin in nature, cold pathogenic factors contract while damp creates stickiness. Lying down compounds damp stagnation, making the patient feel worse; while heat and warmth dissipates the cold, which then helps the patient overcome dampness. Chinese herbal formulas that tonify the earth element or spleen, which improves digestion, administered along with herbs that also control the water element, warm the middle burner, dissipate coldness and dry the dampness are selected in this case to resolve back pain from cold damp invasion. Shen Zhuo Tang modified may be prescribed to resolve the back pain resulting from cold and damp. Included are Gan Jiang, Gan Cao, Fu Ling, Bai Zhu, Rou Gui, Ze Xie, Du Zhong and

Gou Ji. If the pain radiates to the lower limbs, remove Gan Jiang, add Du Huo, Fang Feng, Dang Gui, Shao Yao, Xi Xin and Niu Xi.

There are no herbs for releasing exterior in this prescription; Gan Jiang and Rou Gui are used to expel cold dampness, while the bitter and warm properties of Bai Zhu dry dampness. Gan Cao harmonizes the middle burner and tonifies the spleen; Fu Ling and Ze Xie reduce dampness. All the herbs combined warm the spleen and resolve the internal dampness, benefiting the earth and controlling water. Du Zhong and Gou Ji enter the kidney meridian and tonify kidney yang. Back pain radiating to the lower limbs indicates that cold dampness in invading the meridians, Du Huo and Fang Feng for releasing exterior are added to expel wind and reduce dampness in the low back and legs. Dang Gui and Shao Yao are used to tonify blood and nourish tendons. Xi Xin is used to warm and open the meridian blockage while Niu Xi's guiding properties direct the herbs downward to soothe the tendons and invigorate the collaterals.

In cases of low back pain due to cold and dampness, the excessive dampness, constrains the earth element (spleen); and the external cold dampness invasion injures the spleen yang. Acupuncture points that strengthen the spleen's function of controlling transportation and transformation of water dampness help resolve this condition. The yuan-source point of the spleen meridian and back-shu point of spleen with local moxibustion warm and strengthen the spleen yang, dissipate cold and reduce dampness. Yuan source point, Taibai (SP3); back-shu point, Pishu (BL20); may be administered along with Sanyinjiao (SP6) and Ashi points in this case. Taibai (SP3) is the earth point of the spleen meridian and functions to strengthen the spleen's capacity to transform dampness. Taibai (SP3), together with Pishu (BL20), the entry site of the spleen meridian qi, makes up the powerful back-shu and yuan-source combination.

When low back pain due to cold dampness presents with coughing, the *Yellow Emperor's Classic of Medicine: Plain Questions, On Coughing*, suggests needling back-shu points for zang diseases. Tonifying Taibai (SP3) strengthens the spleen and transforms damp, while warming the spleen, or earth element. Sanyinjiao (SP6) is the meeting point of liver, spleen and kidney meridians and functions to strengthen the spleen, transform dampness and is a powerful point to treat diseases of cold dampness invading the kidneys. Applying moxibustion to Ashi points located in the low back area can further dissipate cold dampness.

2. Back Pain due to Damp Heat

Clinical indications that back pain is due to damp heat, include pain along the spine in the lower back accompanied by heat sensations along the pathway of pain, joints may appear red and swollen. Warmth and pressure will exacerbate the condition and the patient will be restless, thirsty, pass scanty yellow urine and will tend to be constipated. The tongue will have a yellow and greasy coating and the pulse will show excess and will be soggy and rapid.

Pathogenic damp heat accumulations may obstruct the meridians and easily affects the joints, causing redness and swelling. Pain along the spine in the lower back results. Heat is a yang pathogen; damp heat burns up body fluids and cuts-off the supply of body fluid from being disseminated upwards, the lack of fluids combined with heat in the upper jiao then create restlessness and thirst. Damp heat tends to pour downward, creating scanty, turbid and yellowish urine. This pattern may be treated by herbal formulas that strengthening the yin while reducing dampness, such as Si Miao Wan which includes Cang Zhu, Huang Bai, and Yi Yi Ren.

In general, the low back is considered to be the mansion of the kidneys. In most cases of low back pain, the kidneys need to be strengthened. Huang Bai's bitter and cool nature strengthens the yin and clears heat. In order to control kidney water, the spleen must be strengthened. Cang Zhu's bitter and acrid properties serve to strengthen the spleen while drying dampness. Yi Yi Ren expels dampness and fortifies the spleen. Niu Xi invigorate blood, opens blockages in the meridians while guiding the herbs downward.

Acupuncture along the urinary bladder meridian helps transform dampness and clears the excess heat. Shenshu (BL23), Weizhong (BL40) and Xiaochangshu (BL27) are prescribed. In this prescription, Shenshu (BL23) is the generating site of the kidney meridian qi and functions to clear damp heat in the lower burner. Weizhong (BL40) is the he-sea and earth point of the urinary bladder meridian and is the connecting point of the kidney and spleen meridians. It serves to strengthen the spleen, transform dampness and clear heat. Weizhong (BL40) is also named as Xuexi (blood cleft). *Interpretation of Meridian Points* notes that Weizhong (BL40) is used to clear pathogenic heat in the qi and blood, and often used to remove dampness and invigorate blood in the lower back. Bloodletting on Weizhong (BL40) is most applicable to this pattern. Together, Shenshu (BL23) and Weizhong (BL40) are an exterior/interior and back-shu/he-sea combination. They reduce fu while reinforcing zang organs. Along with

Xiaochangshu (BL27), back-shu of the small intestine (which is the fu organ of the fire element), this prescription will clear fire in the small intestines to assist to expel damp heat in the lower burner.

3. Back Pain due to Blood Stasis

After injury, blood stasis obstructs the meridians and collaterals impairing the flow of qi and blood. Clinical manifestations indicating that back pain is due to blood stasis include: pain at fixed sites, pain like being poked by needles, history of injury, pain worse with pressing or moving, pain worse at night and better in the daytime, dark bowel movement, clear urine, dark blood, dark and purple tongue with dark spots and a choppy pulse.

This pattern may be treated by tonifying the blood while nourishing the yin, moving the qi and relieving pain. A Chinese herbal formula such as Huo Xue Wi Wu Tang may be administered. It includes Dang Gui, Chuan Xiong, Sheng Di Huang, Shao Yao, Rou Gui, Tao Ren, Hong Hua, and Yan Hu Suo. If the patient has limited range of motion of the head and neck, add Mu Xiang, Hui Xiang, and Gan Cao to the prescription. In this prescription, Dang Gui is the main herb for the blood; it opens the liver meridian while tonifying and invigorating the blood. Sheng Di Huang opens the kidney meridian and tonifies the blood while nourishing the yin. Chuan Xiong regulates qi and blood, opens the liver meridian and circulates the qi in blood. Chi Shao regulates the yin in the blood, it opens the spleen meridian and harmonizes the blood to stop pain. These four herbs unique properties are combined to treat various blood related diseases. Tao Ren, Hong Hua and Yan Hu Suo function to eliminate blood stasis and stop pain. Stagnated blood in the meridians and collaterals improves with warmth. This is accomplished by Rou Gui, which warms the kidney yang. Back pain caused by injury creates disharmony of the meridian qi, leading to qi stagnation and blood stasis. Mu Xiang, and Xiao Hui Xiang are used to move the qi, then invigorate the blood. Once the blockage is removed, the pain is relieved.

Acupuncture also will relive back pain due to blood stasis by moving and harmonizing the qi and blood. Local acupuncture points on the bladder meridian are used to stop the pain along with distal points that eliminate blood stasis. Ashi points in the lower back are selected for the application of round-sharp needles with cupping. Bloodletting with three-edge needles is applied to Weizhong (BL40). In this treatment protocol, Ashi points are selected from the pain sites and shallow needling with round-sharp needles plus cupping is performed. Cupping sucks out the stagnated blood and new blood is generated. Weizhong (BL40) is bled to remove the stagnated blood in the low back. The combination of applying blood-letting techniques at distal point Weizhong (BL40) and local Ashi points clear the stagnated blood.

4. Back Pain due to Kidney Deficiency

Back pain due to kidney deficiency is generally chronic, manifesting with soreness and weakness which may be relieved by pressure and kneading; this kind of back pain tends to be aggravated by prolonged standing and over-strain. Breathlessness, low-pitched ear ringing, weak back and knees, frequent urination, seminal emission, pale or dark complexion, exhaustion, pale tongue, and a deep, weak pulse may also be present. Kidney yang deficiency tends to have more cold signs such as feeling cold especially in the low back and spine; cold joints, especially knees; pale urine; aversion to cold and a curled body. Red cheeks, slight red face, heat in the palms, red tongue with very little coating, thin and rapid pulse are typical symptoms of kidney yin deficiency plus heat.

The low back is considered to be the mansion of the kidneys. Kidneys control the bones and marrow. Deficiency of kidney essence and lack of nourishment in the spine, creates feebleness and weakness. Kidney deficiency may exhibit with lack of persistence in a patient. Deficient and deep kidney pulses will accompany.

In cases of back pain due to kidney yin deficiency, nourishing yin and tonifying the kidneys with herbal prescriptions such as Liu Wei Di Huang Wan will help restore the patient. Liu Wei Di Huang Wan includes Shu Di Huang, Shan Zhu Yu, Shan Yao, Fu Ling and Mu Dan Pi. If the patient experiences chest heat, crimson tongue and thin pulse, Gui Ban, Zhi Mu and Huang Bai can be added. When the patient complains of breathlessness and frequent urination, Rou Gui, Du Zhong and Bu Gu Zhi may be added.

Liu Wei Di Huang Wan is a leading formula to tonify the pure yin, moisten the lower burner and anchor yang. It strengthens the water element, which belongs to the kidneys. It is often used in cases yin deficiency, which manifest with five-center heat, a crimson tongue and thin pulse. Gui Ban, Zhi Mu and Huang Bai may be added to increase yin-nourishing capacity, dry dampness and strengthen the kidneys. Breathlessness and frequent, pale, clear urination indicate kidney yang deficiency. Rou Gui, Du Zhong and Bu Gu Zhi are added to assist the yang, warm the kidneys, benefit the fire element and eliminate yin factors suppressing yang.

Acupuncture may be used to replenish the water element and tonify the kidneys. The combination of back-shu point, Shenshu (BL23), and earth point, Taixi (KI3) are combined to address this pattern. Moxibustion may be added in cases of kidney yang deficiency. Fuliu (KI7) may be added to treat kidney yin deficiency, while Sanyinjiao (SP6) may be added for abdominal swelling. Zhongfeng (LR4) and Daimai (GB26) are added for low back pain with hypochondriac and abdominal discomfort or pain. In this treatment protocol, Shenshu (BL23) is the transporting site of the kidney meridian qi, and Taixi (KI3) is the yuan-source point for the kidney meridian. They are combined to nourish yin and tonify the kidneys. Moxibustion is added for kidney yang deficiency patients in order to assist yang and warm the kidneys. Kidney meridian belongs to the water element, and Fuliu (KI7) is the metal point on the water channel. The kidney meridian and lung meridian have a connection in that metal (lung) generates water. Fuliu (KI7) is selected for kidney yin deficiency when the lung is also affected. Pain affecting the abdomen and range of motions of movement is associated with the liver meridian; in this case, Zhongfeng (LR4) of the liver meridian and Daimai (GB26) of gallbladder meridian are paired.

5. Low Back Pain Due to Wind Cold

Low back pain due to wind cold may manifest suddenly; characterized by limited range of motion affecting the four limbs, the pain may radiate to the neck and upper back, or even to the hip and joints all over the body. Aversion to cold ranges from mild to extreme depending on strength of the pathogen and the patient's constitution. The patient's whole back may feel chilled and he may be sensitive to drafts. This kind of back pain is relieved with warmth. The tongue may have a thin, white coat; the pulse may be wiry, tight, slow and floating.

The bladder meridian of foot taiyang starts at the inner canthus of the eye, Jingming (BL1), ascends to the anterior hairline on the forehead, intersecting Toulinqi (GB15) and Shenting (DU24). It then continues posteriorly, 1.5 cun parallel to the midline of the scalp, the BL channel meets the DU at vertex point Baihui (DU20); after connecting with Baihui (DU20), the meridian continues to travel 1.5 cun parallel to the DU meridian to the nape of the neck at Tianzhu (BL10); from BL10, the meridian separates into two external branches; the 1st (medial) branch descends along the posterior aspect of the neck, intersecting Dazhui (DU14) and Taodao (DU13), then descends alongside the spine, 1.5 cun lateral to the midline, through the lumbar region; a sub-branch separates in the lumbar region, descends along the sacrum, crosses the buttock and descends to the popliteal fossa of the knee at Weizhong (BL40). The 2nd (lateral) branch separates at the nape of the neck and descends to the medial aspect of the scapula; descends parallel to the vertebral column, three cun lateral to the midline, to the gluteal region; crosses the buttock to intersect Huantiao (GB30), then descends along the lateroposterior aspect of the thigh to meet the other branch at Weizhong (BL40) in the popliteal fossa. The main meridian descends along the gastrocnemius muscle on the posterior aspect of the leg; continues to descend posterior to the lateral malleolus Kunlun (BL60); then follows the lateral aspect of the 5th metatarsal bone to terminate at Zhiyin (BL67), 0.1 cun proximal to the lateral corner of the nail of the small toe, where it joins with the kidney meridian.

When wind cold obstructs the bladder meridian, low back pain may manifest. In mild cases, stiffness and pain of the back occurs. In severe cases, tight pain pulls along the spine, as if the neck is pulled, low back is cut, and chest is broken off. The contractive nature of cold invasion leads to the impaired movement of the limbs. Cold wind and cold currents invade the low back, and aversion to cold develops. Cold pain in the back may be dissipated with warmth.

Clinically, this pattern can be treated by expelling the wind and dissipating cold with herbal formula Du Huo Ji Sheng Tang, which consists of: Du Huo, Sang Ji Sheng, Qin Jiao, Fang Feng, Xi Xin, Dang Gui, Shao Yao, Chuan Qiong, Shu Di Huang, Du Zhong, Niu Xi, Ren Shen, Fu Ling, Gan Cao and Gui Xin. In this prescription, Du Huo is used to dissipate cold and expel dampness in the low back and legs. Du Huo in combination with Qin Jiao and Fang Feng is used to stop bi pain. The Four-substance Decoction (Dang Gui, Shao Yao, Chuan Qiong, Shu Di Huang) is used to nourish and regulate blood, open the meridians and stop pain. Xi Xin functions to dissipate wind cold and stop pain. Du Zhong, Niu Xi and Sang Ji Sheng tonify and nourish the kidneys and liver, assist the yang, dissipate cold and stop pain. Gui Xin is used to warm the meridians and blood vessels, dissipate cold and expel dampness.

An effective acupuncture protocol for cases of low back pain due to wind cold damp invasion may include: Shenshu (BL23), Mingmen (DU4), Fengchi (GB20) and Yangfu (GB38). Moxibustion may be added to Shenshu (BL23) and Mingmen (DU4) to expel wind, dissipate cold, warm the meridians and remove blockages. In this treatment protocol, Shenshu (BL23) and Mingmen (DU4) are classic points for warming the meridians and expelling wind cold. Fengchi (GB20) is the meeting point of hand shaoyang, foot shaoyang and yangwei meridians and is an essential point for dissipating wind. Yangfu (GB38) is the fire point of the gallbladder meridian foot shaoyang. *Explanations of Meridian Points* by Yue Hanzhen states that wind, cold, fire and all external pathogens can be removed by needling this point.

6. Low Back Pain due to Phlegm Dampness

Low back pain due to phlegm dampness manifests as fixed pain in the back with a shape such as a strip, diamond, or triangle located at the sacrum. This type of pain is chronic and enduring, leaving the body fatigued. The patient's complexion is yellow and lackluster and the tongue will have a greasy, sticky coat. The pulse will be slippery and congested.

A patient with low back pain due to a damp phlegmy constitution combined with an externally contracted invasion of damp phlegm will tend to produce lumps of phlegm in the lower back. Damp phlegm is sticky and slow to resolve; making the pain chronic and enduring. Internally, dampness congests the spleen, impairing the transformation function. Over time, the Zang and Fu, meridians and collaterals, four limbs, sensory organs and nine orifices become malnourished; lassitude ensues and the four limbs and complexion take on a withered appearance.

Chinese herbal formula Er Chen Tang modified may be prescribed to resolve this pattern by drying the dampness and dissolving the phlegm. The formula contains Fu Ling, Chen Pi, Ban Xia, Gan Cao, Du Huo, Cang Zhu, and Mu Li. In this prescription, the acrid and warm nature of Ban Xia dries dampness and dissolves phlegm. Chen Pi regulates qi and dries dampness, while transforming phlegm dampness by promoting movement of qi. Fu Ling strengthens the spleen and dissipates dampness. Zhi Gan Cao harmonizes all herbs in the prescription. For back pain, Du Huo is necessary to guide the herbs to move downward in order to dissipate wind and transform dampness in the lower jiao and legs. Cang Zhu strengthens the spleen and dries dampness. Mu Li enters the kidney meridian, softens hard masses and resolves nodules and lumps while strengthening bones and benefiting the kidneys. The combination of herbs in this decoction dissolve phlegm, transform dampness, regulate meridians and remove blockages.

Acupuncture protocols that focus on strengthening the spleen, dissolving phlegm, dissipating nodules and opening the meridians are effective in relieving back pain due to phlegm dampness. Taibai (SP3) and Fenglong (ST40) are selected, along with local points at the sites of the lumps. Vertical and direct needling is applied to the lumps without twisting and rotating until the needle reaches the bottom of the lumps, then twisting and rotating and lifting and thrusting are applied. Lifting and thrusting is repeated through the depth of the pathogenic accumulation, The technique involves obtaining qi, and then directing the needle in five different directions (Hegu needling). Hegu needling is a technique used to strengthen the spleen, dissolve phlegm and dissipate nodules. Taibai (SP3) is the earth and yuan-source point of the spleen meridian, reinforcing this point can strengthen the spleen and dissolve phlegm. Fenglong (ST40) which is the luo-connecting point of the stomach meridian, combined with Taibai (SP3) make up the yuan-source and luo-connecting combo, providing substantial power to strengthen the spleen and dissolve phlegm. Additionally, Fenglong (ST40) is an essential point for treating any phlegm disease.

7. Low Back Pain due to Strains

Low back pain due to strain is fixed on both sides of the spine and is not relieved by lying down. Pain is reduced after getting up in the morning and moving around. Mild exercise and physical activities improve back pain due to strain. Working in the same position for prolonged periods of time places undue burden on the low back, leading to sub-optimal qi and blood circulation. Physical activities move stagnant qi; stuck blood then follows the qi, resulting in alleviation of pain and improved circulation of qi and blood.

Acupuncture treatment applied to Ashi points soothes the tendons and invigorate the collaterals. Fen Ci (needling between muscles), a technique from the Yellow Emperor's Classic of Medicine, soothes the tendons and invigorates collaterals, channel qi and blood in cases of muscle-strain-induced back pain. Mild stimulation tends to be effective.

8. Low Back Pain due to Sprains

Low back pain arising after an injury sprains the low back, manifesting with sharp pain when postural adjustments are made, on deep inhalation or with coughing or sneezing. No obvious Ashi points can be identified as the locus of pain in these cases. After the injury, the qi stagnation combines with blood and obstructs the meridians and collaterals. Pain is exacerbated by activity because some of the peripheral collaterals are empty or deficient.

Acupuncture treatment is used to open the meridians and invigorate the collaterals, move qi and invigorate blood, and often performed with distal needling and physical movement. Zanzhu (BL2) is needled when the pain is located on both sides of the back. Renzhong (DU26) is needled if the pain is located on the spine of the back. Mild needling or needling at the collaterals is performed at the location of the pain. Bloodletting on Weizhong (ST40) is administered to remove stagnation from the bladder channel. Yang Ci (a technique from the *Yellow Emperor's Classic of Medicine*) as described previously, on the local area and cupping can also be applied.

The patient is directed to walk with two feet separate. Distal needling on Zanzhu (BL2) or Renzhong (DU26) with reducing technique by twisting and rotating needles while the patient's moves the low back helps relieve stagnation at the injured site. Shallow needling on sensitive points with reducing technique by twisting and rotating while the patient's moves the painful area of the low back also helps resolve the stagnation and speeds healing. Yang Ci is one of the twelve techniques in the Official Needling from the *Yellow Emperor's Classic of Medicine*: Spiritual Pivot. One needle is inserted in the center, with four needles on the sides. This technique has evolved into plum blossom needling with bloodletting and cupping.

Twenty-six patterns from the *Yellow Emperor's Classic of Medicine* and eight patterns from Yang Jiasan's summarization provide some advanced examples of acupuncture and Chinese medical approaches in the treatment of low back pain. That does not necessarily mean that each individual case fits into one of these patterns as the following case histories attempt to illustrate.

Case Reports from China's Leading Practitioners

In the above two sections, classical approaches from the *Yellow Emperor's Classic of Medicine* and a contemporary approach represented by Yang Jiasan have been introduced. Even though these approaches are fairly comprehensive, the following case studies provide a glimpse into the tremendously diverse and virtually unlimited field of options within the acupuncture and Chinese medicine cabinet. These varied approaches may be dispensed for the purpose of healing back pain at the root as well as the branch. The following ten cases offer a sampling of how standardized approaches may be adapted to fit each unique case. These real-life applications more closely reflect the dynamic art-form Chinese medicine takes in practice. Consistent with human life, experiential knowledge allows for the resolution of known illnesses while the creative application of reliable principles allows for solutions to seemingly new or previously incurable conditions to emerge.

1. Yu Shuzhuang's Case [3]

A 46-year-old woman had suffered from low back pain for years, more severe on the right side. Marked pain occurred when standing and pain was aggravated with movement. The pain prevented her from lying flat. Other symptoms included poor appetite, dizziness, dream-disturbed sleep and fidgeting. Her tongue was pale red with a dry coating. Acupuncture had been applied to Kunlun (BL60) and Houxi (SI3) without success. Then she told the doctor that she had a prolapsed uterus (II) for three years with a bearing-down sensation in the lower abdomen. The Chinese medicine pattern was diagnosed as deficiency of the spleen and kidney with concurrent sinking of qi. The treatment principle chosen in this case was to tonify the kidney and spleen in order to strengthen the qi. The acupuncture prescription included Guanyuan (RN4), Zigong (Extra), Sanyinjiao (SP6) and Qugu (RN2). A needle was inserted at Guanyuan (RN4) and extra point Zigong was needled towards Qugu (RN2). After arrival of qi the patient felt an upward contraction of the uterus. The reinforcing method was applied to Sanyinjiao (SP6). One treatment alleviated the pain. The above points and Qugu (RN2) were used to lift the uterus to its normal position. Six treatments cured the prolapse of the uterus and alleviated the low back pain.

2. Peng Jingshan's Case [3]

A 47-year-old male patient came in for back pain. The main symptom was lumbago due to lumbar sprain, accompanied by pain and numbness of the left leg and limitation of movement. The X-ray showed obvious protrusion of the third and fourth intervertebral disc. Examination by a surgeon revealed an injury of the piriformis muscle. All the symptoms remained even though massage was applied and drugs were taken. He could not walk, turn the body or go upstairs, because he could only elevate the left leg 50 cm and the right leg 45 cm (above the surface of the bed). The pulse was deep and slow with a weak quality in the Chi region. Marked changes, such as thin pale-colored capillaries, were seen in both the ophthalmic middle and lower jiao areas. The diagnosis was deficiency of yang qi due to injury of the Du meridian. Middle and lower jiao orbital areas were needled bilaterally. After the first treatment, the left leg could be elevated 67 cm and the right leg 63 cm. After the second treatment, he could walk a little with the help of others, as the pain was greatly diminished. After the third treatment, he could walk slowly without anyone's help, since the pain and numbness were getting better. Altogether five treatments were given. Then he could raise both of his legs 74 cm above the surface of the bed.

3. He Puren's Case [3]

A 32-year-old female patient presented with back pain. For quite a few days she had lumbago. But on the day before consultation the condition suddenly became worse. She could not move her waist. No trauma and deformity were seen on physical examination. She had a thin white tongue coating and deep tight pulse. Chinese medicine defined this pattern as obstruction of the meridians by pathogenic wind and cold and malnourishment of the kidney by blood. Weizhong (BL40) and Renzhong (DU26) were punctured to bleed. After one treatment the patient could move her waist and walk with a stick. Five treatments completely cured the case. Shenshu (BL23) was used in the last two treatments.

4. Wang Pinshan's Case [4]

A 38-year-old female patient had suffered from low back pain for five years since the delivery of her baby. The disease was treated as pathogenic wind-dampness, strain, deficiency of the kidney and trauma with no effect. After working for one hour, she had to lie down and have a rest. Her appetite, urination and bowel movement were normal. Menstruation was normal and the amount of the leucorrhea was abundant. Upon examination, her pulse was slow, and her tongue body was pale-red with a thin coat. Her complexion was sallow, speech was clear. She displayed tenderness at Zulinqi (GB41) and Mingmen (DU4) points. According to pattern differentiation, the Dai Meridian was affected with meridian qi stagnation causing lumbar pain. The downward draining of damp-heat had led to the production of excessive leucorrhea. In this case, the pathogenesis was in the Dai Meridian, and the position of the disease affected the lumbar region. A treatment plan was made to dredge the meridians and normalize the flow of qi.

Intradermal needling at Mingmen (DU4) was altered with the intradermal needling at Zulinqi (GB41), with needle retention lasting fifteen minutes. Every five minutes, the needles on both sides were twirled and rotated for one minute. After the treatment, the pain in the lumbar region ceased immediately and the patient could move her waist freely, however, there was still tenderness. After the second treatment, the patient was tired. After the third treatment, the amount of leucorrhea was greatly reduced and there was still a tenderness reaction after the fourth treatment. The tenderness disappeared when two more treatments were given and all related symptoms were resolved. For over a month, no attack of lumbago was experienced.

The key point to master in the acupuncture clinic is to understand pathogenesis, to find out the exact position of the disease and to perform a proper manipulation. These three points are so important that none of them can be missed. When we say "to master the pathogenesis", it means that we should trace the disease according to the physical condition of the patient, the predisposing cause of the disease, the duration of the disease, the transformation of the syndrome and translate the meridian information. "To find out or to localize the position of the disease" refers to the localization of pathogenic position, the diseased area and the corresponding needling points. Manipulation includes the order of the needling, the intensity of the stimulation, and applying reinforcing and/or reducing after the arrival of qi. The needling should vary with different patients. For a strong build, the needling should be deep and retention of the needle is preferable. For the patient who is thin, the needling should be shallow and quick. For babies, the needling should be shallow with quick insertion. Therefore, the strength of the stimulation should correspond to the syndrome complex. Without the four diagnostic methods, the eight principles, the differentiation, the manipulation and the point selection the acupuncture clinic loses the TCM theoretical guidance; without the meridian information and meridian differentiation the acupuncture clinic loses the guidance of the meridian doctrine.

5. Yang Yongxuan's Case [4]

A 46-year-old male patient has complained of lower back pain due to sprain for one week. He had a history of strain for many years. The pain was worse when coughing and turning the body. Oral and external applications of herbal medicine did not relieve the pain. Lower back pain was accompanied by motor impairment and he looked tired. The patient's tongue-coating was thin but sticky and his pulse was thready and rolling. This patient was diagnosed with an acute lumbar sprain causing injury to the Governor Vessel, or sea of yang. Qi stagnation and blood stasis obstructed the channels and collaterals, resulting in pain. The treatment principle adopted in this case was to move the obstruction and dispel blood stasis. Acupuncture protocol called for reducing by rotation at points Shuigou (DU26), Weizhong (BL40), Qihaishu (BL24), with cupping after needling Qihaishu (BL24). The patient was treated at a frequency of one session every other day.

The patient gradually improved and was symptom-free after four treatments. This kind of acute lumbar sprain is commonly seen in the acupuncture department. Yu Long Ge (Jade Dragon Song) advises to reduce Renzhong

(DU26) for spinal pain and Weizhong (BL40) can be used to treat diseases of the lumbar region. Here, Shuigou (DU26) is used to regulate the reversed qi of the Governor Vessel; Weizhong (BL40) is used to regulate the qi of the Bladder Channel; needling and cupping Qihaishu (BL24) warms and regulates qi and blood in the lower back. The pain is alleviated when the obstruction is removed.

6. Zhu Bing's Case [4]

A 50-year-old female patient who had been suffering from lower back pain for eight months presented with recurring attacks of lower back pain, worse with exertion. X-ray confirmed she had retrograde degeneration of the lumbar vertebrae. She was afraid of the cold; her extremities were cold and her urine output had increased. Upon examination, she displayed tenderness at L4 and L5. Lifting the legs produced pain as well. She had a pale tongue with white coating and a thready pulse. In Chinese medicine, this patient's retrograde degeneration of the lumbar vertebra was classified as lower back pain due to kidney deficiency. More specifically, her fear of cold, cold extremities, increased clear urine, pale tongue, white coating, and thready pulse implied kidney yang deficiency. A treatment plan was devised to tonify the kidneys and circulate channel qi. The daily acupuncture prescription included Shenshu (BL23) Dachangshu (BL25), Zhishi (BL52), L2-5 Jiaji (EX-B2). Shu Ci (Shu-point acupuncture) method was also used, followed by cupping.

The pain was relieved after six treatments and completely eradicated after another twelve treatments. Shenshu (BL23) was selected to reinforce the kidneys; Dachangshu (BL25) to strengthen the lumbar region and knees and regulate the channel qi in the lower back; Zhishi (BL52) to replenish the kidney yin and to strengthen the lumbar region; and L2-5 Jiaji (EX-B2), to treat the retrograde degeneration of the lumbar vertebra. The Jiaji points were punctured deeply to 1.5 cun. Cupping was performed to promote the blood circulation, and regulate channel qi in the local area, as pain improves with improved circulation of qi and blood.

Shu Ci (Shu-point acupuncture) was used in the case. One of the needling methods mentioned in the *Yellow Emperor's Classic of Medicine*, where the technique is described as follows: "Shu Ci is to insert the needle as deep as to the bone for treating bone bi (osseous pain), which belongs to the kidneys."

7. Cheng Xinnong's Case [4]

A 22-year-old male patient complained of pain in the back and lumbar region for a duration of one week. The pain ensued after being exposed to wind immediately after sweating. He presented with pain in the back and lumbar region, a tense feeling in the back, aversion to wind, accompanied by irritability, insomnia, yellow urine, and constipation.

The patient's tongue tip was red, and there were cracks in the center; the coating was white and dry. His pulse was superficial and tight. Constitutionally, the patient was weak; his sweating seemed to be a main contributing factor in the disharmony between the Ying and Wei. The invasion of wind cold then obstructed the channels and collaterals of the lower back, resulting in pain. His symptoms of tension in the back and aversion to wind further indicated that the back pain was due to wind cold. The accompanying symptoms reflected signs that the wind and cold was interfering with the normal dispersion of heat in the body.

The patient's Chinese medicine diagnosis, lower back pain with disharmony between the Ying-nutrient and Wei-defense was treated by dispelling wind and cold, regulating Ying and Wei, removing obstruction from the channels and alleviating pain. Acupuncture points Dazhui (DU14), Fengchi (GB20), Yaoyangguan (DU3), Jianwaishu (SI14), Shenshu (BL23), Lieque (LU7), Hegu (LI4), Neiguan (PC6), Shenmen (HT7), Dazhui (DU14), Fengchi (GB20), Hegu (LI4), Taichong (LR3), and Neiting (ST44) were reduced. On other points, the even method was applied. Four treatments completely relieved the patient's pain. In this case, clearing the internal heat, dispel the external cold, regulating the Ying-nutrient and Wei-defense systems, and removing obstruction of the channels and collaterals effectively stopped the pain.

8. Cheng Xinnong's Case [4]

A 29-year-old male patient had been suffering from lower back pain for two months. He complained of lower back pain without known cause. On examination, the patient had a dull pain in the lower back, sometimes worse, sometimes better, radiating to the sacral region, accompanied by yellow urine and frequent urination. The patient had a dark complexion without luster. He had a purplish tongue with toothmarks on the borders, a white tongue coating and rolling pulse, weak in the chi position.

The kidneys are located in the lower back region. When kidney qi is deficient, or cold-damp invades, qi and blood will be obstructed in circulation, causing pain. The kidneys control urine and stools, and their channel is externally-internally related with that of the urinary bladder. When the urinary bladder it is too weak to store urine, there will be frequent urination.

In Chinese medicine, the patient was diagnosed with lower back pain due to invasion of cold-damp. The treatment strategy focused on tonifying kidney qi, dispelling cold-damp and removing obstruction from the channels. Acupuncture was applied to Shenshu (BL23), Yaoyangguan (DU3), Mingmen (DU4), Zhibian (BL54), Weizhong (BL40), Feiyang (BL58), Zusanli (ST36), Sanyinjiao (SP6) and Taixi (KI3). Moxibustion was applied at Shenshu (BL23) and Yaoyangguan (DU3). Mingmen (DU4), Zusanli (ST36) and Taixi (KI3) were reduced. The even method was applied at other points.

The lower back pain was greatly relieved after four treatments, although a heavy sensation remained in the sacral region. All symptoms disappeared after ten treatments. In this case, Taixi (KI3), Shenshu (BL23) Yaoyangguan (DU3), Mingmen (DU4), Zhibian (BL54), and so on were used to reinforce the kidney qi and remove the obstruction of channels and collaterals; while Zusanli (ST36) was used for strengthening the acquired foundation.

9. Ji Xiaoping's Case [4]

A 44-year-old male patient had complained of lower back pain for fifteen years. The pain resided in the lower back and legs, sometimes worse, sometimes better, and was aggravated when he was tired. X-ray and MRI examinations reported protrusion of the L4-L5 intervertebral disc. The patient had received block therapy for a total of more than 600 sessions. The therapy served to alleviated pain temporarily, but did not cure it; he then turned to acupuncture.

On examination, the patient complained of pain in the right side of the lower back, buttocks and on the lateral side of the legs, which was aggravated when tired. He experienced numb sensations on the lateral side of the legs, and he had small swellings at the Jiaji (EX-B2) areas of L4-L5 with severe tenderness radiating to the lateral side of the legs. The patient had a purple tongue with dark spots on it, a thick white coating and a string taut and hesitant pulse.

The cause of the patient's pathology was determined to be obstruction of meridian qi. As Huatuo Jiaji points are the distribution areas of the major collaterals of the urinary bladder meridian, and the buttocks and lateral side of the leg are the distribution areas of the gallbladder meridian, blockage in this area, reflects an obstruction of the urinary bladder and gallbladder meridian qi. Prolonged obstruction had led to blood stasis as well in this case. The swellings at the Jiaji (Ex-B2) areas of L4-L5, accompanied by severe tenderness, purple tongue and hesitant pulse all support a diagnosis of blood stasis. The treatment principle consisted of removing obstructions blocking the meridians and collaterals, circulating the qi and activating the blood. Reducing method was applied to Shiqizhui (Extra), Jiaji (Extra) of L4 and L5, Dachangshu (BL25), Weizhong (BL40), Huantiao (GB30) (right side), Yanglingquan (GB34) and Waiqiu (GB36). The needles were retained for twenty minutes at each bi-weekly treatment. After three acupuncture treatments, the patient's pain was greatly relieved, and after seven more treatments, his pain and numbness disappeared completely. A one-year follow-up found no relapse.

In this case, the patient's low-back pain and leg pain, stemming from obstruction of the meridians and collaterals manifested without disease of the Zang Fu organs. Of the possible syndrome differentiation approaches, such as by the Eight Principles, Zang Fu, Meridians and Collaterals, etc., this patient was diagnosed and treated according to differentiation of the Meridians and Collaterals, as his symptoms were not in the Zang Fu. In his case, the fifteen years of pain, combined with swelling and tenderness at the Jiaji area, purple tongue, and hesitant pulse all support a diagnosis of blood stasis. The correct diagnosis of both qi and blood stagnation led to the success of treatment.

10. Wang Juyi's Case [5]

A female patient aged 38-year-old came into the acupuncture office. The patient had chronic back and leg pain. The pain had been getting worse over the past six weeks.

The patient had a history of back pain. She got better after being treated in the hospital, but now complained of cold and soreness of the left lower leg, impaired sensation, cold heels, numbness of lateral side of the feet, and walking was impaired. The patient had a white tongue coating and her pulse was deep and slippery. X-ray revealed that there were herniated disks at L4-5, L5 and S1. Meridian diagnosis indicated an abnormality in the hand taiyang meridian and foot taiyang meridian. Differentiation of meridians indicated that the disease was located in the tendomuscular structure of the foot taiyang. Foot taiyang meridian as well as the governing meridian were selected for treatment. The acupuncture points for needling were Zhiyin (BL67) with bloodletting performed at Houding (DU19).

On the second visit, the patient reported that all symptoms had been relieved by the first treatment. She was treated at Zhibian (BL54), Weizhong (BL40) on the left side and Dingjiejie (Extra) on the right side.

On the third visit, the patient reported that the pain of the left lower leg had disappeared; however, the numbness on the back side of the thigh and soreness on the lateral side still returned when walking or standing for a long time. Dingjiejie (Extra) on the right side and Jinggu (BL64) were needled.

After the third treatment, all symptoms were resolved.

In this case, the patient had herniated discs at L5 and S1 accompanied with cold left limb and numbness of the left foot. The symptoms manifested from a disease of the tendinomuscular structure of the foot taiyang. The numbness of the left lateral foot indicated deficiency of blood. Bloodletting on Zhiyin (BL67) functioned to induce the yang and open the collaterals, promoting the flow of qi and blood. Two needles were inserted at Houding (DU19): one was oriented downward against the meridian, the other pointing toward the left side of the meridian. The needles were stimulated at Houding (DU19) with the practitioner's knee on the low back of the patient. After rotating the needles, the patient was asked to walk. The patient noticed a huge difference compared with how her back had felt when she walked in.

Zhibian (BL54) and Weizhong (BL40) were added because the patient's disease was located in the tendinomuscular structure of the foot taiyang. According to *A Collection of Outstanding Treatises in Acupuncture and Moxibustion (Zhen Jiu Ju Ying),* Zhibian (BL54) is indicated for back pain, and Weizhong (BL40) is indicated for knee pain and heaviness of the low back along the spine with heaviness of the low back and difficulty in lifting objects. Abnormal reaction at extra point Dingjiejie, located on the right side of Houiding (DU19), indicates response at Houding (DU19). Needling Houding (DU19) and Dingjiejie (Extra) were found to be beneficial in this case.

In this case, when the low back was injured, the tendinomuscular structure changed, as did the acupuncture points. Acupuncture points are located between the skin, collaterals, muscles, tendons and bones. Once tissues at the points are damaged or changed, the associated acupuncture points change as well. Just as when an earthquake or flooding thunderstorm occurs upstream of a long river, earth, sand and stones falling off from either of the two sides of the valleys will block the river. The water from the upper stream will continue to pour downstream, flowing around the blocked valley, which slows down the current, affecting the upper stream. Low back pain arising from a herniated disc is similar to a blocked river. The changed position of Houding (DU19) in relation to Dingjiejie (Extra) reflects the disruption in the source to blockage downstream. To clear the blockage, the patient was asked to stomp when the needles were rotated on Dingjiejie (Extra). This action restored the correct position of the tendinomuscular structure of the foot taiyang.

Soreness, formation of lumps, and blockage of collaterals are indications of diseases of tendinomuscular structures. Needling the sites of soreness or the sites of lumps are recommended. In this case, a lump around Jinggu (BL64) had been discovered when the meridians were assessed. A lump at Jingu (BL64) indicates a blockage of qi and blood of the tendinomuscular structure of the foot taiyang. According to *A Collection of Outstanding Treatises in Acupuncture and Moxibustion (Zhen Jiu Ju Ying)* Jinggu (BL64), is indicated for sharp headache, impaired movement of low back, stiff neck and difficulty of moving the head due to back pain.

Protocols from Leading Acupuncture Practitioners

1. Peng Jingshan's Treatment Protocol [6]

The primary prescription for low back pain includes points Weizhong (BL40), Shenshu (BL23), Mingmen (DU4) and Chengshan (BL57). Add Houxi (SI3) and Renzhong (DU26) for severe pain located on the spine; add Feiyang (BL58) and Kunlun (BL60) for severe pain located on both sides of the spine; add Zhaohai (KI6) and Yanggu (SI5) for kidney deficiency; apply moxibustion on Mingmen (DU4) and Qihai (RN6) for kidney yang deficiency; apply bloodletting on Weizhong (BL40), then needle Fengmen (BL12) and Feishu (BL13) for wind dampness; add Zhongdu (LR6) and Ququan (LR8) for abnormality of the liver meridian; and add Yanglao (SI6) and trigger point lateral to Shousanli (LI10) for injury due to sprain.

Contralateral needling is applicable in this case. A central pain point exists for most pain conditions. This point needs to identified and located correctly. Then, the opposite point corresponding to this central pain point needs to be identified. For example, if the pain point is on the back, then the contralateral point is one the front. If the pain point is on the front, then the contralateral point is one the back. If the pain point is on the lower back, then the contralateral point is on the abdomen. If the pain point is on the abdomen, then the contralateral point is one the lower back. The pain point may be located on the body trunk or on the four limbs. The more precise this point is located, the more effective the needling result. The contralateral point of Jiuwei (RN15) is Zhiyang (DU9), and the contralateral point of Shenjue (RN8) is Mingmen (DU4).

For example, if the pain spot is located at five centimeters below Mingmen (DU4) and six centimeters on the left side, the contralateral point is located at five centimeters below Shenjue (RN8) and six centimeters on the left side. The appropriate needling techniques are applied on the contralateral point.

2. Zhou Shudong's Treatment Protocol [7]

Zhou Shudong's Treatment Protocol for back pain is symptom-based. This is summarized from his manuscript, The Poetry of Golden Needle Plum Flower, which is a comprehensive acupuncture needling technique book crafted in the early twentieth century for family use, but published in 1982.

- Back pain accompanied with pain propagating to the head along the spine: Bloodletting on Weizhong (BL40)
- Back pain radiating to shoulder, neck, hips, accompanied with blurry vision and incontinence: Weizhong (BL40);
- Back pain with cold back and feet: Yangfu (GB38) and Yinshi (ST33);
- Back pain with impaired movement of the lower limbs and difficulty in turning around: Ciliao (BL32);
- Back pain with difficulty in coughing and tendon spasm with coughing: Yangfu (GB38);
- Back pain radiating the upper back and with difficulty in standing: Chengshan (BL57);
- Back pain associated with hip pain, difficulty in sitting up: Kunlun (BL60);
- Back pain with difficulty in holding objects up, cold feet and atrophic feet: Pucan (BL61) and Shenmai (BL62);
- Back pain with difficulty in sitting up, foot pain and difficulty in stretching: Diji (SP8);
- Back pain with heat sensations, feeling like a log is attached to the back, incontinence in severe cases: Diji (SP8);

- Back pain with heat up: foot meridians of terminal yin and greater yin, Diji (SP8);
- Back pain with feeling like the back is broken, difficulty in sitting up: Shugu (BL65), Jinggu (BL64), Kunlun (BL60), Shenmai (BL62), and Pucan (BL61);
- Back pain radiating to the abdomen, with lower volume of menses: Shangliao (BL31), Ciliao (BL32), Zhongliao (BL33), and Xialiao (BL34);
- Back pain with subcutaneous pricking feeling, difficulty in sitting up and turning around: Yanglingquan (GB34);
- Back pain with feeling of arrow being on the bow: foot meridian of terminal yin, Ligou (LR5);
- Back pain radiating to the abdomen and hip and testis and with difficulty in sitting up: Pangguangshu (BL28);
- Back pain with hip pain, radiating to abdomen, incontinence: Juliao (GB29) and Yinbao (LR9);
- Back pain with difficult bowel movement: foot meridian of lesser yin, Yongquan (KI1);
- Back pain with difficult bowel movement, diarrhea after meals, cold on the back and hip: Zhongliao (BL33);
- Back pain with heat and wheezing: Yongquan (KI1) and Weizhong (BL40);
- Back pain radiating to the shoulders, with difficulty in coughing and tendon spasm with coughing: Ganshu (BL18);
- Back pain on the spine, radiating to the abdomen: Heyang (BL55);
- Back pain on the spine, radiating to the penis or virginal area with cold feeling: Chengfu (BL36);
- Back pain with a cold feeling in the sacral area, difficulty in urination: Zhibian (BL54);
- Back pain on the spine, indigestion, and hard abdomen: Zhishi (BL52);
- Back pain with stiff spine, rebellious qi moving upward and hiccups: Shentang (BL44);
- Back pain radiating to the inside spine with cold sensation: Fuliu (KI7);
- Back pain with cold and stiff spine: Yinshi (ST33), Changqiang (DU1);
- Back pain with fullness and distention of the abdomen: Taichong (LR3), and Yinbao (LR9);

- Back pain with difficulty in turning the head: Zusanli (ST36), Yinshi (ST33), Yangfu (GB38), and Ligou (LR5);
- Back pain with difficulty in sitting up and fullness in the back: Jingmen (GB25);
- Back pain radiating to the hips, with blurry vision, feeling the low back is broken, and impaired tongue movement: Jiaoxin (KI8);
- Back pain with difficulty in raising feet: Shenmai (BL62);
- Back pain on the spine, with difficulty in urination and fullness of abdomen: Taichong (LR3);
- Back pain with difficulty in sitting up: Foot meridian of lesser yang;
- Back pain caused by hip injury: Jianjing (GB21);
- Back pain connected with abdominal pain: Mingmen (DU4);
- Back pain with difficulty in standing up and sitting up: Yinlingquan (SP9), Jingmen (GB25), and Xingjian (LR2);
- Back pain with knee spasm: Yinjiao (RN7);
- Back pain with hip pain, stiff spine and difficulty in turning: Yaoshu (DU2);
- Back pain with stiffness in both lower back and upper back: Feishu (BL13)
- Back pain with difficulty in turning around: Zhangmen (LR13).

3. Gao Lishan's Treatment Protocol [8]

- Back pain worse with stretching the knees: Tianzhu (BL10);
- Back pain radiating to the abdomen: Tianshu (ST25);
- Back pain worse with coughing: Yanglingquan (GB34)
- Back pain manifested with walking: Moxibustion on the points of left, right, upper and lower one cun from the Ashi point;
- Back pain radiating to the upper back: Ganshu (BL18);
- Back pain radiating to the leg: Zhibian (BL54);
- Back pain caused by wind cold: Houxi (SI3) with reducing method;
- Back pain caused by sprain injury with stasis blood: Weizhong (BL40) with bloodletting.

In combination with herbal medicine treatment:

- Back pain with kidney deficiency: Liu Wei Di Huang Wan;
- Back pain with cold retention: Shu Feng Ding Tong Wan;
- Back pain with dampness: Er Miao Wan;
- Back pain with qi deficiency: Bu Zhong Yi Qi Wan;

- Back pain with blood deficiency: Yang Xue Rong Jin Wan;
- Back pain with blood stasis: Die Da Wan or Qi Li San.

Clinical Evidence: Individual Clinical Trials

Acupuncture and traditional Chinese medicine treat every body system; yet, back pain continues to be a popular topic in research. Data from more than one hundred clinical trials on acupuncture and back pain have amassed worldwide, making back pain the most researched condition in the field. The following section presents a summary of a few compelling clinical studies.

In China, acupuncturists often complete a full western medical education and Chinese medical degrees simultaneously. One such doctor's practice in Germany hosted a randomized controlled trial comparing acupuncture to conventional interventions for the treatment of chronic low back pain. The trial [9] was single-blinded and comprised of one hundred and fifty outpatients assigned to either standardized or individualized acupuncture groups. Those in the condition-specific, standardized group received acupuncture at Shenshu (BL23), Qihaishu (BL24), Zanzhu (BL2), Weizhong (BL40), Kunlun (BL60), Yanglingquan (GB34), and Taixi (KI3). Pattern differentiation determined the point selection for those in the individualized group. All patients received between ten and fifteen bi-weekly treatments depending on symptoms.

Pain severity was rated daily and graphed, with 0 mm representing no pain, and 100 mm representing the maximum pain possible; the total area under the curve mapped over the eight-week duration was then compared between groups. Overall pain averages for those who had received individualized acupuncture according to pattern differentiation were not significantly different than those for the standardized acupuncture group, 1768.7 vs. 1482.9, respectively ($P= 0.080$). The researchers found the results consistent with earlier German studies, and concluded that standardized and individualized treatments were equivalent in terms of reducing chronic low-back pain. The confirmation that standardized treatments are effective for chronic low back pain led researchers to suggest that a multicenter noninferiority study be done to assess the feasibility of the widespread use of standardized acupuncture for chronic low back pain in a conventional care setting.

Yamamoto developed a signature scalp acupuncture method for acute, non-specific low back pain. A recent Brazilian study [10] was conducted to determine the efficacy of Yamamoto's method on pain as well as medication use, functionality and quality of life. Eighty patients meeting the criteria were randomized into either a non-insertion sham acupuncture or Yamamoto acupuncture group. Each received Yamamoto or sham acupuncture for twenty-eight days.

Cumulative Visual Analogue scores showed a significant pain reduction from day fourteen among those who received Yamamoto acupuncture compared with those who received sham acupuncture. This trend continued through study completion, twenty-eight days later. However, the pre-determined clinically relevant difference was not achieved between groups. Those in the intervention group also gained significant improvements over controls in functionality and SF-36 pain and vitality scores at days fourteen, twenty-one and twenty-eight ($p<0.05$). Patients who received Yamamoto acupuncture also displayed significant improvements in SF-36 mobility ratings throughout; while SF-36 functional capacity scores at days twenty-one and twenty-eight were also significantly more elevated in the treatment group ($p<0.05$). Regarding the need for medication, those who received Yamamoto acupuncture needed significantly less anti-inflammatory medication ($p=0.004$) throughout. Moreover, the overall improvement rating was greater in the intervention group ($p<0.001$). Researchers concluded that Yamamoto's innovative scalp acupuncture reduced pain and the use of anti-inflammatory medication, and improved functionality and quality of life for patients suffering from acute, non-specific low back pain.

A Chinese study [11] recently evaluated the efficacy of electric-thermal bian-stone therapy compared to moxibustion in cases of low back pain due to cold-dampness. Forty-one patients were randomized to receive either electric-thermal bian-stone therapy or moxibustion. For a course of ten days, patients received either intervention daily or on every other day at Shenshu (BL23) and Weizhong (BL40). The symptom and physical signs score of low back pain and the score of cold-damp syndrome were observed before and after patients receiving treatment. Both interventions were found to be successful in reducing symptoms, diminishing low-back pain and dissipating the cold-damp syndrome (all $P<0.01$). Syndrome scores decreased similarly in both groups, mean scores dropping from 37.04% to 22.85% and from 47.29% to 23.89% in the hot-stone and moxibustion groups respectively (all $P > 0.05$). Researchers concluded that electric-thermal bian-stone therapy is as effective as moxibustion in treating low back pain due to cold-dampness. They also remarked that bian-stone interventions are more convenient, safer and cause less pollution.

Pregnant women often suffer from low-back pain through most or all of the pregnancy. Pregnancy-related back pain often resolves or improves within six months post-partum; however, some women then go on to develop chronic back issues. To determine the efficacy of dry cupping at BL23 on back pain in women after delivery, an RTC [12] with 100 women was performed. The women were randomized into either the cupping or control group. Researchers discovered that women who had received the cupping protocol reported a near 50% reduction in mean VAS pain intensity rating immediately following the procedure; that score then dropping by 10% after twenty-four hours; with mean cupping averages falling to 1.4 two weeks after the intervention, (from the original intensity mean of 7.8). McGill pain questionnaire scores showed a similar progression, with means falling from 31.8 to 9.0 to 7.5 and finally to 3.6. These differences observed among the various follow-up scores were found to be significant (P=0.01). Researchers concluded that cupping therapy is beneficial in lowering back pain in post-partum women.

Degenerative articular disease and related pain is arguably the most prevalent condition affecting the elderly in Turkey. Usually treated with pain medication and physical therapy, concurrent medical and nutritional concerns within this population can present challenges in utilizing prescription pain killers for relief. To expand helpful options, researchers [13] assessed the potential benefit of acupuncture for back-pain and knee-pain in the elderly. Twenty-four women of average age 69, and eight men, of an average age of 73 years received acupuncture every two days. Ten treatments were provided in all, in which needling Yintang (Extra), Shenmen (HT7), Hegu (LI4), Taixi (KI3) and Zhaohai (KI6) significantly lowered pain. Average back pain fell from 8.8696 to 2.1739, while knee pain also dropped significantly. Researchers concluded that results validate the use of acupuncture as a viable treatment option for elderly patients with knee and /or back pain.

Cost-benefit assessment research [14] was recently conducted in Korea to determine the feasibility of the general use of acupuncture for patients with chronic low back pain. Outpatients who had received at least one regular acupuncture session were observed over a three-month follow-up interval. Of the 105 participants, significant condition-specific and preference-based benefits were achieved. Monthly average individual cost of treatment was $146, $231 for three months; while a reduction was seen in other medical costs related to chronic low back pain. Researchers concluded that this inexpensive method of treatment relieved pain, restored functionality and improved quality of life. They found that the study results supported the findings of previous European trials, however the power of this study was assessed to be relatively weak due to design. They recommended a larger-scale cohort or practice registry may allow for a more compelling argument as to the economy of acupuncture's use for chronic low back pain.

Electro-acupuncture is known to benefit many cases of back and nerve pain. To zero-in on the most advantageous electrostimulation parameters for eliciting a response, researchers [15] compared the frequency and intensity differentials. Patients received one of three electro-acupuncture stimulations at one of three acupoints. Acupuncture was administered either at Quanliao (SI18), Quchi (LI11) or and the back acupoint Dachangshu (BL25). Electrostimulation intensity and frequencies of 3.3 and 33 Hz, 12.5 and 66.7 Hz, and 3.3 and 3.3 Hz were provided according to group. Researchers found that the EAS values were significantly reduced at 10 to 30 compared with those at 0 min. The researchers overall found that the duration of needle sensation increased with greater electrostimulation frequency. Intense electro-stim was found to cause too much discomfort on the facial point.

Patients with persistent, unrelenting, low-back pain are often in need of immediate, substantial relief. To gather scientific data as to the safety and efficacy of a solitary wet cupping treatment in these cases, researchers [16] in Saudi Arabia conducted an outpatient RCT. Eighty patients who had been suffering from persistent non-specific low back pain for a minimum duration of three months were randomized into either the intervention or control group. Those in the intervention group received a series of six wet cupping treatments over the course of two weeks on two of the three points selected for treatment: Shenshu (BL23), Qihaishu (BL24), and Dachangshu (BL25). During the study, acetaminophen was the only medication allowed for all participants. Researchers found statistically significant benefits among those who had received the intervention compared with the control group. NRS improved in the treatment group versus the controls, 29.2 versus 57.9. Better PPI scores were achieved in the treatment group, 1.17 versus 2.3. Better ODQ scores were also seen among those who received the wet cupping procedure, 19.6 versus 35.4. Gains lasted for two weeks beyond the intervention. Researchers found an insignificant additional benefit of decreased acetaminophen use in the wet cupping group; however, it was not significantly different than use in the controls. No adverse events were observed. Researchers concluded that wet cupping in cases of persistent non-specific low back pain is indicated for short-term (two-week) alleviation of pain and improved mobility. Researchers also mentioned the need for placebo-controlled trials to more accurately gauge specific intervention benefit.

The emergency department frequently sees cases of low back pain. Acute, severe low back pain is not well-researched as of yet. To evaluate the efficacy and safety of acupuncture for treating ER patients with acute low back pain, a clinical pilot [17] was launched. Forty-five suitable patients received a standardized acupuncture protocol while fourteen served as controls, receiving sham acupuncture consisting of seeds being pasted near acupoints. The study revealed that after just fifteen minutes of acupuncture, visual analogue pain scores among those receiving the intervention showed a significant decrease (P value <0.001). Heart-rate variability remained unaffected in both groups and no adverse events were observed. Researchers found the study provides support for acupuncture's use in reducing low back pain in acute ER cases.

The increased use of dry needling for patients with low back pain has inspired researchers to define the characteristics of those patients who may respond most favorably. Seventy-two patients with low back pain due to mechanical issues received one bilateral dry needling treatment at the lumbar multifidus muscles [18]. Researchers discovered that patients who displayed increased low back pain with the multifidus lift test, or with passive hip flexion when lying supine increased the likelihood of positive response to dry needling. Positive beliefs about acupuncture/dry needling also correlated strongly with positive treatment response. In patients whose low back pain was exacerbated by standing, coincided with leg pain, or in those who perceived a sense of excessive mobility in the lumbar spine showed less favorable response to dry needling. Researchers concluded that patients whose low back pain was positive to the multifidus lift test were the most likely to improve with dry needling. Findings suggest that pain during muscle contraction may be a strong indicator for dry needling; future research is needed in this area to confirm.

Acupuncture's role in low back pain treatment is controversial, especially concerning priority in relation to other options and coordination of care. Research on patient preference has found that acupuncture's use may be limited according to willingness-to-pay. A discrete choice study [19] was undertaken to better understand preferences among Chinese patients from September 2011 to August 2012. This study was unique in that outpatients from the 'traditional medicine department' at a traditional Chinese medicine hospital and the 'rehabilitation department' at a Western medicine hospital in Guangdong Province of China participated. Preference for either acupuncture, low frequency infrared therapy or neither was assessed via questionnaire. Preference did not depend on expected usefulness of receiving the treatment and it was noted that the gender of the prospective patient being female and higher out-of-pocket payment significantly decreased chance to receive treatments. De qi was revealed as the most telling predictor of efficacy. Efficacy, maintenance duration, onset of efficacy, and the out-of-pocket cost determined greatly the preference levels. Willingness to pay $618.6 and $592.4 USD per course for acupuncture and infrared therapy respectively, demonstrated patients' demand for effective pain management care. Researchers noted there may be other factors influencing patients' preference to receive treatments as yet to be determined.

Neuroimaging provides a rare opportunity to gain visual insights regarding acupuncture's influence on brain activation. To illuminate how acupuncture affects specific areas of the brain in patients with acute low back pain, baseline functional magnetic resonance imaging (fMRI) scans [20] were made and compared with scans taken during acupuncture or sham acupuncture stimulation of Weizhong (BL40). The scans showed a correlation between the pain state and greater regional homogeneity (ReHo) in the pain matrix, limbic system, and default mode network (DMN), which coincided with lower ReHo values in the frontal gyrus and temporal gyrus compared with the O, pain status, and DMN. Pain state was also found to elicit activation of the attentional and somatosensory systems. Acupuncture was found to more likely to deactivate than activate compared to sham acupuncture. Researchers concluded that several brain pathways contribute to the analgesic effects of acupuncture, the neuroimaging implying acupuncture has a definitive effect directly on brain function.

A qualitative study [21] via interview was conducted to learn more from those directly experiencing chronic low back pain. Eleven individuals who had received acupuncture engaged in audio-recorded interviews which were then transcribed. Researchers determined that reclaiming control by regaining a sense of well-being represented a healing quality of experienced by those undergoing acupuncture care. Gaining a sense of sanctuary, trust and establishing a working relationship were also deemed to be important aspects of the acupuncture experience. An aesthetically appealing healing environment, confidence in the practitioner and participation in the decision-making process were all found to influence the patient's experience. The researchers ascertained that full consideration of the patient's situation leads to providing an understandable, cohesive plan and options reflective of the patient's viewpoint and priorities that allows for a positive experience. Researchers stipulated that the application of these findings may be limited to private practice in affluent countries. As other populations and settings were not included in this study, further research is needed to determine the span of applicability.

Mainstream health care emphasizes cost-effectiveness in rationalizing the incorporation of new strategies and interventions. The cost-benefit ratio concerning acupuncture care for low back pain was analyzed in a recent study. Meta-analyses revealed a significant improvement in low back pain among those who had received both acupuncture and conventional care compared to those who had undergone only conventional treatment. In cases where acupuncture was combined with conventional interventions, an insignificant improvement occurred from weeks twelve to sixteen, compared to conventional intervention with sham acupuncture. When patients received only acupuncture, significant improvement compared with conventional interventions was seen at week eight, which disappeared at weeks twenty-six and fifty-two.

To measure the cost-benefit of acupuncture versus conventional care in the treatment of low back pain, the incremental cost-effectiveness ratio of acupuncture treatment was assessed according to (A$) per disability-adjusted life-year (DALY) saved. Results [22] were compared with standards set forth by the World Health Organization, which deems very highly cost-effective interventions to be those that cost less than gross domestic product per capita per quality-adjusted life-year (QALY) gained or DALY averted. This value would have been less than approximately $A52,000 in 2009. In this study, acupuncture as an adjunct to conventional treatment in the care of patients with chronic low back pain was found to be highly cost-effective. Its value assessed at $48,562 per DALY avoided. In cases where comorbid depression diminished equally with pain, treatment cost was assessed at $18,960 per DALY avoided. Acupuncture alone fell short of cost-effectiveness requirements; however, the lessening of comorbid depression increased its value tremendously. As acupuncture often relieves many related and unrelated symptoms (such as depression), cost-benefit analysis may have to take these into consideration in order to determine truer cost-benefit ratios. Even without full consideration of the complex sets of symptoms relieved by acupuncture care, the WHO cost-effectiveness threshold values were met in this study, leaving researchers to rate acupuncture as a cost-effective method of treatment for patients suffering from chronic lower back pain.

The cost versus benefit of implementing acupuncture for chronic low back pain was also researched in Korea [23]. One hundred and five outpatients who were treated with acupuncture at least once throughout the duration of the study were assessed. The cost averaged $146 (US) for one month and $231 (US) per three months. Additionally, a reduction in other medical costs related to the condition was seen. Researchers concluded that acupuncture was found to be a cost-effective method of alleviating chronic low back pain, increasing functionality, and improving quality of life; with significant benefits seen in condition-specific measures. Also considered in assessment were preferences patients provided through questionnaires. Researchers found the results supported findings of research from European countries, however the power of this study was deemed to be relatively weak due to small population. They suggested a cohort registry according to practice may more accurately reflect the cost-effectiveness of acupuncture for low-back pain.

Clinical Evidence: Systematic Reviews and Meta-analysis

Low back pain can result from sudden injury, or may develop gradually over time. Its high rate of prevalence and ability to stop one from working can have a cumulative deleterious effect on the economy. The best way to manage non-specific low back pain is not obvious as many variables are involved. Recently published guidelines and the inclusion of acupuncture for chronic pain by many health insurance plans, show an acceptance of the demand for acupuncture by patients with low back pain. A Medline search [24] produced seven relevant randomized controlled trials spanning the last decade. Three studies found that acupuncture's analgesic effect was significantly greater than sham acupuncture, standard care and no treatment controls. An additional two studies also found that acupuncture significantly reduced pain after eight weeks and at three months compared to standard care or no treatment. Three studies found significant reductions in pain and disability compared with sham acupuncture in a six-to-twelve-month period. Researchers concluded that the comprehensive literature review provides some promising, yet limited data to support its benefits over no treatment. More research is still needed to determine specific applications as some results conflicted.

Strict methodology guidelines have not been followed in most research on Tuina. To arrive at a better understanding of the real benefit of this form of therapy for low back pain, researchers [25] recommended focusing on improving methods and including long-term follow-up. Compiled results from twenty of the available RCTs on Tuina-focused integrative Chinese medical therapies among Chinese and English databases showed that Tuina significantly decreased pain and debility; with a greater improvement seen when combined with Chinese herbal medicine or acupuncture or Tuina plus acupuncture. The trials assessed did not find significant pain reduction when Tuina was applied in conjunction with moxibustion or hot packs.

Cupping therapy has been used for the treatment of chronic conditions including low back pain. Cupping styles include dry cupping, wet cupping (with controlled bleeding), cupping with retention, moving cupping; shaking-cupping; quick cupping; and balance-cupping. Since there is no consensus on the role of cupping therapy in the treatment of low back pain, the authors [26] reviewed the medical literature in an attempt to test its effectiveness in low back pain and to further examine this method. The systematic research started with an English and Chinese language literature search of PubMed from 1980 through 2013. The keyword search terms "cupping therapy", "low back pain", "lumbar sprain", "lumbar myofascitis" and "lumbosacral pain" in combination were used. Identified studies were assigned a level of evidence according to the Oxford Centre for Evidence-Based Medicine 2011 levels of evidence. 29 citations were identified: one randomized controlled trial (level I evidence), 4 six non-RCTs (level II evidence), 20 case reports (level IV evidence) and two mechanism-based studies (level V evidence). In the RCT, the effective rate of the wet-cupping group was similar to that of the waiting-list group ($p>0.05$). Interventions in both groups decreased pain, disability and acetaminophen dosage, but a significant decrease in pain intensity according to the McGill pain questionnaire ($p<0.01$) and reduced consumption of acetaminophen ($p=0.09$) were seen in the wet-cupping group. Of the six non-RCTs, one showed that the visual analogue scale (VAS) score and the Oswestry disability index in the balance-cupping group were significantly lower than in the group with cupping with retention and diclofenac ($p<0.05$), but there was no difference between the cupping with retention group and the diclofenac-only group ($p>0.05$). The other studies demonstrated that the effectiveness of cupping in decreasing VAS, reducing recurrence rate and improving quality of life was better than Western medication. Although evidence level I and II studies on the effectiveness of cupping treatment in low back pain have been reported, aspects such as manipulations, sites and dosage of cupping and Western medication in the comparison group are not uniform. Although RCTs provide a higher quality of evidence, the authors included non-RCTs in this study because the limited number of RCTs did not provide convincing evidence.

The study shows that cupping therapy is promising for pain control and improvement of quality of life, and minimizes the potential risks of treatment. Further studies to determine the potential role of cupping therapy in the treatment of low back pain are highly recommended.

Low-back and/or pelvic pain are experienced by a majority women during pregnancy. Pain tends to increase with advancing stages of pregnancy due to weight gain, pressure and hormonal fluctuations. The pain often interferes with work, much needed sleep and activity in general. To compare efficacy of interventions for this group, twenty-six RCTs including 4093 pregnant women with low back or pelvic pain were gathered from Cochrane databases. Researchers [27] found that, although study quality was lacking, low back pain and debility tended to respond significantly positively to exercise. Water-based exercise was found to significantly diminish time away from work due to pain. Although study quality was low, analgesic effect and functionality between two kinds of pelvic support band, between osteopathic manipulation and standard care or sham ultrasound did not demonstrate significant differences. Researchers found that a therapeutic pillow may help alleviate pain during the night compared with a standard pillow. Acupuncture was found to significantly alleviate evening pain better than exercise; both were better than usual care. Low-quality evidence from single trials suggested that adding a stabilizing belt while exercise lessened pain although functionality was not affected. Acupuncture was also found to be significantly superior to sham acupuncture for alleviating pain in the evening and decreasing debility; however, pain averages were not significantly improved. Pain in the evening was found to improve to the same degree with either deep or superficial acupuncture. Exercise from eight to twenty weeks also reduced lumbar and pelvic pain; however, a sixteen-to-twenty-week training program did not prevent pelvic pain more than standard care. Although study quality was low, researchers found that exercise significantly reduced time away from work, alleviated pain and decreased debility. Low-quality trials also showed significant pain relief and improved functionality in women receiving orthopedic manipulation; they also found that combined intervention approaches that included manual therapy, exercise and education, or conventional care significantly improved function. Acupuncture relieved pain and improved functionality better than conventional interventions or physiotherapy; and it was found that these effects were greater when acupuncture began at twenty-six weeks' gestation, than when started at twenty weeks. Auricular acupuncture also significantly improved pain and debility to a greater degree than sham acupuncture. Only minor, short-term adverse effects were reported.

These studies deemed moderate in quality found that compared to conventional care alone, evening pelvic and lumbar pain was significantly alleviated by term-specific acupuncture or exercise. Acupuncture's analgesic effect on those suffering from pelvic pain in the evening was also found to be significantly superior to exercise. Conventional care prevented pelvic and lumbar pain as well as a sixteen-to-twenty-week training program. Among studies with low-quality ratings, low back pain and disability were significantly improved by exercise. Bias and spotty data were to blame for low-quality ratings of many single trials; data pooling was inhibited by lack of homogeneity. Analgesic effects of conventional care modalities seemed to be improved with the inclusion of physiotherapy, osteopathic manipulation, acupuncture, combined interventions, or the wearing a supportive pelvic belt during exercise. When acupuncture began at twenty-six weeks' gestation rather than twenty weeks, pain in the evening and debility were slightly reduced, however improvements were greater than with physiotherapy. No significant differences were found among the use of varied belts, exercise, neuro emotional technique or spinal manipulation. No significant differences in outcomes were seen between superficial and deep needling when treating women suffering from pelvic pain in the evening. Due to lack of quality and data in general, researchers proposed the findings may or may not be supported by future research. They also vied for consensus on categorizing pregnant women with low back and pelvic pain according to symptom differentiation in future research.

To get a sense of the overall impact of acupuncture on nonspecific chronic low back pain, researchers consolidated the existing data through May 2012. This review [28] was unique in that the employment of traditional acupuncture theory was essential for inclusion in this analysis. Thirty-two studies met criteria for a systematic review; twenty-five also presented data appropriate for meta-analysis. Researchers found that immediately following acupuncture, pain was reduced by an average of 16.76%. ($P = 0.05$) compared with sham acupuncture; while function averages were improved by close to one point compared with no treatment. Functionality also tended to increase when acupuncture was combined with conventional care. Electroacupuncture also improved functionality more than conventional care alone. Compared to medications such as non-steroidal anti-inflammatory drugs, muscle relaxers, and pain-killers and conventional care, acupuncture produced clinically irrelevant statistically significant differences between the controls and those receiving intervention. Studies on transcutaneous electrical nerve stimulation showed the intervention produces as much improvement as acupuncture. Researchers concluded that the consolidated results suggest that acupuncture has a potential to relieve pain and reduce debility in patients with nonspecific chronic low back pain. Heterogeneity and the low methodological quality restricted the researchers from forming a strong opinion at this point.

Acute nonspecific low back pain has been widely treated with acupuncture and traditional Chinese medicine, both historically and in recent times. In a recent systematic review [29] of eleven RCTs from scientifically credible sources, the effects of acupuncture compared to other interventions was assessed for acute and subacute cases of low back pain. Results showed that acupuncture was superior to nonsteroidal anti-inflammatory drugs in symptom reduction. Results varied when comparing acupuncture analgesic effects to those of medication. Functionality and disability ratings were similar in acupuncture and sham acupuncture groups; although scores indicated a greater benefit was derived from acupuncture in terms of pain. Among the trials included, few side effects were noted. Researchers concluded that the preliminary findings favor acupuncture as a method of reducing symptoms and acute low back pain. Further study with improved methods were suggested to verify positive findings.

Research on traditional medical interventions in East-Asian countries was evaluated in relation to current Clinical Practice Guidelines. After reviewing the research and guidelines, Cho et al. [30], found the current guidelines lacked evidence for acupuncture and related modalities, such as cupping and manual therapy. However, research found supported a moderate recommendation for the use of acupuncture in cases of chronic LBP. Limited evidence in the use of acupuncture for (sub)acute LBP prevented researchers from making a firm decision regarding acupuncture's use in these cases. In (sub)acute and chronic cases, researchers weakly recommended cupping and manual therapy. There was not enough data for researchers to recommend moxibustion and Chinese herbal medicine. When comparing the evidence with the Clinical Practice Guidelines, researchers concluded that the current guidelines were not closely based on the evidence for traditional medical interventions. Researchers proposed that with the growth of research in the areas of acupuncture, cupping, and manual therapy, the results generated be applied concordantly to the establishment of Clinical Practice Guidelines.

Neck pain and low back pain, occurring independently or together, have been experienced at one time or another by most people. These both have been treated in China by Traditional Chinese medicine practitioners for thousands of years. To consolidate scientific evidence on the effects of acupuncture for low back and neck pain, studies through August, 2013 were reviewed [31]. Among seventy-five randomized controlled trials on chronic neck or low back pain, researchers found that acupuncture was somewhat more effective than sham-acupuncture in producing an immediate post-treatment analgesic effect in cases of chronic neck pain, and acute and chronic low back pain. They also determined that cupping may reduce pain compared to a waitlist in cases of chronic neck pain; and may be superior to medications in cases of chronic low back pain. In the review, researchers found there were no serious or life-threatening adverse effects. Researchers concluded that acupuncture and related modalities such as acupressure and cupping may be beneficial in the short-term reduction of pain and debility in cases of chronic low back pain. Related modalities such as gua sha, tai chi, qigong, and Chinese manipulation techniques seemed to have some positive effects, however, more research is needed to form a firm conclusion. The efficacy of tuina and moxibustion were not determined due to lack of quality data. The researchers did regard the TCM modalities to be relatively safe as no serious negative effects were observed.

In order to sift through inconsistencies in the research on low back pain management with acupuncture, researchers compiled data from sixteen systematic reviews. Researchers[32] deemed the most studies in this area to be of low methodological quality. They also rated the external validity as weak. In cases of acute low back pain, inconsistencies were found when comparing analgesic effects with sham acupuncture although findings suggest they have similar benefits regarding function. In cases of chronic low back pain, short-term analgesic effects and functionality improvements were consistent when compared with acupuncture as an adjunct to conventional care or no treatment. Researchers concluded that acupuncture alone or together with standard interventions provides short-term analgesic effects and improves functionality in chronic low back pain. Internal and external validity were assessed to be in need of improvement to increase confidence of findings in these cases.

Clinical studies on the efficacy of acupuncture for patients with low back pain were collected from English and Chinese journals published between 2002 and 2012 and compared. In the forty-seven English, and 115 Chinese studies, researchers[33] found that the English studies tended to be broader in scope, while the Chinese studies maintained a higher level of focus. Researchers also found that interpretations and perspectives varied between the English and Chinese studies. How each group defined terms and prioritized focus and study design also differed. Researchers suggested contradictions be resolved to improve acupuncture research and advance the field.

Chapter Two

Acupuncture for Knee Osteoarthritis

Introduction

People all over the world suffer from osteoarthritis. Osteoarthritis of the knee has become so common, that if you have not already had your knees replaced, the rest of society may think there is something wrong with you. Aches, pains and stiffness of the joints is considered normal; and, if you do happen to swiftly jaunt up a flight of stairs, passers-by may be stunned. Unfortunately, societies are easily programmed, and when a particular disease or condition becomes an acceptable standard, it becomes ingrained and as much a part of current culture as any popular trend. Any visionary knows that when something is held in mind strongly and consistently, the belief system solidifies; when an illness is supported by a whole population, the likelihood that the condition will manifest physically increases exponentially.

The process that most cultures go through to rid themselves of particular conditions or diseases, tends to be through education. When a condition is sufficiently understood, with the aid of medicine, change of lifestyle or shift in attitude or mental focus, the prevalence of a particular condition tends to decline. Many illnesses that were thought to be a normal part of human life have thus disappeared. Infectious diseases, that in the past plagued all of mankind, have been effectively eradicated in the United States. So many conditions that used to wipe out entire civilizations have been overcome to the degree that life expectancy has been extended far beyond what it was just a century ago. People may live entire lifetimes in relatively good health without ever experiencing or suffering from serious illness. Education, medical innovation, change of habit or lifestyle along with a shift in attitude and mental focus is just as likely to heal current highly prevalent conditions, such as osteoarthritis.

Osteoarthritis is a condition in which the cartilage protecting the ends of adjacent bones gradually wears away; when completely depleted, bones may scrape against each other with movement or continual pressure may lead to fusion, as in the spine. Hands, knees, the big toe, hips and spine are common joints afflicted with degenerative arthritis, or osteoarthritis (OA). This condition, a result of wear and tear combined with endogenous pathogenic factors and compounded by reinforced belief systems now affects approximately 27 million Americans.

Cartilage facilitates smooth, fluid motion, allowing articulating bones to move together or slide past each other. It absorbs shock during impact and cushions bone ends. When cartilage deteriorates, pain, swelling and inflammation may restrict movement. The development of spurs causes further irritation, and when brittle bones chip, the floating bits may add to discomfort. An accumulation of cytokines (proteins) and enzymes due to the inflammatory response of the body may flood the affected joint, further damaging the cartilage.

Osteoarthritis may be present at any stage of the lifespan, especially in athletes that continually place immense pressure on joints, or those who engage in repetitive movements, such as those that affect the finger joints. Those with highly acidic internal conditions, such as occurs in diabetes, alcoholism and the development of gout may present with osteoarthritis earlier than others. People who believe that osteoarthritis is a normal part of aging may develop osteoarthritis, (most commonly after age 65), especially if all their friends have it and they watch TV, which continually bombards and programs the elderly with endless advertisements.

To get a grasp on the statistical relevance of the condition, 50% of adults experience symptoms of knee OA at some point during life, 25% of adults are expected to experience symptoms of hip OA by age 85 and more than 10% of those 60 years or older have OA of the hand.

Pain and stiffness, especially upon waking or after being sedentary for a period of time marks the condition. As symptoms tend to follow a gradual progression, they may not be attended to until most of the cartilage is already gone. Painful swelling of joints may get worse, especially when exacerbated by movement or an extended period of activity, or at the end of the day. Common symptoms may include: limited range of motion that improves with regular movement, clicking or cracking sounds with joint movement.

Manifestations in various body parts may take on specific characteristics. Osteoarthritis of the hips may produce pain in the groin or buttocks and occasionally along the inner knee and/or thigh. Knee osteoarthritis is often described as a grating sensation during movement. Spurs are common in osteoarthritis of the fingers; the joints may be swollen; tender and red. pain is frequently noticed at the base of the thumb. When osteoarthritis affects the big toe, sharp or throbbing pain and tenderness may come and go at the base of the big toe. The other toes and the ankles may be swollen as well.

Etiology of Osteoarthritis

Currently, osteoarthritis is considered a disease of the joint. Contributory factors may include:

Genetic Influence: A rare defect in the production of the protein in cartilage, collagen, has been identified as a risk-factor for osteoarthritis. Those with the defect, may develop osteoarthritis earlier-on in the life cycle; possibly, as early as age 20. Other genetic anomalies may manifest as suboptimal joint articulation, leading to an accelerated wearing away of cartilage. The FAAH gene, associated with pain hypersensitivity, is higher in those with knee OA.

Body Constitution: Excess weight over time, especially when combined with muscle weakness, leads to inordinate pressure on the hips and knees. Interestingly, those who are overweight tend to have a greater risk of developing osteoarthritis in the hands; this phenomenon possibly due to higher levels of cytokines from an inflammatory response within fatty tissue.

Injury and Overuse: Injuries at or affecting the joints, including fracture or ligament tears as well as surgeries and repetitive movements may contribute to osteoarthritic conditions. Athletes who repeatedly injure the same joints or engage in high-impact sports may accumulate damage within the joints, tendons and ligaments; this, combined with chronic inflammation may accelerate cartilage deterioration. Occupations that require habitually standing for prolonged periods of time, frequent bending and lifting, heavy lifting and detailed finger-work, such as painting, needlework or typing, may deplete cartilage as well.

Other Risk Factors: Concurrent disease of or abnormality of the bones, such as Rheumatoid arthritis; metabolic disorders such as hemochromatosis, (hyperabsorption of iron); or acromegaly, from an over-production of growth hormone all are associated with increased risk for osteoarthritis.

Tests, Physical and Medications

Diagnostic Tests: Osteoarthritis may be diagnosed based on history and physical exam. Although blood tests are generally not of use, there are medical tests that help confirm a diagnosis, such as joint aspiration, in which aspirated fluid is searched for crystalline formations or joint deterioration. This procedure may also be used to rule out other potential conditions, or to diagnose other types of arthritis. X-rays may show abnormalities associated with loss of cartilage. Magnetic resonance imaging (MRI), which may be selected over x-ray as it does not image through radiation, shows the cartilage and provides detail needed to detect early-stage osteoarthritis.

Physical Activity in the Management of OA Symptoms: A moderate amount of movement is recommended to maintain healthy joints. Strength training, especially of intrinsic muscles and ligaments that support joints, and exercises that improve range of motion and fluidity are recommended in cases where weakness is contributing to joint stress.

Pain and Anti-inflammatory Medications: Medicines for osteoarthritis are available as pills, syrups, creams or lotions, or may be injected into a joint, including, pharmacologic analgesics, pain-killers, (including acetaminophen), opioids (narcotics) and atypical opioids such as tramadol. Each of these may alleviate pain for a period of time. Nonsteroidal anti-inflammatory drugs (NSAIDs), such as aspirin, ibuprofen and naproxen may provide relief in cases where inflammation is causing pain. Corticosteroids have stronger anti-inflammatory effects, and may be prescribed orally or may be administered via injection directly into the affected joint. Hyaluronic acid, normally present in joint fluid, lubricates the joint and absorbs impact shock. Deficient in those with osteoarthritis, hyaluronic acid can be injected into the affected joint(s).

Osteoarthritis in Chinese Medicine

Traditional Chinese medicine differentiates types of joint pain, such as the joint pain seen in osteoarthritic conditions, according to specific manifestation of symptoms. As the same diagnosis may present differently in each individual, specificity of diagnosis then allows for specificity of treatment that matches the patient.

Painful Obstructive syndrome, bi syndrome, or *Bi Zheng*, all are Chinese medical terms that reflect conditions similar to those seen in various forms of arthritis; although, the terminology may also describe conditions not meeting the requirements for an arthritic diagnosis. Pain in the joints is generally attributed to the external environmental factor of wind, which combines with damp and/or hot or cold that then transgresses the body's defense system, becoming lodged in the joints, obstructing qi and blood in the related channels and collaterals. Alternatively, the condition may arise as a result of the same pathogenic factors accumulating due to endogenous imbalances.

Bi syndrome is characterized by soreness, achiness and pain in the muscles, joints and tendons accompanied by numbness or heaviness. The joints may also be swollen, retain fluid, or be stiff and lacking in fluid. Painful areas may be warm, cold, dry or moist to the touch depending on pathogenic factors involved. The joints may also be deformed.

Pathogenesis & Etiology: One becomes vulnerable to external invasions such as those seen in Bi syndromes, when the Zheng qi is weaker than the invading pathogen. Pathogenic wind, cold, damp and heat can then invade the interior layers between the muscles and skin obstructing qi and blood which leads to pain and stiffness.

Differential Diagnosis: To assess whether the Bi syndrome is predominantly due to wind, damp, dryness, heat, cold or any combination, distinctions in signs and symptoms are listed: Wind Bi, also called Wandering Bì, like the wind is not fixed to a particular anatomical location, and will move from joint to joint; soreness and itchiness may also predominate. Cold Bi also called Painful Bì is dominated by intense consolidated pain, contraction and stiffness or rigidity. Damp Bi or Fixed Bì can be described as heavy, dull and achy, swollen, edemic, and numb. While Heat Bì tends to be painful, red, swollen and warm.

Complicating Factors: When the condition becomes chronic, more severe blockages or systemic symptoms may arise; such as, when the accumulation of damp and phlegm blocks the qi and blood leading to stasis. Lack of ability of blood and qi to reach certain areas may then lead to local depletion. The condition itself is associated with underlying liver and kidney deficiencies and/or deficiencies of blood and essence which may further be depleted as the condition progresses.

Treatment Principles: According to traditional Chinese medicine, each type of pathology requires a different treatment approach.

When the condition is in the acute or excess stage, the excess is expelled, channels and collaterals are opened and pain is relieved. Each pathogen is overcome, then, by specific means. Wind is expelled and blood is generally tonified. When blood circulation is abundant there is no space for wind to invade and course through channels. Cold is scattered while yang is fortified.

Dampness can be dissolved while the Spleen is tonified to reinforce its ability to maintain proper moisture balance. In cases of heat Bi, heat is cleared and yin aspects may be tonified. When the disease becomes chronic, underlying deficiencies are tonified such as the qi, blood, essence; and commonly, the liver, and/or kidney. Pathogenic factors are also eliminated through appropriate methods and pain is relieved.

TCM Pattern Differentiation & Treatment

Wind Bi: Wind Bi is characterized by soreness and pain that does not remain fixed at any location. Like the wind, it moves from joint to joint, resulting in difficulty when flexing or extending joints. The person may be averse to wind and cold and may experience fever and or chills. The tongue is generally unremarkable although may be stiff. The pulse tends to be floating and wiry. The acupuncture protocol will then seek to expel wind, scatter cold, dissolve dampness, unblock channels and collaterals and relieve pain. Excessive acupuncture points can then be reduced, such as reducing method: Fengmen (BL12), Geshu (BL17) and Xuehai (SP10). Additional points may be added for whole-body pain, such as Houxi (SI3), Shenmai (BL62), Dabao (SP21), Yangxi (LI15), Quchi (LI11), Hegu (LI4), Yangchi (SJ4), Yanglingquan (GB34), Xuanzhong (GB39), Jiexi (ST41).

Cold Bi: Cold Bi can be extremely painful to the point of agony. Pain is fixed, joints are stiff and contracted; the condition is worse with cold and better with warmth. The tongue tends to be stiff, retracted, may be bluish or pale; the coating may be moist and white. The practitioner will scatter excess cold, warm the channels and collaterals, expel wind, dry dampness and alleviate pain. Acupuncture plus moxibustion may be applied with deep insertion and reducing method at excess points; while tonifying Shenshu (BL23), and Guanyuan (RN4) to warm the yang.

Damp Bi: Damp Bi patterns are characterized by swollen, heavy, painful joints accompanied by numbness of the limbs. Distention, fullness and swelling edema and fatigue are common. The pain tends to be fixed and slow to change; motion is often restricted due to swelling. The condition tends to be worse with damp or humid weather, bathing or swimming. The tongue may be swollen with toothmarks, wet; and may have a white and greasy coat. The pulse tends to be soft and or slippery. An effective treatment may serve to dissolve dampness, unblock obstructions in the channels and collaterals, expel wind and relieve pain. Acupuncture and moxibustion protocols may include Zusanli (ST36), Pishu (BL20), Shangqiu (SP5), and Yinlingquan (SP9).

Heat Bi: Heat Bi is characterized by red, swollen, and burning joint pain. Skin over the affected area may radiate warmth. Pain tends to be worse with heat and be better with cold. The person may exhibit fever and sweating, thirst, irritability and may have difficulty being still. The tongue tends to be red with a yellow, dry or greasy yellow coat. The pulse may be rapid and slippery. To clear heat and unblock the channels and collaterals, expel wind, and alleviate pain, reducing acupuncture may be applied to points such as Dazhu (DU14) and Quchi (LI11).

Clinical Evidence: Individual Trials

Knee arthritis is one of the mostly researched conditions with acupuncture and related modalities. The following clinical trials are selected to illustrate the breadth of these researches.

High-frequency Electric Stimulation and Point-injection Therapy

Many with knee pain experience relief from acupuncture; however, many patients wonder what possible lasting benefit may be achieved if the cartilage has already deteriorated. To compare benefits of possible treatments, 205 patients received either high-frequency electric stimulation and point-injection therapy (HESPT), warming needle moxibustion or point-injection therapy [1]. The acupuncture plus moxibustion group was prescribed ipsilateral Xuehai (SP10), Neixiyan (EX-LE4), Waixiyan (EX-LE), Dubi (ST35), Zusanli (ST36) and Yanglingquan (GB34), Yinlingquan (SP9) and Sanyinjiao (SP6). Those receiving HESPT were prescribed Ashi points, Liangqiu (ST34), Xuehai (SP10), Neixiyan (EX-LE4), Waixiyan (EX-LE5), Zusanli (ST36), Yinlingquan (SP9), Weizhong (BL40) and Chengshan (BL57); Corydalis decumbens Pers. liquid was then injected into the points and high-frequency electric stimulation was administered. Those in the point-injection group received the same point injections as those in the HESPT group.

HESPT was found to significantly improve pain, stiffness and swelling upon waking. Severity lessened and range of motion also improved more than with the other two methods. Rates of effectiveness were significantly higher as well in those who had received HESPT than the other modalities. In future studies, comparing each modality applied to the same point prescription may isolate the differences between modality rather than point selection. Determining which type of Bi pain each participant has could be important as well, as moxibustion would make hot or dry Bi worse and cold Bi better.

Moxibustion

Moxibustion was compared with placebo to determine safety and efficacy in terms of pain, stiffness and motor ability in those with knee osteoarthritis (OA) [2]. Moxibustion cones or placebo was administered to Neixiyan (EX-LE 4), Dubi (ST35) and Ashi points of 59 osteoarthritis patients. A total of three cones were placed on each point per treatment, treatments were provided at a frequency of three sessions per week for six consecutive weeks.

In the moxibustion group, according to standard measures, osteoarthritis was reduced at the 3rd and 6th week and one week following the final treatment. Although stiffness score was lower in the placebo group at the end of treatment compared with pre-treatment measures, this improvement did not match that achieved in those who received moxibustion. During the six weeks of treatment and at follow-up assessment one week after the final treatment, pain, stiffness and motor ability were more improved than in the placebo group. Those who received moxibustion improved walking speeds to a greater extent than those in the placebo group as well. Researchers also discovered that the point treated was approximately nine degrees Celsius warmer than placebo moxibustion. Although local skin temperature was elevated at the end of treatment compared to before treatment in both groups, this difference was greater among those who had received moxibustion compared with placebo. Moxibustion was thus affirmed as a safe and effective treatment for osteoarthritis patients with pain, stiffness and mobility issues.

Insight into the patient experience was sought in order to supplement statistical data with subjective experience. As part of a larger clinical trial on moxibustion for knee osteoarthritis, participants of a 12-week trial were interviewed. Open-ended questions were asked with the purpose of eliciting more telling information from the patient's perspective. According to responses, participants accepted knee osteoarthritis as part of aging, taking both a physical and emotional toll on life. The majority wanted to continue moxibustion as a long-term means of reducing symptoms and improving overall wellness. Moxibustion was thus found to be of benefit to patients with knee osteoarthritis. In analyzing patient answers to questions regarding the experience, researchers surmised that attitude towards moxibustion played a role in outcome, and those wishing to continue with moxibustion, recognized that the chronic nature of osteoarthritis may need long-term treatment. Researchers [3] also discovered that patient education plays a crucial role in limiting the chance of adverse effects, as patients may suffer through adverse effects of moxibustion, in trying to magnify gains.

Moxibustion seems to improve some signs and symptoms associated with knee osteoarthritis, especially in yang-deficient cold patterns. To assess the effect of moxibustion on knee arthritis in patients not categorized according to traditional Chinese medicine patterns, researchers [4] compared the effects of moxibustion with sham moxibustion. Patients (110) received a six-week course of moxibustion or sham moxibustion applied three-times per week to Dubi (ST35), extra-point Neixiyan (EX-LE 4) and an Ashi point. No adverse effects were noted among either group. Those who received real moxibustion experienced less pain at weeks 3, 6, 12 and 24 than those in the sham group. Physical functionality was also more improved in those who received real moxibustion when assessed at weeks 3, 6, and 12; however, functionality scores were similar at week 24. At conclusion of the double-blind study [4], total findings suggested that a six-week course of moxibustion at local acupuncture points, Dubi, Neixiyan and an Ashi point may reduce pain and increase physical functionality in those with knee osteoarthritis more than placebo for up to 24 weeks after the end of the treatment series. Deemed safe, moxibustion may provide relief to those with chronic knee osteoarthritis.

The impact of moxibustion (the burning of mugwort over acupuncture points or Ashi points) on pain and functionality in chronic knee osteoarthritis (KOA) among 212 South Korean patients was studied. Patients from multiple clinical centers received a four-week course of either moxibustion or conventional care without moxibustion. After five weeks, Korean WOMAC global arthritis values, numerical rating scale (NRS) and timed-stand test were more greatly improved in those who had received moxibustion than those who had not. Researchers also noticed that after five weeks, K-WOMAC scores were diminished in those who had mild rather than moderate-severe osteoarthritis. After 13 weeks, arthritis global scores and pain were significantly reduced in those who had received moxibustion. After five weeks, SF-36 scores reflected improvements in physical component summary, physical pain and functionality as well as social functionality among those who had received moxibustion. Interestingly, although pain and functionality improved, SF-36 scores did not detect mental gains after five or 13 weeks. Adverse effects were reported in less than 10% of moxibustion treatments such as first and second-degree burns, pruritis and fatigue. Researchers [5] concluded that pain, function and quality of life in Korean patients with knee osteoarthritis tend to improve with moxibustion; protective measures to avoid burns or adoption of application techniques with less risk should be considered in future studies.

Acupuncture Versus Western Medication

Palliative medication and pain killers, although they do not cure the condition or prevent further degeneration, are often the treatment of choice among patients. They may provide enough relief to lessen the negative impact of the condition on daily life. Acupuncture, in therapeutic doses may be too consuming in terms of treatment time and cost to the patient, and the restorative extent or ability to prevent further damage is not fully known. To gain a better understanding of the potential benefits of each, 120 cases were administered either acupuncture or western medication, glucosamine hydrochloride [6]. The acupuncture protocol included local points: Neixiyan (EX-LE 4), Dubi (ST35), Yinlingquan (SP9) and Yanglingquan (GB34); along with points according to differential diagnosis. Western Ontario and McMaster Universities Osteoarthritis Index (WOMAC) and Medical Outcomes Study 36-Item Short Form Health Survey (SF-36, Chinese version) were used to assess the therapeutic effect before treatment, after four weeks treatment and in follow-up visit at nine weeks after treatment separately.

Following the four-week treatment period, total effective rate was similar in both groups, 86.7% for those who received acupuncture compared with 88.3% in those who were prescribed medication. Nine weeks following treatment, total effective rate for acupuncture remained high, 83.3%, compared with 61.7% in the medication group. Arthritis indices and overall health outcome measures were all improved in both groups. Similar to effectiveness ratings, no significant differences were seen between groups at the four-week follow-up; while at the nine-week follow-up, those who had received acupuncture-maintained improvements to a greater degree than those in the medication group.

These findings [6] indicate that short-term efficacy of acupuncture according to differential diagnosis is similar to orally administered glucosamine hydrochloride. However, an acupuncture treatment series maintained positive effects to a greater degree than did medication.

Electroacupuncture (EA) Versus Warming Needle Moxibustion on Knee Osteoarthritis Due to Kidney Deficiency and Marrow Insufficiency

Electroacupuncture (EA) or warming needle moxibustion was administered to 74 patients with knee osteoarthritis due to kidney deficiency and depletion of marrow. Local points, Dubi (ST35), Neixiyan (EX-LE 4), Xuehai (SP10), Zusanli (ST 36), and Yanglingquan (GB34) were selected. Either continuous low-frequency (5Hz) electroacupuncture or warm needling moxibustion with two cones per acupoint was applied. Three treatments per week were administered for a period of four weeks. Both treatment methods were deemed effective. The cure-rate and rate of efficacy reached 64.7% in those who received electroacupuncture, significantly greater than the 40.0% achieved by those who had received warming-needle moxibustion. While EA was more effective at diminishing pain, warming-needle moxibustion was better at alleviating stiffness [7].

Electroacupuncture relieved different aspects of knee osteoarthritis due to kidney and marrow deficiency than warming needle with moxibustion at the selected points. Electroacupuncture, in this case was more effective at alleviating pain, while warming needle moxibustion was more effective at resolving joint stiffness. Total efficacy of electroacupuncture was superior to warming needle moxibustion. If the patients in this case exhibited kidney-yin deficiency, rather than kidney qi or yang deficiency, the expectation would be that electroacupuncture would be more effective than warming-needle moxibustion.

Acupuncture as an Adjunctive therapy to Pharmacological Treatment

Pharmacotherapy (etoricoxib) intervention and the combination of acupuncture plus pharmacotherapy were compared as to their effects on chronic pain due to knee osteoarthritis [8]. Patients (120) received one of either of the two interventions or sham acupuncture and pharmacotherapy. Researchers discovered that nearly all outcomes were significantly superior in those who received the combination of mediation and acupuncture than among those who received sham acupuncture and medication, or medication alone. Thus, etoricoxib together with acupuncture may be an effective means of reducing negative symptoms associated with knee osteoarthritis.

Acupuncture in Total Knee Replacement (TKR)

Statistical reports do not always tap into measures that are meaningful to human experience, especially when considering the diversity of priorities, attitude, lifestyle and perception among individuals. According to scientific evaluation, total knee replacement (TKR) is considered a cost-effective means with which to successfully resolve pain due to knee osteoarthritis and restore a reasonable level of functionality. According to patients who have had the procedure, 20% are not satisfied with outcomes one year after surgery that had been deemed successful.

Previous research demonstrated that symptoms of knee osteoarthritis may be alleviated with acupuncture in those with knee osteoarthritis while waiting for surgical intervention. Acupuncture and physiotherapy were assessed in 56 knee osteoarthritis patients for effects on preoperative and postoperative pain and function [9]. Patients received physiotherapy plus acupuncture or a brochure that contained advice for the patient along with standard exercises. Although researchers were not able to establish significant results due to small sample size; interestingly, six of those in the treatment group improved to such a degree that they did not have the scheduled surgery. Comparatively, only one in the control group withdrew due to symptomatic improvement. A larger sample size is necessary to fully assess the effect of acupuncture plus physiotherapy on symptoms in those with severe osteoarthritis of the knee.

Warming-Needle Moxibustion

Moxibustion adds a warming and tonifying effect to acupuncture treatment. To assess the therapeutic impact of warming-needle moxibustion on knee osteoarthritis, 120 patients were administered the intervention or were prescribed Celebrex. Deqi response was achieved in all cases following moxibustion. Treatments were provided once per week for a total of four weeks. The therapeutic effect was evaluated after the four-weeks treatment course. Follow-up assessments were taken three months following end of treatment. After the four-week treatment series, the effective rate in the control group was 78.3%, which further improved, reaching 81.7% at the three-month follow-up. Those who received warming-needle moxibustion, demonstrated significantly greater rates of effectiveness than controls, which reached 96.6% at the end of treatment. This effectiveness rating remained stable at the three-month follow-up. Pain in the treatment group, and in the control group, was significantly diminished after the four-week treatment period and at the three-month follow-up. Overall, researchers [10] concluded that warming-needle moxibustion alleviates pain in patients with knee osteoarthritis as well as stiffness, swelling and mobility issues.

Ultrastructural Acupotomy Therapy

A less common form of treatment, ultrastructural acupotomy therapy, applied to counter-Ashi points (those points, that when pressed, elicit a pain-relieving effect rather than pain) was compared with warming-needle moxibustion in the treatment of knee osteoarthritis. Either treatment was applied to 60 cases, weekly, over the course of one month. For those receiving warming-needle moxibustion, the protocol included local points such as: Dubi (ST35), Neixiyan (EX-LE 4), Zusanli (ST36) and Yanglingquan (GB34). The prescription was provided daily over the course of one month. Pain and range of motion improved in both groups. Researchers [11] found that superior results were seen in those who received ultrastructural acupotomy at the counter-Ashi points than those who received warming-needle acupuncture. The ultrastructural acupotomy therapy at the counter-Ashi points demonstrated a greater level of efficacy in treating osteoarthritis of the knee compared with warming-needle moxibustion acupuncture therapy; as weekly, rather than daily treatments were needed, resulting in greater cost-benefit and convenience.

Local Acupuncture

Conventional acupuncture was provided at local points to assess potential benefits on knee osteoarthritis. The protocol was administered three to four times per week, for four consecutive weeks, and included points such as: Liang-qiu (ST34), Dubi (ST35), Zusanli (ST36), Yanglingquan (GB34) and Yinlingquan (SP9). The Western Ontario and McMaster Universities osteoarthritis index (WOMAC) and the visual analogue scale (VAS) were utilized to numerize relevant outcomes of 73 cases. Researchers found that acupuncture improved every VAS and WOMAC rating. These findings [12] demonstrate that acupuncture reduces knee osteoarthritis pain while improving functionality. Of note, positive improvements were retained at the four-week follow-up.

Warm-Needling in Different Syndromes

In traditional Chinese medicine, arthritis is best treated after determining differential diagnosis, as underlying conditions and pathogenic influences vary, each requiring a different treatment approach. To assess efficacy of warming-needle moxibustion, 197 patients with knee osteoarthritis were diagnosed according to traditional Chinese medicine syndrome and grouped accordingly. The study [13] included wind-cold-damp, yang-deficiency with cold stagnation, blood stasis and depleted essence; 50 cases of each identified pattern. Three courses of warming-needle moxibustion were applied for 10 days each course. To gauge internal changes, levels of interleukin-1 (IL-1), interleukin-6 (IL-6), and tumor necrosis factor-alpha (TNF-alpha) in the synovial fluid were measured before and after the treatment series.

Researchers discovered that symptoms improved, efficacy was established and serum levels associated with the negative impact of arthritis decreased regardless of pattern manifestation. Those with an underlying yang-deficient pattern accompanied by an accumulation of pathogenic cold improved to a greater degree than those expressing other syndromes; while those with blood stasis improved the least among the four groups in terms of symptoms and efficacy.

Osteoarthritis of the knee due to wind-cold-damp pathogenic factors, yang deficiency with accumulated pathogenic cold stagnation, blood-stasis or depletion of essence all improved with warming-needle moxibustion. As would be expected with moxibustion, yang-deficiency with cold improved the most across all measures. Also, not surprisingly, blood stasis improved the least, as blood stasis can be due to injury, heat or cold.

Non-Specific Versus Modern Versus Classical Acupuncture

Diverse forms of needling techniques have been developed since traditional Chinese Medicine first emerged as a medical system. In addition to following protocols as determined through individualized differential diagnosis, diverse modern assessment and point-selection methods have been developed. Some also believe the needling effect in-and-of-itself may provide some benefit. To learn more about the different effects associated with specific needling approaches, 116 patients with knee osteoarthritis from three research institutes received, either traditional acupuncture, semi-standardized acupuncture protocols or non-specific needling.

Researchers found that the effects of traditional Chinese acupuncture according to syndrome differentiation were superior to standard protocols or non-acupoint needling. Knee flexibility improved 10.3 degrees, expressing a significant difference. Standardized acupuncture protocols increased flexibility by less than half the amount as did individualized treatment, approximately 4.7 degrees. Although all interventions improved pain to some degree, the analgesic effect of traditional acupuncture exceeded the other two methods, 73% compared to 64% with standardized protocols and 48% with non-acupuncture point needling. By needling in all three groups, researchers [14] were able to employ a double-blinded method that may be utilized in future research. The findings strongly supported point-specificity of acupuncture.

Collateral Meridian Therapy

Arthritic conditions occur when wind, cold, heat and/or damp can invade the body's defense system and become lodged in the channels and collaterals blocking the flow of qi and blood, causing pain. To assess the benefits of relieving stagnation of the collaterals involved in osteoarthritis of the knee, 28 patients with knee osteoarthritis received either Collateral Meridian (CM) therapy or placebo twice per week for three weeks. During the second and third week or treatment, researchers noticed that those who had received Collateral Meridian therapy reported significantly less pain, and greater functionality. Researchers [15] suggested further research to fully evaluate the benefits of Collateral Meridian therapy in the treatment of knee osteoarthritis.

Electroacupuncture and Cartilage Restoration

The analgesic effects of electroacupuncture have been well-verified; however, the physiological impact on tissues has not. To determine the restorative capacity of electroacupuncture on knee cartilage in those with osteoarthritis researchers conducted a study. Sixty cases of knee osteoarthritis received a four-week series of either electroacupuncture at Neixiyan (EX-LE 4), Dubi (ST35), Heding (EX-LE 2) and Xuehai (SP10) once every other day, or physiotherapy. Both interventions had a significant positive effect on knee functionality except in the area of demand for support. According to T2 values, anterior lateral tibial sub-region was significantly improved in those who had received electroacupuncture; however, significant improvement was not achieved in nine other sub-regions tested. T2 values were not significantly affected by physiotherapy. Overall, results [16] showed that electroacupuncture produced greater functionality gains than physiotherapy and showed that it may promote cartilage renewal.

Long-Term Efficacy of Warm-Needling Moxibustion and Rehabilitation

Patient receiving rehabilitation after an earthquake participated in a trial to assess the benefit of warming-needle moxibustion versus acupuncture on knee osteoarthritis. In both interventions, the same points were used, Neixiyan (EX LE 4) and Dubi (ST 35); all patients also participated in rehabilitation training. Total effectiveness after 20 treatments was 100.0% in 41 patients who received warm-needling moxibustion; benefits were greater than those achieved in the acupuncture groups, which was rated at 85.4%. After the 20 treatments, significant improvements in symptoms, pain and functionality were achieved in both groups; greater reductions in symptoms and pain were achieved in those who received warming-needle moxibustion compared to acupuncture alone. Benefits were stable at the two-month follow-up, improvements in functionality; however, did not remain statistically significant. Overall, rehabilitation plus warm-needling moxibustion [17] was found to be safe and more efficacious than rehabilitation training plus acupuncture without moxibustion for patients with knee osteoarthritis.

Acupuncture Versus Isometric Exercises

As stiffness, pain and limited range of motion predominate in osteoarthritis, regular movement as well as exercises that intend to strengthen the intrinsic tendino-musculature that supports the joints is a reasonable means of diminishing the harmful effects of chronic joint deterioration. To determine the difference in benefits between isometric exercise for knee osteoarthritis and acupuncture, patients who met criteria according to the American College of Rheumatology were randomized to either treatment group. Patients were scored according to intensity of pain and functionality during a four-week course totaling 12 sessions. Quality of life improved in both groups by the end of the treatment course, with no significant differences between groups. Pain was reduced in both groups as well. Total findings [18] suggest that the acupuncture protocol provided and isometric exercises are equivalent in terms of pain reduction and quality of life improvements for those with knee osteoarthritis.

Acupuncture at Neiguan (PC6) and Taichong (LR3) Versus Standard Points

In the practice of acupuncture, a variety of approaches may be applied to the same problem. If one protocol is ineffective, a different protocol may be highly effective. To assess differences in two completely different approaches, the effects of acupuncture point combination, Neiguan (PC6) and Taichong (LR3); were compared with local points for knee osteoarthritis. Neiguan (PC6) was needled on the healthy side while Taichong (LR3) was needled on the affected side; or bilaterally at both points if treating both knees. Yanglingquan (GB34), Yinlingquan (SP9), Neixiyan (EX-LE 4), Dubi (ST35), Zusanli (ST36) and other relevant points on the affected side were needled in those receiving standard acupuncture.

At the end of treatment, researchers [19] found that pain, stiffness, functionality and osteoarthritis scores improved in both groups. Pain was more greatly diminished in those who received acupuncture at Neiguan (PC6) and Taichong (LR3) than standard acupuncture; however, osteoarthritis scores reached a similar level of improvement. Thus, as the analgesic effect of acupuncture at Neiguan (PC6) and Taichong (LR3) was stronger than standard points; the simple, two-point combination was less time-consuming and other osteoarthritis improvements were similar to those achieved with standard acupuncture. Therefore, the simple two-point point combination may be more desirable as a treatment option for knee osteoarthritis.

Resting-State Blood Flow and Moxibustion at Dubi (ST35)

Mechanisms of acupuncture are not fully known; even less is understood regarding moxibustion. To see changes in the brain when moxibustion is applied to Dubi (ST35); and therefore, gain insight into underlying mechanisms, functional magnetic resonance imaging (fMRI) scans were captured of 30 left knee osteoarthritis patients. Resting-state scans, fractional amplitude of low frequency fluctuation (fALFF) and regional homogeneity (ReHo) were assessed. Researchers noticed that moxibustion induced elevations in fALFF within bilateral cerebrum, extra-nucleus, left cerebellum and white matter. Meanwhile fALFF within the precentral gyrus, frontal lobe and occipital lobe declined. Elevations in ReHo were observed within the thalamus, extra-nucleus and parietal lobe; while ReHo within bilateral cerebrum and frontal lobe diminished.

Researchers [20] stated that brain effects associated with the application of moxibustion were congruent with the understanding of how pain and heat signals are transmitted. Activation patterns produced reflect that body systems rather than one single point of the skin were affected. These findings support channel theory. As is true with acupuncture, moxibustion at Dubi (ST35) was found to affect whole brain networks rather than one specific area or structure within the brain.

Stiletto Needle

New and efficient applications of traditional acupuncture practices are constantly being sought to limit time and expense of treatment. One such application, acupuncture with stiletto needle, was evaluated for its effect on pain due to knee arthritis. In seventy-six cases, Jingjin theory, in traditional Chinese medicine, was applied with stiletto needle at the point of pain, Jingjin, in the extra-articular area. Significant improvements were observed in pain, tenderness, functionality and range of motion. Overall effectiveness was measured at 89.5%. Researchers [21] concluded that stiletto needle relieves knee osteoarthritis pain; efficacy evaluation may be improved via objective tenderness measuring device.

Meridian Sinew Release

The widespread prevalence of osteoarthritis and its devastating effects are comparable to those of cardiovascular disease. Management of the condition can be cumbersome and costly, however, there is no cure. Innovative applications of acupuncture-derived techniques, such as "meridian-sinew release," offer some hope to patients diagnosed with this progressive condition. A meridian-sinew scope and meridian-sinew knife were utilized to evaluate the intervention in 90 patients with knee osteoarthritis. Each received either meridian-sinew release treatment, acupuncture or medication. Pain, stiffness, functionality, total symptom and overall changes were assessed after 12 weeks of treatment. General assessments by the patient and practitioner were similar across treatment groups. Significantly greater improvements were observed in pain and stiffness between meridian-sinew treatment and acupuncture and between meridian-sinew treatment and controls. Overall, meridian-sinew release was found to be safe while providing benefit to those with knee osteoarthritis including relief from pain, and improved functionality [22].

Qi Sensation (Deqi)

Deqi is considered to be the most-crucial factor associated with a successful acupuncture treatment. Characterized most often as a dull, heavy ache accompanied by a calming of the mind, researchers used the MGH Acupuncture Sensation Scale (MASS) to assess effects in regard to deqi. Over the course of four weeks, 30 osteoarthritis patients received either high dose, low dose, or sham acupuncture. Both high and low dose acupuncture reduced pain to a greater degree than sham, both achieving significant reduction in osteoarthritic pain and significantly improved functionality than sham acupuncture. MASS and patient ratings correlated in 11 of 12 types of sensations, with heaviness being the most common sensation observed. Perceptions of sensations varied among all acupuncture participants, as did level of soreness and achiness. Low and high dose acupuncture elicited stronger deqi than sham, which correlated with more successful clinical outcomes among knee osteoarthritis patients. This study [23] demonstrated that the MASS may be an accurate measure of deqi response and therefore, useful as an assessment tool in future acupuncture studies.

Knee osteoarthritis, due to its progressively degenerate nature and lack of cure, may bring about mental and physical anguish in those afflicted. The gradual loss of motility and functionality combined with gradually escalating pain intensity and chronicity may wear away not only the cartilage of the affected joint, but motivation and enjoyment of daily life may also deteriorate. There is yet much debate as to how best to economically and effectively manage symptoms in a way that optimally diminishes negative symptoms and impact on life. A comprehensive care plan may provide a combination of benefits not possible to achieve in any one modality alone. To determine the overall impact of providing a course of acupuncture plus exercise-based physical therapy, researchers conducted a randomized, double-blind controlled trial with 214 patients; of note, 66% were African American. Through x-rays, researchers detected Kellgren scores of 2-3 in all patients. Over a 6-12-week interval, patients received 12 exercise-based physical therapy sessions immediately followed by acupuncture. The method of acupuncture included a standardized nine-point protocol for Bi syndrome with either standard needles or non-skin-puncturing needles.

Researchers [24] detected an approximate 30% improvement in osteoarthritis outcomes with the combination of either acupuncture or non-penetrating acupuncture plus physical therapy. It is well-understood that expectation and attitude influence outcomes; this was found to be true in this study, as those who expected acupuncture to alleviate pain correlated with a higher level of subjective gains. Although the majority of participants were African American, with genetic differences and inherited differences in skeletal-musculature, differences were not detected according to race, sex or age. As none of the participants received physical therapy without acupuncture or non-penetrating acupuncture, the effects of each could not be differentiated and no explanation for the equivalency seen between groups could be surmised.

Effects of Different Acupuncture on Different Stages of Osteoarthritis

To determine if different applications of acupuncture are more or less effective at the beginning or later stages of osteoarthritis, researchers conducted a complex study with 180 patients. Three stages with specific characteristics were identified: stagnation, fascia cramping and tendon lesion. Participants at each stage then received either a specific modality according to stage of disease or electroacupuncture. Specific stage-related treatments were provided. During the stagnation phase, tendon meridian acupuncture is applied with electric thermal needling. In the fascia cramping stage, small needle-knife and bleeding were administered. Electroacupuncture at local points was administered during the tendon lesion stage using thermal-electric therapy with silver needles.

Researchers [25] discovered that staging treatments were slightly more effective than standardized electroacupuncture overall; reaching an effectiveness rating of 96.1% in the staging group versus 91.1% among those receiving electroacupuncture. A greater level of remarkable effectiveness was observed in those receiving stage-related treatment (88.9%), compared with those receiving electroacupuncture (62.2%). In acupuncture clinical practice, more remarkable improvements are often easier to attain in the earlier stages of most diseases; concordantly, electroacupuncture achieved less remarkable rates of effectiveness with further progression of the disease. This study showed that with applying stage-related modalities, greater improvements were achieved in knee osteoarthritis.

Heat-Sensitive Moxibustion Versus Non-Heat-Sensitive Moxibustion

Just as deqi is considered an essential response to acupuncture, deqi during the application of moxibustion is also desired for better outcomes. While needle sensation may more commonly elicit a feeling of dull, heavy pressure; a spreading sensation of warmth may be noticed more frequently with moxibustion. This phenomenon was explored via application of moxibustion above and below the right knee at Xi Yan (EX-LE5) and He Ding (EX-LE2). Significant reductions in arthritis measures were observed in the trial group compared with controls which were maintained in the follow-up. Researchers [26], thus determined that deqi response was associated with greater improvement in patients with knee osteoarthritis than when deqi response was not obtained.

Thermal Laser Acupuncture

Diverse imbalances according to traditional Chinese medicine theory may underlie individual manifestations that fall under the diagnosis of knee osteoarthritis. Three common syndromes seen in patients with osteoarthritis of the knee include yang deficiency with cold stagnation, kidney deficiency or blood stasis. Logically it seems that the application of heat as in thermal laser acupuncture may be of greater benefit to patients with underlying cold patterns than those patients with other underlying patterns. Researchers explored the validity of this treatment principle in 52 knee arthritis patients. Thermal laser acupuncture was applied to Dubi (ST35) over the course of six weeks; three-times per week initially, and twice per week the following three weeks. Those patients who were yang-deficient showed significantly greater gains in terms of functionality throughout the treatment series; however, significant differences in pain reduction and relief of stiffness were not observed between groups. The study [27] overall supported thermal laser acupuncture as a safe and effective means for treating knee osteoarthritis especially for those with yang deficient patterns. Those with yang-deficiency knee osteoarthritis experienced greater gains in functionality with thermal laser than those with other underlying patterns.

Periosteal Stimulation Therapy (PST)

Innovations based on traditional Chinese medicine are constantly emerging to address difficult to treat conditions. Building on previous research that established the efficacy and tolerability of periosteal stimulation therapy

(PST) (electrical stimulation of needles inserted near the periosteum); researchers assessed the lasting effects of PST in the management of chronic pain due to severe knee osteoarthritis.

One hundred ninety participants received one of three periosteal stimulation therapies. Either PST (weekly for 10 weeks) followed by PST boosters for six months (weekly for two weeks, then reduced to monthly), control PST (weekly for 10 weeks), or PST (weekly for 10 weeks) followed by control PST boosters for six months.

In addition to standard osteoarthritis measures, researchers also observed changes in physical ability, mental state, quality of life, activity level, need for pharmaceutical intervention and other medical interventions. Findings [28] showed that PST plus control booster results were similar to controls at 10 weeks and after nine months. Those who received PST plus PST booster reached similar gains as controls by week 10; however, those who received boosters reached a significantly greater level of benefit by nine months. Patients with more severe levels of initial symptoms such as depression, ineffectiveness, difficulty in completing normal daily activities, and knee stiffness were less likely to improve. In summary, PST with additional boosters for nine months following a 10-week course of PST was found to be advantageous in reducing pain in those with advanced knee osteoarthritis.

Acupuncture and Moxibustion Versus Medication

Acupuncture, moxibustion and medication each have their advantages in terms of treating knee osteoarthritis. To evaluate relative benefits, acupuncture plus moxibustion was compared with medication. Daily acupuncture was provided for five consecutive days at local Ashi points along with points selected according to traditional Chinese medical pattern differentiation; distal points according to meridian therapy were also included. Strong stimulation was induced with lifting and thrusting; or rotating technique was applied with appropriate tonification or sedation. Techniques applied included "Duanci" or "Shuci" needling at extra and Ashi points. Following acupuncture, heat-sensitive indirect moxibustion was administered at local Ashi points and Shenshu (BL23), the back-shu of the kidney, in order to discover which points were heat-sensitized. After a two-day rest period, another series of daily treatments were given over the course of five days. Glucosamine sulfate capsules were prescribed for those in the medication group plus joint cavity injection. Sodium hyaluronate 25 mg and triamcinolone acetonide acetate 50 mg were the contents of injection initially; sodium hyaluronate 25 mg was injected each subsequent week, for four weeks.

Researchers [29] found that the efficacy was significantly greater for those who received western medication than acupuncture plus moxibustion. The improvement overall in those who received acupuncture and moxibustion was greater than that achieved with medication. Functionality was similar between the two groups at the three-month follow-up; however, functionality in the combined treatment group was more improved than those who had received medication at the sixth-month follow-up. Researchers concluded; overall, that the acupuncture method provided plus moxibustion was safe and effective for patients with knee osteoarthritis and has greater lasting effects than medication.

Combined Modalities Versus Acupuncture

Traditional acupuncture and Chinese medicine include many modalities and methods, the most appropriate in each case are skillfully combined for the best therapeutic impact in clinical practice. To gather scientific evidence of potential optimization, a comprehensive strategy was adopted including fire needles at the painful bones plus cupping plus local Tuina for the treatment of knee osteoarthritis. The combined effect was then compared to the effects of administering acupuncture alone. Fire-needling was administered every other day, while daily cupping and Tuina were also provided. For those in the acupuncture group, standard acupuncture was administered daily including points such as: Dubi (ST35), Neixiyan (EX-LE 4), Xuehai (SP10), Liangqiu (ST34). Each participant received one or two sets of a ten-day course of either treatment intervention.

Both treatment strategies were found to reduce pain; with greater improvements achieved in those who received the comprehensive approach. Comprehensive cure rate was also greater in those who received a combination of modalities than acupuncture alone, 38% (19/50), versus 20.0% (10/50), respectively. Osteoarthritis of the knee improved with either acupuncture or a comprehensive combination of fire needles at painful bones plus cupping plus local Tuina; however, the combined treatment method achieved a greater level of improvement in such indices as joint pain, swelling and functionality [30].

Heat-Sensitive Moxibustion and Serum OPN and MMP-3

Heat-sensitive moxibustion was assessed for its impact on knee pain and serum osteopontin (OPN) and matrix metalloproteinase-3 (MMP-3). Heat-sensitive indirect moxibustion, electroacupuncture (EA) or Chinese herbal medication were administered to 144 patients with knee osteoarthritis. Those in the moxibustion group received a 15-day course of daily indirect moxibustion; applied for 40 minutes each side at bilateral Weizhong (BL40), influential point for acute low-back pain. Those in the electroacupuncture group received a 15-day course of daily electroacupuncture, applied to local points, Neixiyan (EX-LE 4), Dubi (ST35), Xuehai (SP10) and Liangqiu (ST34) for a duration of 30 minutes. Meanwhile, those in the medication group ingested Sanqi Tongshu herbal formula capsules (Panax Notoginseng, etc. for moving the blood and removing blood stasis), three times per day over the course of 15 days.

Researchers found significant reduction in serum OPN of those in the moxibustion and EA groups, as well as significant reduction in serum MMP-3 of the moxibustion group after treatment. Insignificant reduction of serum OPN was observed in the medication group and MMP-3 was insignificantly reduced in the EA group. Moxibustion was found to be more effective than herbal medication at reducing serum OPN and more effective than EA or herbal formula in degree of reducing serum MMP-3. Researchers [31] concluded that heat-sensitive indirect moxibustion alleviates acute knee pain due to osteoarthritis. The mechanisms involved in the analgesic effects of indirect moxibustion may be associated with a lowering effect on serum OPN and MMP-3,

Heat-Sensitive Versus Resting-State Moxibustion

Moxibustion is known to produce deqi sensations described as a spreading feeling of warmth; patients who experience this response are said to be heat-sensitive. To gain insight regarding efficacy, heat-sensitive moxibustion was compared with non-heat-sensitive (resting-state) moxibustion in 60 knee osteoarthritis patients. A 20-day course of indirect moxibustion was applied daily for 45 minutes to local standard points, including: Neixiyan (EX-LE 4), Dubi, (ST35) and Heding (EX-LE 2). If patients noticed heat spreading out from the acupoint in any direction, such as warmth penetrating more deeply from the skin to the underlying tissues, across the skin surface or tissue, or coursing through the channels, deqi in the form of producing a heat-sensitization state was accepted.

After integrating VAS scores at the end of the treatment course and those at the six-month follow-up, researchers determined that those who had demonstrated heat-sensitization to moxibustion reached a significantly less-painful existence than those who did not experience heat deqi. At the end of the treatment series, 46.7% of those in the heat-sensitive group and 16.7% of those in the resting group experienced noticeable improvement. Similar rates of effectiveness were observed in both groups, 33.3% among those who were heat-sensitive compared with 30.0% in those non-heat-sensitive. After six months, the heat-sensitive group reached a rate of effectiveness of 79.2% compared to 42.9% of those in the non-heat-sensitive group. The result [32] suggest that, just as deqi is crucial to efficacy of acupuncture treatment, heat-sensitivity was associated with greater clinical improvements in those with knee osteoarthritis.

Sustained Effects of Acupuncture

Chronic conditions such as knee osteoarthritis often benefit from regular, continuous care; it is not fully known how essential it is to start acupuncture early-on after diagnosis. To gauge potential long-term effect of acupuncture in chronic knee pain, outcomes of those who received acupuncture along with standard medical care soon after diagnosis were compared with those who received a series of acupuncture treatments three months after starting the standard medical protocols. Three years later, 500 patients completed follow-up questionnaires. Researchers found that, arthritis indices were not significantly different between treatment groups.

Researchers [33] noted that 202 of 500 patients continued with acupuncture during the follow-up period. Whether patients continued tended to correspond to having achieved benefits from acupuncture in the beginning. Long-term lowered arthritic score ratings correlated to positive response to acupuncture after the first treatment series. Higher level of education, desire to avoid pharmacological intervention, and engaging in other additional interventions were also associated with better arthritic scores after three years. Although many factors influenced positive outcomes, this study found no correlation in outcomes after three years between those who stared acupuncture immediately with standard medical intervention or three months later. A more telling study might evaluate both short-term and long-term outcomes in those who start acupuncture before other interventions are applied.

Electroacupuncture Versus Manual Acupuncture

When patients are in extraordinary pain or have been in a state of chronic pain for an enduring length of time, the immediate effects of treatment may make a profound difference in restoring a sense of hope. To assess the differences in immediate response of electroacupuncture compared to manual acupuncture, researchers measured induced changes in pain, mobility and muscle strength in 60 patients with knee osteoarthritis. Changes in severity of pain, functionality, maximal isometric contraction and ability to tolerate pain and pressure were measured following one manual acupuncture or electroacupuncture treatment. Severity of pain was significantly lessened by a similar degree in both groups; meanwhile, functionality significantly increased to a similar degree in both groups. Maximum voluntary isometric contraction as well as pressure and pain threshold also changed to a similar degree in both groups. In conclusion, researchers [34] found acupuncture and electroacupuncture to induce equivalent changes in pain, muscle strength, and mobility among knee osteoarthritic patients which may be observed immediately following treatment.

Lateral Wedge Insert Versus Acupuncture

Energetic in nature, acupuncture may influence structural impairments via the invisible support it provides to tissues at the joints and to the whole body's ability to hold itself up. Potential impact of acupuncture on structural issues associated with knee osteoarthritis was compared to that of wearing an insole on medial knee osteoarthritis. Before and after values of pain, functionality and thickness of cartilage at the knee were assessed among 40 patients. Researchers discovered that pain was significantly lessened while functionality was improved by either intervention. Physiologically, femoral and tibial cartilage protecting the affected area, increased in thickness to a non-clinically statistically significant degree in those receiving either intervention. No significant difference between groups was detected regarding any measure. Researchers [35] concluded that acupuncture was equivalently effective as lateral wedge insole for improving pain, functionality, and thickness of cartilage in medial knee osteoarthritis patients. Most impressively, acupuncture was found to influence the regrowth of cartilage in a typically progressively degenerative disorder.

Low-Level Laser Therapy Acupuncture

Non-invasive interventions for knee osteoarthritis are often sought out before more extreme measures such as knee-replacement surgery. Low-level laser therapy at local acupuncture points plus exercise and advice was assessed as a potential non-invasive treatment for patients with knee osteoarthritis. To evaluate response compared to placebo effect, patients received either nine treatments with gallium aluminum arsenide laser or placebo laser at local acupuncture points. At six weeks and at six months following completion of the intervention series, those who had received the active laser treatment were experiencing a significant reduction in pain compared with placebo. During the last of nine treatments, and at six months following the treatment series, functionality was significantly greater in those that had received the active intervention than those that had received the placebo. Thus, locally applied low-level laser acupuncture in addition to advice and exercise effectively reduced pain and improved functionality of knee osteoarthritis patients [36].

Acupuncture Needle-Knife Therapy and Bleeding

Knee osteoarthritis (KOA) is associated with an elevation in inflammatory cytokines. These, and other toxins may be reduced in the blood via needle-knife therapy, an acupuncture modality in which a small amount of blood is drawn to activate a healing response from the body. Osteoarthritic knee stiffness, pain and functionality were compared as was total change and clinical cure rate among 233 cases who received either needle-knife therapy or acupuncture. Biochemical markers common in arthritic joints, synovial cytokines, such as interleukin (IL)-1β, IL-6 and tumor necrosis factor-α (TNF-α) were also compared before and after treatment. Researchers found that symptom scores significantly diminished in those who received needle-knife therapy among those with stage I-IV knee osteoarthritis; symptom scores were also significantly diminished in stage I-III knee osteoarthritis patients who received acupuncture. Significantly higher effectiveness rates were observed among those who had received needle-knife treatment during stage III and IV of knee osteoarthritis therapy than those who had received acupuncture. Markers indicating breakdown of IL-1β, IL-6 and TNF-α were observed to a greater degree in the needle-knife treatment group than acupuncture group. This study [37] suggests that needle-knife therapy improved clinical symptoms in knee osteoarthritis patients, possibly via influence over inflammatory synovial cytokines.

Yamamoto New Scalp Acupuncture

Much of the pain and discomfort associated with osteoarthritis derives from progressive deterioration of cartilage protecting the joints. Effective scalp acupuncture protocols have been developed for pathologies associated with the brain and neurological system, such as recovery from stroke, MS and paralysis or other sensorimotor disorders. To assess potential effects of scalp acupuncture on osteoarthritis in Egyptian women, a novel treatment, Yamamoto New Scalp Acupuncture was studied at the Female Outpatient Pain Clinic, of the National Research Centre, in Cairo. Needles were inserted into the Yamamoto New Scalp Acupuncture points and retained for 20 minutes in 30 women with osteoarthritic chronic pain. Initial pain scores prior to treatment ranged from 3-10 on a numerical scale, 1-10; scores were reduced to 0-8 after treatment. Researchers further determined that pain scores following scalp acupuncture scores were significantly associated with location of pain. Pain was significantly lowered in those with osteoarthritis of the cervical spine, compared to those with osteoarthritis of the low back (lumbosacral spine). Overall results [38] showed that Yamamoto New Scalp Acupuncture immediately reduces pain of Egyptian women living with osteoarthritic chronic pain.

Auricular Electroacupuncture and Moxibustion with Lingxian Herbal Paste

Traditional Chinese medicine modalities may be applied in endless combinations to increase efficacy and personalize treatments. Although research is growing on specific modalities, little research exists on each possible combination. Lingxian herbal paste is one topical formula that is commonly used in the practice of traditional Chinese medicine to alleviate pain. Its effects on knee osteoarthritis when combined with auricular electroacupuncture and isolated moxibustion was assessed. Ninety patients received either knee irradiation with TDP-lamp, electroacupuncture or auricular plus isolated moxibustion with Lingxian herbal paste. For those receiving auricular electroacupuncture, the protocol applied included: Xi (AH4), Pizhixia (AT4), Shenmen (TF4) and other relevant points. Lingxian was applied to local Ashi points of the knee and standard local points for knee pain such as Yanglingquan (GB34), Dubi (ST35), Zusanli (ST36), Neixiyan (EX-LE 4) and Heding (EX-LE 2). For those receiving electroacupuncture only, the point protocol was the same as those in the combined treatment group. A total of 30 treatments were provided approximately once per week for each group.

All treatments significantly lowered physical signs and symptoms of knee osteoarthritis at assessment one week following the treatment series; with superior improvements observed in those who received the combination intervention. The combination of electroacupuncture and Lingxian herbal paste also more greatly reduced pain. The cure-rate of the combination group doubled that of both other groups, reaching 40.0%, compared with 17.2% in in the electroacupuncture group and 20.0% in the TDP group. Total efficacy of the combined therapy group, thus exceeded efficacy of both of the other treatment interventions. The evidence [39] overwhelmingly supported the combination of auricular electroacupuncture plus isolated moxibustion with Lingxian herbal paste at local standard knee points as a treatment for knee osteoarthritic pain. Total scores and efficacy were superior to local electroacupuncture or TDP irradiation.

Post-Surgical Electroacupuncture

The benefits of post-surgical acupuncture have led to its inclusion in many health insurance plans. To define the role of adjunct electroacupuncture following arthroscopic debridement among knee osteoarthritis patients, researchers assessed effects on 78 patients. Patients received either arthroscopic debridement plus post-operative electroacupuncture or served as controls, receiving surgery without post-operative electroacupuncture. Those patients were treated only with arthroscopic debridement. All the patients also received physiotherapy consisting of rehabilitative exercises. At the final follow-up, 12-30 months after surgery, significant improvements in pain and all Lysholm scores except for support demand were significantly better in both groups compared to pre-surgical values in both groups. Pain scores were significantly more reduced in those who had received electroacupuncture than those who did not. Significant between group differences were also noted in terms of Lysholm limp, pain, swelling, stair-climbing and squatting. Thus, researchers determined that electroacupuncture synergistically improves pain and clinical symptoms associated with knee osteoarthritis, when administered after arthroscopic debridement. These findings [40] support electroacupuncture during the recovery phase following osteoarthritic knee surgery.

Cortical Thickness and Functional Neuronal Connectivity

Imaging studies have shown that the analgesic effects of acupuncture may be due the influence of acupuncture on activation patterns and functional connectivity in specific neural networks. To assess the impact of acupuncture cortical thickness and functional connectivity throughout a series of acupuncture treatments on patients with knee osteoarthritis, six sessions were provided over a course of four weeks. Resting-state functional magnetic resonance imaging (fMRI) scans were captured of 30 patients at initiation and periodically throughout the course of treatment. Researchers assessed that significantly greater improvements were observed in terms of pain and osteoarthritis outcome scores in those who received real acupuncture versus sham acupuncture. During the course of treatment, significant reduction in cortical thickness at the left posterior medial prefrontal cortex occurred in those who received sham acupuncture compared with sessions as compared with true acupuncture. Using this area as a seed network, significantly greater resting-state functional connectivity was observed between the seed area and the rostral anterior cingulate cortex, medial frontal pole and periaqueduct grey in those who received true versus sham acupuncture. Researchers [41] surmised that the analgesic effects of acupuncture in patients with knee osteoarthritis may be associated with a protective mechanism that serves to prevent cortical thinning; thereby, preserving functional connectivity in brain areas moderating pain.

Laser Acupuncture Versus Acupuncture

The effects of laser and needle acupuncture were compared according to their ability to treat chronic knee pain of 282 patients over 50 years of age in Australia. Family physician acupuncturists administered laser acupuncture, acupuncture, sham acupuncture or no acupuncture to each patient during a course of 12 weeks. Upon analysis at 12 weeks, researchers found that acupuncture and laser acupuncture did not significantly lower pain or improve functionality compared to sham; however, both methods moderately diminished pain compared with controls after 12 weeks. These gains were not observed after 12 months. After 12 months, findings revealed that true acupuncture more effectively increased functionality than controls; this difference was also not detected at the 12-month follow-up assessment. No serious adverse events occurred in either group. Researchers [42] concluded that acupuncture and laser acupuncture offered no significant long-term relief of pain or improvement of functionality for chronic patients older than 50 years.

RCT Quality Regarding Warming-Needle Moxibustion

Although warming-needle moxibustion studies have shown a potential benefit in some cases of knee osteoarthritis, the best methods of investigating this topic are not well-established. To gather information on the quality of randomized controlled trials (RCTs) on the topic, Chinese and American databases were searched. The Consolidated Standards for Reporting of Trials Statement 2010 (CONSORT 2010) and Standards for Reporting Interventions Controlled Trials of Acupuncture 2010 (STRICT A 2010) were then used to evaluate 37 selected RCTs. Researchers reported that less than approximately half of the studies stated a randomized sequence of methods. Sub-adequate methods were applied in nine studies. Only one disclosed how blindedness was achieved. One study calculated sample size and 62.16% used adequate statistical methods. Thirteen studies included background information and justification for the RCTs, while three shared information on patients who did not complete the study. RCT limitation were shared in 8.11%. Intentional analysis was also absent from all studies. Overall, researchers rated the 37 studies as being of moderate to low quality. Researchers concluded that better RCT design, analysis and description of the studies are needed. Researchers [43] recommended that CONSORT 2010 and STRICT A 2010 be applied to future studies to raise the standards of acupuncture RCTs.

Comparison of Moxibustion Protocols

Moxibustion may be applied in various ways to immeasurable combinations of acupuncture points, Ashi points or channels for varying effects. In patients diagnosed with knee pain due to yang-deficiency with cold accumulation, two moxibustion approaches were compared. Patients received a protocol for knee osteoarthritis due to yang-deficiency with cold-accumulation; or moxibustion applied to local points without addressing the underlying differential diagnosis. Patients received either mild doses of moxibustion at standard local acupuncture points, Neixiyan (EX-HE4) and Waixiyan (ST35), once daily for 7days, rested for one day, then received another 7-day course; or mild moxibustion of EX-HE 4 and ST35 daily for 7 days, followed by one day of rest, then moxibustion at Yaoyangguan (DU3) and Mingmen (DU4) daily for 7 days. Both groups also received routine acupuncture stimulation of EX-HE 4, Waixiyan (ST35), Yanglingquan (GB34), Kunlun (BL60), etc.

Both treatments were effective at significantly reducing pain intensity, morning stiffness, arthrocele; meanwhile, functionality was also significantly improved in both groups. Those who received syndrome specific treatment in addition to local points achieved a higher degree of improvement in these measures over those who did not. Effectiveness rating for those who received syndrome specific treatment reached 89.66% compared to 70%

among controls. Thus, mild moxibustion at local points Neixiyan (EX-HE 4) and Waixiyan (ST35), plus points to treat the underlying syndrome, Yaoyangguan (DU3) and Mingmen (DU4) was found to be clinically superior in treating patients with knee osteoarthritis due to yang-deficiency with cold accumulation than moxibustion at local acupoints only [44].

Moxibustion and Quality of Life

Moxibustion was assess for potential effects on quality of life in those with knee osteoarthritis. In a double-blinded RCT, differences between moxibustion and sham moxibustion were compared among 150 patients. Treatments were provided at a rate of three times per week over a course of six weeks. SF-36 values were used to assess quality of life from baseline through 12 weeks after baseline. Of the original 150 patients, 136 completed the study. Significantly greater improvement in overall health were obtained the true treatment group as opposed to sham at weeks six and 12. Moxibustion significantly increased vitality compared to sham at week 12. Severe adverse effects were not observed in any participant. Researchers [45] concluded that a 6-week course of true moxibustion more significantly improves general health and vitality in knee osteoarthritis for up to 12 weeks compared with sham moxibustion.

Heat-Sensitive Moxibustion

In China, moxibustion is commonly applied for many deficient and cold conditions. Considered to be more efficacious when heat-sensitivity is achieved, and when the underlying syndrome is of a deficient and cold nature, these effects have not been not well-studied. To gather more scientific data on heat-sensitive moxibustion on knee osteoarthritis, researchers evaluated effects on pain and physical activity. In a multi-center, randomized controlled trial (RCT), 432 patients received either heat-sensitive moxibustion conventional moxibustion or conventional sodium hyaluronate injection. Upon analysis researchers [46] found that heat-sensitive moxibustion was more effective than conventional injection. Conventional moxibustion and the conventional injection were equal in all measures. Heat-sensitive moxibustion was thus found to be superior to conventional moxibustion across all outcomes.

Acupuncture on Neural Network Connectivity and Pain

To delve into the mechanisms underlying the therapeutic effects of acupuncture on knee osteoarthritis, researchers assessed changes in functional connectivity throughout a treatment series. Acupuncture was provided at a rate of six treatments over a course of four months; during which, resting state functional magnetic resonance imaging (fMRI) scans were obtained from 30 patients. Researchers found significantly greater reduction of pain in those who received true acupuncture as compared with sham acupuncture. According to imaging evidence, functional connectivity of both the right frontoparietal network (rFPN) and the executive control network (ECN) with the rostral anterior cingulate cortex/medial prefrontal cortex was strengthened in those who had received the true acupuncture treatment series. Greater connectivity in these brain networks suggests that acupuncture influences the descending pain circuitry. Improved connectivity between the rFPN and the left insula was found to significantly correlate with reduction in pain. True acupuncture was also found to induce activations in the left operculum/insula. These findings [47] imply that mechanisms involved in the analgesic response to acupuncture may be related to optimizing functional connectivity in the rFPN and ECN and the descending pain mediating pathway. In conclusion, the therapeutic value of acupuncture for knee osteoarthritis was verified.

Acupuncture Plus Shock-Wave

The role of acupuncture plus shock-wave intervention was assessed in treatment of knee osteoarthritis. Patients received either acupuncture or acupuncture plus low-, medium- or high-frequency shock-wave. Acupuncture was applied to Xuehai (SP10), Liangqiu (ST34), Yanglingquan (GB34), Waixiyan (ST35) and Ashi-point with even-method for 15-20 minutes; seven treatments total were provided at a rate of every other day. Shock waves were then delivered to these same points of those in the combined treatment group.

At the end of the treatment series, all experienced significant reductions in pain and improved motility compared to baseline values. Of the four acupuncture applications, acupuncture plus medium-frequency shock-wave was found to elicit the strongest deqi response and produce the greatest reduction in pain and improvements in mobility. Thus, acupuncture at local points plus shock wave, especially when delivered at a medium frequency, was verified for its therapeutic benefit in those with knee osteoarthritis [48].

True Versus Sham Acupuncture

Chronic pain takes a toll on the body and mental state of those afflicted. Research suggests that certain areas of the brain in those with chronic pain exhibit a greater level of dysregulation. These areas are distinct from brain regions associated with acute pain. To assess the influence of repeated acupuncture treatment on areas normally dysregulated in those with chronic pain researchers conducted a study. The behavioral patterns observed in those with chronic pain, such as mental fixation on the pain; emotional rumination; continually expressing resentment, regret and loss; constant expectation of pain and avoiding anticipated pain correlate with specific brain connectivity differences in those with chronic pain. Areas that are especially implicated in chronic pain include the periaqueductal gray (PAG), medial frontal cortex and bilateral hippocampus. Researchers found that abnormal connectivity in these brain areas correlates with pain severity. Additionally, acupuncture-induced reduction in pain was found to reflect functional modulation of connectivity in the affected brain areas. These findings [49] reveal that repeated acupuncture treatments may restore proper regulation of connectivity within emotional processing centers and those networks related to perception, memory and learning; thus, releasing mental-emotional patterns that have become ingrained in the chronic pain patient.

Clinical Evidence: Systematic Reviews and Meta-Analysis

Acupuncture

Randomized controlled trials (RCTs) on acupuncture, sham acupuncture, standard care or waiting list were reviewed as to compile evidence of effects on knee osteoarthritis. Meta-analysis was them conducted across 14 RCTs of 3,835 patients. Consolidated results revealed that acupuncture immediately reduced pain and improved functionality to a greater significant degree than sham acupuncture. In the long-term, acupuncture relieved pain and restored functionality to a less significant degree than in the short-term. However, acupuncture was found to more significantly reduce pain and restore function compared to standard care or waiting list. Acupuncture was therefore found to be superior to sham control or standard care at improving functionality while relieving pain [50].

Moxibustion

The collective knowledge from randomized clinical trials (RCTs) was gathered to assess the role of moxibustion in patients with osteoarthritis. Eight trials, although weak in methodology, were reviewed. Of six RCTs comparing the effects of moxibustion and conventional oral pharmaceuticals in patients with knee osteoarthritis, meta-analysis revealed a positive effect of moxibustion on response rate. Collective results of two RCTs after meta-analysis indicated that moxibustion did not influence response rate after two months. Overall, moxibustion may consistently reduce symptoms in patients with knee osteoarthritis. However, low number of RCTs and high risk of bias, limits generalizability and reliability of this assessment [51].

Pattern Differentiation

The practice of traditional Chinese Medicine relies on syndrome differentiation to assess and treat patients in the most effective manner. The Cochrane Database was searched for systematic reviews to get a sense of scientific consensus on pattern differentiation efficacy compared to other acupuncture protocols. Of 44 trials, seven meta-analyses found similar mitigation of symptoms with standardized acupoint protocols or treatment based on syndrome differentiation in acute stroke, depression, epilepsy, migraine, and osteoarthritis. The remaining 3 meta-analyses revealed that standardized protocols evoked stronger analgesic effects in osteoarthritis than protocols according to pattern differentiation or sham control. Overall, acupuncture protocols were equally effective with or without syndrome differentiation. Large, well-designed trials were recommended to evaluate potential distinction between efficacy of syndrome differentiation and other types of acupuncture. A holistic health assessment may show the particular advantages more clearly than evaluation based on a few obvious external symptoms [52].

External Validity of Acupuncture

External validity, popular acupoint protocols and treatment plans regarding acupuncture research studies on osteoarthritis knee pain were assessed. Reporting and performance were analyzed among 16 randomized controlled trials (RCTs). Reporting reflected the acupuncturist's background, location of the study, level of detailed description of treatment, patient characteristics, results, adverse effects and between-group statistical analyses. Performance reflected treatment relevance to patient condition, controls used and outcomes.

The treatment described in each RCT was then compared with typical treatment in clinical practice, treatment as described in acupuncture literature and response to questionnaires by acupuncturists in Thailand. After analysis, trials were rated at 31-100% external validity concerning reporting and performance. Statistics were reported in 44%, while patient satisfaction and quality of life were provided in 31% of trials. Research and practice were found to be similar in terms of point prescriptions, number of treatments and frequency. Liangqiu (ST34), Waixiyan (ST35), Zusanli (ST36), Sanyinjiao (SP6), Yinlingquan (SP9), Xuehai (SP10), Yanglingquan (GB34), Xiyan and Ashi points were most frequently selected, with treatment duration tending to last for 20 minutes. Most often, 10-15 total treatments were provided with bi-weekly administration. Researchers summarized that external validity of acupuncture RCTs for osteoarthritic knee pain were sub-par in reporting of trial location, acupuncture provider and statistics. According to researchers [53], most trials applied relevant controls and explored relevant outcomes while administering treatments representative of those provided in clinical practice.

Cost-Effectiveness

Chronic pain can become expensive in terms of money, time and inability to earn the same income prior to diagnosis. Acupuncture may reduce the negative impact of some chronic pain conditions on many levels. More and more insurance companies have responded by offering acupuncture coverage for chronic pain. As decisions regarding coverage, especially among government-controlled entities such as Medicare, require economic evaluations of medical benefits, researchers aimed to, through systematic review, compare cost-benefit of acupuncture in the treatment of chronic pain.

Health and economics databases and the written literature was searched for information regarding the economic impact of acupuncture in chronic pain. According to seven analyses, acupuncture was found to be effective; however, more expensive than standard treatment. The cost per gain in each quality adjusted life year (QALY) was estimated to be £2527 - £14,976. The UK National Institute for Health and Clinical Excellence generally holds the maximum pay-out to be approximately £20,000 - £30,000. One trial implied that acupuncture may be clinically beneficial and reduce costs in cases of migraine. Heterogeneity of acupuncture providers, acupuncture treatment plan, and region of the world was observed among the eight trials. Thus, acupuncture was deemed to be cost-effective for some types of chronic pain [54].

Cost-Effectiveness

Comprehensive assessments such as cost-effectiveness analysis (CEA), cost-utility analysis (CUA), cost-benefit analysis (CBA) and randomized controlled trials (RCTs) have attempted to determine the value of acupuncture treatment of various illnesses, diseases, injuries, etc. To provide an overview, researchers compiled available analyses on the topic. The 17 studies were comprised of nine cost-utility analyses (CUAs) which assed benefits in terms according to quality-adjusted life years (QALYs); and eight cost-effectiveness analyses (CEAs) in which effectiveness of treatment depends on changes in clinical symptoms. No cost-benefit analyses (CBAs) were included in the review. Every cost-utility analysis (CUA) demonstrated that acupuncture is cost-effective compared with waiting list control or conventional care alone. The benefits were noticed when acupuncture was provided as a solitary treatment or combined with other modalities. The incremental cost-effectiveness ratio (ICER), summarizing the cost-effectiveness of acupuncture compared with other interventions in Germany, ranged from €3011 per Quality-Adjusted Life Years (QALY) in cases of dysmenorrhea, to €22 298 per Quality-Adjusted Life Years (QALY) in cases of allergic rhinitis. The incremental cost-effectiveness ratio among UK studies ranged from £3855 per Quality-Adjusted Life Years (QALY) in osteoarthritis patients to £9951 per Quality-Adjusted Life Years (QALY) among headache sufferers. In cost-effectiveness analyses (CEAs) of European and Asian studies, acupuncture was found to improve clinical symptoms at comparatively low cost. As researchers [55] determined that all of the cost-utility analyses (CUAs) were well-designed with a low risk of bias, and all revealed acupuncture to be cost-effective, these results carry sufficient weight. Although CEAs were not as well-designed or as free from bias, they still reached a similar conclusion, that acupuncture was relatively cost-effective. As not all medical conditions are included among the studies, the positive results reported here cannot be assumed to be applicable to every condition in every part of the world.

The Value of Acupuncture in Chronic Pain

Chronic pain is difficult to treat, many sufferers try clinic after clinic, treatment after treatment, and when obvious relief is not immediately noticed continue to seek out different approaches to resolve the endless agony. This can lead to endless expense with virtually no benefit. According to imaging research, brain networks become conditioned to the chronic pain-state, making improvements in the condition imperceivable to the patient. It may be that continued, regular treatment with modalities that restore normal functionality of brain networks affected by chronic pain (different than those involved in acute pain) offer the best hope for patients with chronic pain. More research is needed in this area, however; acupuncture may positively influence networks related to chronic pain.

Although chronic pain may accompany many enduring disease states, researchers assessed relative cost-benefits of acupuncture treatment for back and neck pain, osteoarthritis, headache, and shoulder pain. A systematic review of approximately 30 randomized controlled trials (RCTs) of 17,922 patients, demonstrated that among all selected types of chronic pain, acupuncture was more cost-effective than sham and no-acupuncture controls. When outlying RCTs favoring acupuncture were removed from analysis, effect sizes were found to be similar among all conditions. Acupuncture alleviated pain to a greater degree than sham controls in those with chronic back and neck pain, osteoarthritis, and headache. Acupuncture was also determined to be more effective than non-acupuncture controls in treating chronic pain from these three conditions. These results [56] were determined to be robust, leading researchers to conclude that acupuncture is effective for chronic pain. Significantly greater benefits achieved with true acupuncture compared to sham acupuncture attest that acupuncture produces genuine therapeutic effect and is not just a placebo.

Acupuncture Versus Physical Therapy

Physiotherapy is commonly recommended for patients with knee osteoarthritis, as moderate movement generally helps the condition. Some patients receive acupuncture in addition to physiotherapy or choose acupuncture in lieu of other treatments. Researchers conducted a systemic review and meta-analysis to assess the relative benefits of each in terms of reducing pain associated with knee osteoarthritis. RCTs (114) on pain due to knee osteoarthritis in a total of 9,709 patients were included in the review. Meaningful analysis was difficult, as most trials did not include long-term benefits and few were of adequate quality; bias also played a role, mostly due to lack of blinding. Compared to conventional care, interferential therapy, acupuncture, TENS, pulsed electrical stimulation, balneotherapy, aerobic exercise, sham acupuncture, and muscle-strengthening exercises were all found to significantly alleviate pain. Additionally, acupuncture was found to produce significantly greater relief than muscle-strengthening exercises. Researchers [57] concluded that acupuncture showed greater short-term analgesic impact on knee osteoarthritis than physical treatments. Lack of quality research limits the confidence of these assessments regarding all physical interventions.

Sham and Non-Sham Controls

Recent review finds acupuncture a more effective chronic pain analgesic compared with sham and non-sham controls. As many different types of sham and non-sham controls are used in acupuncture studies, the relative differences between placebo effects and acupuncture are difficult to gauge; differences may vary with each type of control.

Researchers attempted to compare relative differences between sham and non-sham controls in 29 trials on chronic pain due to headache and migraine; osteoarthritis; and back, neck and shoulder pain. Sham controls included: non-needle sham, penetrating sham needles and non-penetrating sham needles. Non-sham controls included conventional care and protocol-guided care. Researchers [58] found acupuncture to produce significantly greater improvement regardless of control used. Less difference was seen when penetrating sham needles were used. Researchers removed outlying acupuncture data that reported massive acupuncture effects. (Although scientific research tends to consider large differences in results abnormal, in clinical practice, highly variable response to acupuncture is considered normal, as some patients respond remarkably while others may exhibit very little response; there really is no ability to predict how much benefit any given patient may derive.) When non-sham controls were used, the difference in effects was greater between acupuncture and non-specified routine care than protocol-guided care. Overall, acupuncture was found to be significantly more effective than any control. The difference in effects was less pronounced when penetrating needles were applied to sham points, suggesting that this technique does produce some benefit and is not an appropriate true control.

Acupuncture and Osteoarthritis

Researchers [59] reviewed acupuncture and osteoarthritis trials to assess comprehensive effects. Trials (12) of 1763 osteoarthritis patients were gathered from reputable sources and assessed for bias. Pooled data assessed relative effects of acupuncture, sham acupuncture, no treatment or conventional care. Although lack of clarity and high level of bias among most trials was noted, pooled data revealed that acupuncture significantly diminished severity of pain, increased functionality and improved quality of life. A series of acupuncture treatments over more than four weeks reduced severity of pain to a greater degree than shorter courses of acupuncture treatment. While the differences are less than those demonstrated in other reviews, improvements in severity of pain, functionality and quality of life were confirmed; therefore, acupuncture is a valid treatment for pain related to osteoarthritis.

CHAPTER THREE

ACUPUNCTURE FOR *IN VITRO* FERTILIZATION (IVF)

Introduction

Acupuncture is a millennia-old medical modality which has the objective of regulating the balance and flow of energy (Qi) in the body through the insertion of needles into specified points distributed along energy channels or meridians all over the body. IVF is a process involving fertilizing a female's egg with male sperm outside the body and then implanting the resulting embryo into a uterus. Applying acupuncture to the *in vitro* fertilization (IVF) process was a recent medical innovation in the West [1]. This marriage of an ancient medical tradition with a contemporary medical development has the potential to affect a wide population of infertile couples. Infertility in humans is defined as the inability to conceive a baby after one year of unprotected intercourse. Ten to fifteen percent of couples in the United States are infertile. Infertility may be due to a single factor in one of the partners, or a combination of factors in one or both partners that may prevent a pregnancy from occurring. Currently, about 17% of couples in industrialized countries seek medical advice for infertility [2].

IVF, as a documented medical process, began in 1978 with the *Birth of Louise Brown* by Edwards and Steptoe. In the United States, IVF treatment for infertility began in the 1980s, spread during the 1990s, and became a standard of care in the 2000s. Currently, over 150,000 treatment cycles have been documented. According to the Centers for Disease Control and Prevention, IVF treatments produced an average increase of one to two percent per year in positive outcomes, pregnancy or babies, from 1985 to 2001. Since 2001, this annual gain has disappeared [3]. Applying acupuncture to IVF programs represented an innovative effort to enhance the rate of improvement for IVF. This innovation is generally credited to Dr. W. Paulus and his colleagues, working at the Christian-Lauritzen-Institut in Ulm, Germany.

For couples struggling with infertility, *in vitro* fertilization (IVF) is an option if either one has been diagnosed with one of the following conditions: endometriosis, low sperm counts, problems with the uterus or fallopian tubes, problems with ovulation, antibody problems that harm sperm or eggs, the inability of sperm to penetrate or survive in the cervical mucus, or an unexplained fertility problem. It was estimated that in 2002-2003, 932,000 IVF and related cycles were performed worldwide, resulting in an estimated 232 000 babies being born in 2003 [4]. The United States has among the highest IVF success rates worldwide, with about 30% of treatment cycles resulting in a live birth. This is due to a combination of factors, including few restrictions on the number of embryos transferred and the routine use of embryo selection [4, 5].

Since the publication in 2002 of the clinical trials conducted by Dr. Paulus and others, and the research studies which followed, acupuncture has become the most commonly used adjuvant, complementary therapy among couples seeking treatment at fertility clinics in the United States. Acupuncture has been used extensively to treat infertility by means of *in vitro* fertilization and embryo transfer (IVF-ET). Acupuncture application to IVF protocols has become one of the most contested areas in clinical acupuncture research. Most of the studies done in this area suggest a positive effect of acupuncture in infertility treatment, although non-supportive evidence appears once in a while.

In this chapter, we collected nineteen studies in our narrative report, eleven of which are original clinical trials, six of which are systematic reviews or meta-analyses, and one of which is a theoretical and methodological exploration. Examining these studies, we can see both the positive responses and the negative responses to acupuncture application to IVF procedures. Creative design of the clinical trials, different acupuncture protocols, and the validity of sham acupuncture emerged as critical issues in these studies. These important issues warrant further investigation. Through the interplay of narrative report and critique, we can see the evolution of clinical studies on the application of acupuncture to IVF procedures.

The Paulus Protocol: A Quiet Revolution

Acupuncture applied to the IVF process started with the seminal work of Dr. W. Paulus and others at a research institute in Ulm, Germany. In their pioneering work, published in *Fertility and Sterility* in 2002, Paulus, *et al.* [1] attempted to evaluate the effect of acupuncture on the pregnancy rate in assisted reproduction therapy (ART) by comparing a group of patients receiving acupuncture treatment shortly before and after embryo transfer with a control group receiving no acupuncture. In their prospective randomized study conducted in fertility centers, 160 patients who were undergoing ART and who had good quality embryos were randomly divided into two groups: embryo transfer group with acupuncture (n = 80) and embryo transfer group without acupuncture (n = 80). Acupuncture was performed in 80 patients in the first group 25 minutes before and after embryo transfer. In the control group, embryos were transferred without acupuncture treatments. The acupuncture operations followed the following protocol (it will hereinafter be referred to as the Paulus Protocol): before the embryo transfer, the following points were needled: Neiguan (PC6), Diji (SP8), Taichong (LR3), Baihui (DU 20), and Guilai (ST29). After the embryo transfer, the following points were needled: Zusanli (ST36), Sanyinjiao (SP6), Xuehai (SP10), and Hegu (LI4). In addition, small stainless needles (0.2X13mm) for auricular acupuncture were applied at the following points, without rotation: ear point 55 (Shenmen), ear point 58 (Zigong), ear point 22 (Neifenmi), and ear point 34 (Naodian). Two needles were inserted in the right ear, the other two needles in the left ear. The four needles remained in the ears for 25 minutes. The side of the auricular acupuncture was changed after embryo transfer. The patients in the control group also remained lying still for 25 minutes after embryo transfer. All treatments were uniformly performed by the same well-trained practitioner. In this study, clinical pregnancy was defined as the presence of a fetal sac during an ultrasound examination six weeks after embryo transfer. The results showed that clinical pregnancies were 34 of 80 patients (42.5%) in the acupuncture group, while pregnancy rate was only 21 out of 80 patients (26.3%) in the control group. The study concluded that acupuncture is a useful tool for improving pregnancy rate after ART.

The significance of this paper was remarked upon by Paul C. Magarelli, MD, PhD, FACOG [3]: "China's Cultural Revolution marked a move from the past into a new plan for the future. A small paper published in 2002 in *Fertility & Sterility* by Paulus, *et al.* showed a similar, though relatively silent revolution." The Paulus protocol and its clinical results provided the impetus for further studies and brought significant follow-ups in the study of acupuncture applications to IVF. We have selected a number of them for review. These studies were conducted in different ways and investigated different aspects of the IVF process. *Fertility and Sterility*, an international journal for obstetricians, gynecologists, reproductive endocrinologists, urologists, basic scientists and others who treat and investigate problems of infertility and human reproductive disorders, and the American Society of

Reproductive Medicine's journal, became the main platform for these publications.

Dieterle, *et al.* [6] at the Division of Reproductive Endocrinology and Infertility, Department of Obstetrics and Gynecology, University of Witten/Herdecke, Dortmund, Germany conducted a randomized, prospective, controlled clinical study at the university IVF center to determine the clinical effect of luteal-phase acupuncture on the outcome of IVF/intracytoplasmic sperm injection (ICSI). They recruited two hundred and twenty-five infertile patients undergoing IVF/ICSI. These patients were randomly assigned into two groups. In group I, 116 patients received luteal-phase acupuncture according to the principles of traditional Chinese medicine. In this group, the patients were needled at Guanyuan (RN4), Qihai (RN6), Guilai (ST29), Neiguan (PC6), Xuehai (SP10), and Diji (SP8) after embryo transfer. At the same time, a particular Chinese medicinal herb seed from the plant *Caryophyllaceae* was placed on the patient's ear points including ear point 55 (Shenmen), ear point 58 (Zigong), ear point 22 (Neifenmi), and ear point 33 (Pizhixia). These seeds remained in place for two days and patients were asked to press/stimulate the seeds twice daily for ten minutes. All patients received a second acupuncture treatment three days after embryo transfer. In this treatment, Hegu (LI14), Sanyinjiao (SP6), Zusanli (ST36), Taixi (KI3), and Taichong (LR3) were needled. In addition, the same ear points with the same herb seeds were positioned and stimulated in the opposite ear twice daily. The medicinal herb seeds were removed after two days. In group II, 109 patients received placebo acupuncture. In group II, the following acupuncture points were needled after embryo transfer and again three days later: Sidu (SJ 9), Xiaoluo (SJ12), Fengshi (GB31), Zhongdu (GB32), and Yanglingquan (GB34). Patients in group II also received acupuncture treatment for 30 minutes. At the same time, the following ear points were used: ear point 17 (Shangzhi), ear point 14 (Fengsi), ear point 8 (Sisheng), and ear point 53 (Jian). Equal numbers of needles were applied to both group I and group II. Clinical and ongoing pregnancy rates were assessed. The clinical pregnancy rate and ongoing pregnancy rate were 33.6% and 28.4%, respectively, in group I. The clinical pregnancy rate and ongoing pregnancy rate were 15.6% and 13.8%, respectively, in group II. Both clinical rates in group I were significantly higher than in group II. The study concluded that luteal-phase acupuncture has a positive effect on the outcome of IVF/ICSI. The efficacy of acupuncture for IVF luteal-phase was demonstrated.

It is interesting that Westergaard, *et al.* [7] conducted a trial that combined acupuncture with IVF and ICSI during embryo transfer, following a protocol similar to the Paulus protocol, and demonstrated that acupuncture on the day of embryo transfer significantly improves the reproductive outcome of IVF/ICSI, compared with no acupuncture. Repeating acupuncture two days after embryo transfer provided no additional beneficial effect. Westergaard *et al.* recruited 273 couples for the study and they were randomized into three groups: 1) a control group with no acupuncture (87 patients); 2) ACU 1: a group that received acupuncture on the day of embryo transfer (95 patients); 3) ACU 2: a group that received acupuncture on the day of embryo transfer and again two days later (91 patients). ACU 1 received acupuncture treatments before and after embryo transfer. ACU 2 received the same treatment as ACU 1 but had an additional treatment two days after the embryo was transferred. The idea of the additional treatment again two days later was to enhance blood flow to the uterus and increase the endometrial effect of acupuncture on ICSI and IVF reception of the embryo closer to the day of implantation. All patients in the three groups followed the same standard clinical hormone protocol. It was confirmed that the three groups did not differ on demographic and confounding variables including patient age, BMI, length of infertility, average number of stimulation days, consumption of FSH during stimulation and the average number of oocytes obtained, fertilized, cryopreserved, and number of embryos that could be transferred. The study found a significant increase in positive pregnancy test results, clinical pregnancy rate, and ongoing pregnancy/delivery outcome in the ACU 1 group when acupuncture treatment was used in conjunction with IVF or ICSI. The positive pregnancy test rate (P=.044) for the three groups was 24/87 (28%) for the control group, 40/95 (42%) for the ACU 1 group, and 36/91 (40%) for the ACU 2 group. The clinical pregnancy rate (P=.038) was 21/87 (24%) for the control group, 37/95 (39%) for the ACU 1 group, and 33/91 (36%) for the ACU 2 group. The ongoing pregnancy/delivery rate (P=.049) was 19/87 (22%) for the control group, 34/95 (36%) for the ACU 1 group, and 24/91 (26%) for ACU 2 group. Both ACU 1 and ACU 2 groups were compared with the control group. Clinical and ongoing pregnancy rates were significantly higher in ACU 1 group compared with the control group (39% vs. 26% and 36% vs. 22%, respectively). The clinical and ongoing pregnancy rates in the ACU 2 group (36% and 26%, respectively) were higher than in the control group, but the difference did not reach statistical significance. The researchers concluded that acupuncture on the day of embryo transfer significantly improves the reproductive outcome of IVF/ICSI, compared with no acupuncture, but repeating acupuncture two days later provides no additional beneficial effect.

The Paulus protocol study [1] implied that acupuncture performed onsite before and after embryo transfer improved *in vitro* fertilization (IVF) outcome in patients with good-quality embryos. This claim was challenged by Craig, *et al.* [8] in a multi-center, prospective, randomized study in 2007. The objective of Craig's team was to evaluate whether acupuncture before and after embryo transfer would alter pregnancy rates in patients undergoing IVF regardless of embryo quality if the treatment was performed offsite. They recruited 107 patients undergoing IVF and they were randomized to acupuncture vs. control group. The two groups were statistically similar with respect to age, peak estradiol, number of oocytes retrieved, fertilization method, fertilization rate, number of embryos transferred, and the proportion with blastocyst transfer (P=NS). The acupuncture group received acupuncture at an offsite location for 25 minutes before and after embryo transfer using a modified Paulus protocol in which the Paulus protocol was modified by adding Qihai (RN6) before and Taixi (KI3) after transfer. We will call this procedure the "Craig protocol." The Craig protocol included the following acupuncture points before embryo transfer: Baihui (DU20), Qihai (RN6), Guilai (ST29), Diji (SP8), Neiguan (PC6), Taichong (LR3); Shenmen and Brain on the left ear; and Uterus and Endocrine on the right ear. After transfer, the points used were Hegu (LI4), Xuehai (SP10), Zusanli (ST36), Sanyinjiao (SP6), Taixi (KI3); Uterus and Endocrine on the left ear; and Shenmen and Brain on the right ear. The control group underwent embryo transfer without acupuncture or other intervention. The treating physician who determined the IVF protocol was blinded as to assigned group. The outcome measures included a positive quantitative hCG, clinical pregnancy as manifested by fetal cardiac activity, and live birth. Of the 107 patients randomized, 94 completed the study (10 IVF cycles canceled, 3 patients withdrew). The study result showed that the percentage of patients with a positive pregnancy test was higher in the control group (78.3%) than the acupuncture group (52.1%). The difference is significant ($P<0.01$). Also, the clinical pregnancy rate was higher in the control group (69.6%) than in the acupuncture group (43.8%); $P<0.03$. In contrast to Paulus and other studies, this study concluded that acupuncture before and after embryo transfer was associated with lower biochemical and clinical pregnancy rates when compared to the control group. They questioned the value of acupuncture in patients undergoing IVF and recommended further study to be done.

In a recent study by Hullender Rubin, *et al.* [9], Craig's test using the modified Paulus protocol was challenged again. In their retrospective chart review study conducted at a private infertility clinic, the researchers, one of whom was using the Craig protocol at an infertility clinic between 2005 and

2007, reviewed clinic records to evaluate the effect of the Craig protocol in both donor and non-donor IVF cycles in terms of four outcomes: (1) live births; (2) biochemical pregnancies; (3) adverse outcomes; and (4) live births in non-donor cycles across age groups established by the Society for Assisted Reproductive Technology. Patients underwent fresh, donor (N=70) or non-donor (N=402) IVF-ET. The main outcome measure is the live births (LB) beyond 24 weeks' gestation. There were no differences in LB across age groups (odds ratio [OR]=1.04, 95% confidence interval [CI] 0.68-1.57), biochemical pregnancies (OR=0.60, 95% CI 0.27-1.33), or adverse outcomes (OR=0.63, 95% CI 0.31-1.26) in non-donor IVF cycles. Live births were higher in the acupuncture group (relative risk=1.31, 95% CI 1.02-1.71) in donor cycles. This observational study found that the Craig protocol was not associated with lower IVF live births. Actually, higher live births in donor cycles were associated with the Craig protocol. These findings encouraged more rigorous randomized studies.

The First Wave of Systematic Reviews and Meta-analysis (2008-2010)

A systematic review is a critical assessment and evaluation of all clinical trials that address a particular clinical issue such as acupuncture intervention during IVF. The researchers use an organized method of locating, assembling, and evaluating a body of literature on the subject under investigation using a set of specific criteria. A systematic review typically includes a description of the findings of the collection of research studies. The systematic review, including a quantitative pooling of data from all the individual studies, is called a meta-analysis. After five years of extensive clinical research on acupuncture application to the IVF process triggered by the Paulus study of 2002, systematic reviews and meta-analyses started appearing in the scientific and medical literature. In this first wave of systematic reviews and meta-analyses, seven studies were published in the mainstream journals, three of which show a beneficial effect in applying acupuncture during IVF and four of which could not confirm the beneficial effect of acupuncture during IVF. The three showing supportive evidence are Manheimer, *et al.* [10] (seven trials with 1,366 patients) published in *BMJ* in February 2008, demonstrating that acupuncture given around embryo transfer improved the rates of clinical pregnancy, ongoing pregnancy, and live birth in women undergoing IVF; Ng, *et al.* [11] (ten trials with 2,003 patients) published in *Fertility and Sterility* in July 2008, demonstrating that the IVF pregnancy rate was significantly increased, especially when the acupuncture was administered on the day of embryo transfer; Cheong, *et al.* [12] published in the Cochrane Database of Systematic Reviews in 2009 (thirteen trials with 2,300 patients), demonstrating that acupuncture performed on the day of embryo transfer increased live birth rates, but not CPRs, or showed no beneficial effects on pregnancy outcomes when acupuncture was performed around the time of oocyte retrieval. The four reviews showing no supportive evidence for acupuncture application to IVF are: El-Toukhy, *et al.* [13] published in 2008 (thirteen trials with 2,500 patients); Cheong, *et al.* [14], published in 2010 (fourteen trials with 2,670 patients); El-Toukhy, *et al.* [15], published in 2009 (fourteen trials with 2,870 patients); and Sunkara, *et al.* [16], published in 2009 (fourteen trials with 2,870 patients). Two of these studies are presented below: Manheimer's supportive study and El-Toukhy's non-supportive study. Reviewing these studies demonstrates the tendency for inconclusiveness in regard to clinical recommendations at this early stage of research.

Manheimer *et al.* [10] initiated the first systematic review and meta-analysis for acupuncture on IVF to evaluate whether acupuncture improves rates of pregnancy and live birth when used as an adjuvant treatment to embryo transfer in women undergoing in vitro fertilization. Seven clinical trials from Medline, Cochrane Central, Embase, Chinese Biomedical Database, hand searched abstracts, and reference lists were included. All eligible studies were randomized controlled trials that compared needle acupuncture administered within one day of embryo transfer with sham acupuncture or no adjuvant treatment, with reported outcomes of at least one of the following outcome measures: clinical pregnancy, ongoing pregnancy, or live birth. Two reviewers independently agreed on eligibility; assessed methodological quality; and extracted outcome data. For all trials, the authors requested additional data not included in the original publication from the investigators, such as live births. Meta-analyses included all randomized patients in the seven trials with 1366 women undergoing *in vitro* fertilization. Little clinical heterogeneity was identified. Trials with sham acupuncture and no adjuvant treatment as controls were pooled for the primary analysis. The review and analysis indicated that applying acupuncture to the IVF process was associated with significant and clinically relevant improvements in clinical pregnancy (odds ratio 1.65, 95% confidence interval 1.27 to 2.14; number needed to treat (NNT) 10 (7 to 17); seven trials), ongoing pregnancy (1.87, 1.40 to 2.49; NNT 9 (6 to 15); five trials), and live birth (1.91, 1.39 to 2.64; NNT 9 (6 to 17); four trials). The unavailability of outcome data on live births for three of the included trials hindered the odds ratio analysis for live birth rate. The pooled odds ratio for clinical pregnancy more accurately represented the true combined effect from these trials. The authors believed that the results were robust to sensitivity analyses on study validity variables and preliminary evidence suggested that acupuncture given with embryo transfer improved rates of pregnancy and live birth among women undergoing *in vitro* fertilization.

The second review [13] looks at the randomized studies that have reported pregnancy outcome in women who received acupuncture during their *in vitro* fertilization (IVF) treatment cycle. The study was to conduct a systematic review with meta-analysis of the trials of acupuncture during IVF treatment on the outcomes of clinical pregnancy and live birth rates. Their searches included Medline, Embase, Cochrane Library, ISI Proceedings and SCISEARCH. They include all randomized controlled trials that evaluated the effects of acupuncture compared with no treatment or sham acupuncture in women undergoing IVF-intracytoplasmic sperm injection treatment. Standard procedures for study selection, quality appraisal and data extraction were performed independently and in duplicate. The study conducted sensitivity analysis, where the meta-analysis was restricted to trials in which sham acupuncture was used in the control group. The study used meta-regression analysis to explore the association between study characteristics and pregnancy rates. They identified thirteen relevant trials which included a total of 2500 women randomized to either acupuncture or a control group. Among them, five trials (n = 877) evaluated IVF outcome when acupuncture was performed around the time of transvaginal oocyte retrieval, while eight trials (n = 1623) reported IVF outcome when acupuncture was performed around the time of embryo transfer (ET). The study reported the following five findings: 1. Meta-analysis of the five studies of acupuncture around the time of egg collection did not show a significant difference in clinical pregnancy (relative risks [RR] = 1.06, 95% CI 0.82-1.37, P = 0.65). 2. Meta-analysis of the eight studies of acupuncture around the time of ET showed no difference in the clinical pregnancy rate (RR = 1.23, 95% CI 0.96-1.58, P = 0.1). 3. Meta-analysis from five of the eight studies of acupuncture around the time of ET with available live birth data showed no significant increase in live birth rate with acupuncture (RR = 1.34, 95% CI 0.85-2.11). 4. No significant association between any of the studied covariates and clinical pregnancy rate was found ($P > 0.05$ for all covariates), using meta-regression. This study concluded that current available literature does not provide sufficient evidence that adjuvant acupuncture improves IVF clinical pregnancy rate.

One contribution to this first wave of systematic reviews and meta-analysis was from an acupuncture college. Anderson *et al.* [17] at Pacific College of Oriental Medicine provided a positive picture in an overview of the use of acupuncture as an adjunct therapy for *in vitro* fertilization (IVF), including an evidence-based evaluation of its efficacy and safety and an examination of possible mechanisms of action. Their scope of literature includes the publications PubMed, the Science Citation Index, The Cochrane Library, the New England School of Acupuncture library databases, and a cross-referencing of published data, personal libraries, and Chinese medicine textbooks. They found limited but supportive evidence from clinical trials and case series which suggest that acupuncture may improve the success rate of IVF and the quality of life of patients undergoing IVF and that it is a safe adjunct therapy. Because most studies reviewed had design limitations, and the inconsistency of acupuncture interventions employed with traditional Chinese medical principles, the conclusion should be interpreted with caution. The literature review suggests four possible mechanisms by which acupuncture may improve IVF success rates. One of the possible mechanisms, neuroendocrinological modulations, suggests that acupuncture could change the way a woman's nervous system and endocrine glands interact. This is supported by the facts that the endocrine glands are in charge of hormone secretion, and that hormone imbalances can be the cause of infertility. The other three possible mechanisms are increased blood flow to the uterus and ovaries that improves the success rate of implantation; improved cytokine balance in which acupuncture could help balance the body's level of cytokines, which are involved in immunity and imbalance of certain cytokines has been attributed to infertility; and reduction of stress, anxiety and depression in which the elimination of one or all of these has been shown to increase the chances of pregnancy. The review suggests that more high-quality randomized, controlled trials incorporating placebo acupuncture controls, authentic acupuncture interventions, and a range of outcome measures representative of both clinical outcomes and putative mechanistic processes are required to better assess the efficacy of acupuncture as an adjunct for IVF treatment.

The inconclusiveness of the above reviews represented the status of this early-stage research. Researchers' dissatisfaction with the lack of conclusive findings resulted in more studies on acupuncture application to the IVF process. The variety of research findings developed from the additional studies brought surprises to researchers, practitioners and readers.

More Advanced Clinical Trials

A randomized double-blind study [18] conducted in the Department of Obstetrics and Gynecology at the University of Hong Kong was published in 2009. The objective of the study was to compare real acupuncture with placebo acupuncture in patients undergoing IVF treatment. Three hundred and seventy patients were randomly assigned to either real or placebo acupuncture according to a computer-generated randomization list on the day of embryo transfer (ET). All the patients received 25 minutes of real or placebo acupuncture on the same acupuncture points before and after ET. The acupuncture points used before ET were: Neiguan (PC6), Diji (SP8), Taichong (LR3), Baihui (DU20) and Guilai (ST29). After ET, acupuncture was performed at Zusanli (ST36), Sanyinjiao (SP6), Xuehai (SP10) and Hegu (LI4). For the patients in the placebo acupuncture group, Streitberger's placebo needles [19] and Park's placebo device [20] were used. Streitberger's placebo needle was developed to appear indistinguishable from a real acupuncture needle, but the needle tip is blunt and the shaft telescopes into the handle when downward pressure is applied. The handle of the needle is made of stainless-steel wound into a regular tube shape which gives consistent resistance to movement of the needle. The needle diameter is 0.35 mm and its length is 70 mm including handle. The Park placebo device consists of two tubes. The guide tube holds the needle perpendicular to the skin and is fitted within the Park tube, a larger tube fixed to the ring base, so that the standard guide tube slides freely within the Park tube. A silicon base rests under the ring base and adheres to the skin with double-sided tape. The practitioner positions the needle perpendicular to the skin and taps the handle of the needle in a precise imitation of the insertion of a real acupuncture needle. Park's placebo device is too short to penetrate the skin. The appearance of Streitberger's placebo needle was the same as the needle used in the real acupuncture group, but the Streitberger's placebo needle was not fixed into the handle, and the tip of the needle was blunt. When the needle was pushed forward against the skin, it slid into the handle and the whole needle appeared shortened. The Streitberger's placebo needle also gave patients a pricking penetration sensation. The patients were evaluated in terms of endometrial and subendometrial vascularity, serum cortisol concentration, and their anxiety level before and after real and placebo acupuncture. Results revealed that the overall pregnancy rate was significantly higher in the placebo acupuncture group than that in the real acupuncture group (55.1 versus 43.8%, respectively, $P = 0.038$). Further, no significant differences were found in rates of ongoing pregnancy and live birth between the two groups. The study observed reductions of endometrial and subendometrial vascularity, serum cortisol concentration, and anxiety levels following both real and placebo acupuncture, although no significant differences were found in the changes in all these indices between the two groups. Researchers observed that placebo acupuncture was associated with a significantly higher overall pregnancy rate when compared with real acupuncture.

To test the validation of a scientific discovery, one criterion is that it must be reproducible. Domer *et al.* [21] from Boston IVF, Inc., in Waltham, Massachusetts, replicated the 2002 Paulus protocol on the efficacy of acupuncture in increasing pregnancy rates (PR) in patients undergoing IVF to determine whether such an increase was due to a placebo effect. This was a prospective, randomized, controlled, single blind trial conducted in a private, academically affiliated infertility clinic. One hundred-fifty patients scheduled to undergo embryo transfer participated in the study. Patients were randomly assigned to either the acupuncture or control group. Acupuncture patients received the treatment protocol described in Paulus' 2002 study [1]. Patients in the control group simply rested quietly. Questionnaires on anxiety and optimism were completed by all patients. The IVF staff was blind to patient assignment. Clinical PRs, anxiety, and optimism were assessed. The patients in both the acupuncture and control groups had similar demographic characteristics including age and psychological variables before randomization. A finding of this study is that no significant differences in PRs were discovered between the two groups. However, another significant finding of this study was that acupuncture patients reported significantly less anxiety post-transfer and reported feeling more optimistic about their cycle and enjoyed their sessions more than the patients in the control group. This study concluded that the use of acupuncture in patients undergoing IVF didn't increase the pregnancy rate, but that patients were more relaxed and more optimistic.

A prospective cohort clinical study led by Magarelli [22] was performed as collaboration between a private practice reproductive endocrinology and infertility clinic and a private practice acupuncture consortium. Researchers attempted to determine whether changes in serum cortisol (CORT) and prolactin (PRL) are affected by acupuncture in acupuncture-treated IVF patients. Sixty-seven reproductive-age infertile women undergoing IVF participated in this study. Blood samples were obtained from all patients and serum CORT and serum PRL were obtained prospectively. Patients were assigned to a control group (IVF with no acupuncture treatment) and a treated group (IVF with acupuncture treatment) according to the Cridennda/Magarelli protocol, which is a combination of the Stener-Victorin protocol [23] and the Paulus protocol [1]. In the Cridennda/Magarelli protocol, patients are treated with the electroacupuncture procedure (nine treatments) before egg retrieval, and are treated with pre-embryo-transfer acupuncture within 24 hours before and one hour after ET. In the acupuncture treatment, four needles were located bilaterally: Shenshu (BL23) and Pangguangshu (BL28), at the thoracolumbar and lumbosacral levels of the erector spinae, and were stimulated with high frequency (100 Hz) pulses of 0.5 ms duration. The intensity of stimulation was low, giving non-painful paraesthesia. Four needles were located bilaterally: Sanyinjiao (SP6) and Chengshan (BL57), in the calf muscles, and were stimulated with low frequency (2 Hz) pulses of 0.5 ms duration. The intensity of stimulation was sufficient to cause local muscle contractions. Serum levels of CORT and PRL were measured and synchronized with medication stimulation days of the IVF cycle (e.g., day 2 of stimulation, day 3, etc.). Reproductive outcomes were obtained according to Society for Assisted Reproductive Technology protocols, and results were compared between those patients without acupuncture treatment and those patients treated with acupuncture. The study found that the CORT levels in the acupuncture group were significantly higher on IVF medication days 7, 8, 9, 11, 12, and 13 compared with the controls; and PRL levels in the acupuncture group were significantly higher on IVF medication days 5, 6, 7, and 8 compared with the controls. The study concluded that there existed a beneficial regulation of CORT and PRL in the acupuncture group during the medication phase of the IVF treatment with a trend toward more normal fertile cycle dynamics.

Some IVF-related studies explore the psychological aspects of acupuncture treatments. It is a concern among many that IVF, as an accepted and effective treatment for infertility, is contributing to, rather than lessening, the overall psychosocial effects of infertility. Psychological and counseling interventions have been recommended as supplementary treatments to patients undergoing IVF treatments. With acupuncture being increasingly used as an adjunct to IVF, a study was conducted by de Lacey, *et al.* [24] to investigate the experience of infertile women who had used acupuncture to improve their fertility in South Australia. Twenty women were drawn from a cohort of women who had attended a minimum of four acupuncture sessions. Among the eight women interviewed with a semi-structured questionnaire, six had sought acupuncture during IVF treatment, and two had begun acupuncture to enhance their fertility and had later progressed to IVF. From the descriptive content analysis, four major categories of perceptions about acupuncture in relation to reproductive health were identified: (a) Awareness of, and perceived benefits of acupuncture; (b) perceptions of the body and the impact of acupuncture upon it; (c) perceptions of stress and the impact of acupuncture on resilience; and (d) perceptions of the intersection of medical treatment and acupuncture. This study confirms that acupuncture is perceived by infertile women to have an impact to their health. The small size of the study is a limitation. The study suggests that further studies of acupuncture as an adjunct to IVF should systematically explore the issues of wellbeing, anxiety, personal and social resilience and women's identity in relation to sexuality and reproduction.

In 2010, Balk *et al.* [25] conducted an observational prospective cohort study that assessed the stress relief effect of acupuncture on women undergoing IVF. The study compared the stress levels of women undergoing IVF who received acupuncture therapy with a control group who did not receive conjunctive acupuncture. The Perceived Stress Scale (PSS) was used to measure the stress levels of the participating women. 10 questions related to chronic ongoing stress along with stress from expectations of future events, both of which have a close correlation to women's desire to conceive through IVF were included in the PSS. A questionnaire was filled out by all the women in the study before embryo transfer and again after embryo transfer. The change in the stress level before and after embryo transfer was the main outcome variable. Protocol of the study consisted of the acupuncture group filling out the initial PSS form with acupuncture treatment to follow. Embryo transfer was performed after acupuncture treatment. Following embryo transfer, acupuncture treatment was performed again and then the second PSS form was filled. The Paulus protocol was used in the acupuncture treatment. Protocol for the control (non-acupuncture) group was required to fill out the initial PSS form with embryo transfer to follow. After the embryo transfer, the second PSS form was completed. 57 women were included in the study, with 17 in the acupuncture group and 40 in the non-acupuncture group. Women in the acupuncture group reached pregnancy at a higher rate than those in the non-acupuncture group. Pregnancy success rate in the acupuncture group was 64.7% ($p=0.13$). Donor egg IVF with acupuncture resulted in a pregnancy success rate of 75.0% ($p=0.71$) while non-donor egg IVF with acupuncture success rate was 55.6% ($p=0.28$). The overall pregnancy rate in the non-acupuncture group was 42.5% ($p=0.13$). Donor egg IVF without acupuncture resulted in a pregnancy success rate of 66.7% ($p=0.71$) while non-donor egg IVF without acupuncture success rate was 35.5% ($p=0.28$).

This study indicated that women whose PSS scores decreased by two or more points had increased pregnancy rates when compared to women with lower reductions or increases in stress scores. Women who received acupuncture treatment had lower stress scores both pre-ET and post-ET compared to those who did not. Women with decreased perceived stress scores compared to baseline had higher pregnancy rates than those who did not demonstrate this decrease, regardless of acupuncture status. The study concluded that the acupuncture regimen was associated with less stress both before and after embryo transfer, and it possibly improved pregnancy rates. Lower perceived stress at the time of embryo transfer may play a role in an improved pregnancy rate.

Acupuncture can be applied in different technical ways. Transcutaneous electrical acupoint stimulation (TEAS) is one of them. A prospective, randomized, single-blinded placebo-controlled clinical trial conducted at research and laboratory facilities in Beijing [26] was designed to evaluate TEAS on pregnancy rates (PR) in women undergoing embryo transfer (ET). A total of 309 patients who were less than 45 years old and underwent cryopreservation embryonic transplant or fresh cycle IVF, with or without intracytoplasmic sperm injection (ICSI), were recruited to the study. The patients were randomly allocated to three groups: Group I (mock TEAS treatment, n=99): 30 minutes after ET; Group II (single TEAS treatment, n=110): 30 minutes after ET; and Group III (double TEAS treatments n=100): 24 hours before ET and 30 minutes after ET. For patients allocated to Group II, TEAS was administered 30 minutes after ET. At acupuncture points Zusanli (ST36) and Taixi (KI3), Shenshu (BL23) and Guanyuan (RN4), self-sticking skin electrodes of 2.9X2.9 mm were placed. The parameters of TEAS were frequency 2 Hz, pulse width 0.6 ms, intensity 10–12 mA, lasting for 30 minutes. For patients in Group III, extra TEAS was given 24 hours before ET on bilateral acupuncture points: Diji (SP8) and Guilia (ST29), Zigong (EX-CA 1) and Xuehai (SP10). The parameters were 2 Hz, 15–20 mA, and 30 minutes. For patients in Group I, 2 Hz intermittent (10 seconds on and 20 seconds off) TEAS at 5 mA (designated as i5mA) was used for 30 minutes, on the same acupuncture points as for Group II. The i5mA intensity represents an extremely weak stimulation level, but patients still have a sense of intermittent stimulation. The i5mA intensity has been approved as a successful placebo (psychologically effective yet physiologically inert) treatment modality. The outcomes were measured by clinical PR, embryo implantation rate, and live birth rate. The study showed that the clinical PR, embryo implantation rate, and live birth rate of group I (29.3%, 15.0%, and 21.2%, respectively) were significantly lower than those in group II (42.7%, 25.7%, and 37.3%, respectively) and group III (50.0%, 25.9%, and 42.0%, respectively). The results indicated that TEAS significantly improved the clinical outcome of ET.

Do "true" acupuncture and "sham" acupuncture produce measurable differences in IVF outcomes? Numerous studies in the 2008-2010 timeframe indicated that the answer is yes. However, even though the evidence supported a difference in outcomes, this question was still being raised and occasionally tested. Researchers [27] at the Division of

Reproductive Endocrinology and Infertility, Department of Obstetrics and Gynecology, Northwestern Feinberg School of Medicine, Chicago, Illinois, conducted a randomized controlled trial, double-blinded with an independent observer to evaluate the influence of "true" versus "sham" acupuncture on pregnancy rates (PRs) in women undergoing IVF, and presented a disappointing answer. They recruited one hundred-sixty patients who were younger than 38 years old, undergoing IVF with or without intracytoplasmic sperm injection. Patients were randomly assigned to the true acupuncture or sham acupuncture group and underwent acupuncture 25 minutes before and after embryo transfer (ET). The acupuncture protocol for the patients in the true acupuncture group was as follows: before ET, patients were needled at Qihai (RN6), Diji (SP8), Taichong (LR3), Guilai (ST29), and Baihui (DU20). After ET, these patients were needled at Zusanli (ST36), Sanyinjiao (SP6), Xuehai (SP10), and Hegu (LI 4). Auricular acupuncture was performed unilaterally at the following points: shenmen, sympathetic, uterus, endocrine, before ET. The same auricular points were needled on the other side after ET. The patients in the sham acupuncture group were treated on predetermined point locations before and after ET. Auricular acupuncture was performed unilaterally before ET at the following points: knee, heel, allergic area, mouth. The side of the auricular acupuncture was changed after ET. Outcomes were measured by clinical PR and clinical symptoms during ET. The study found that the clinical PR was 45.3% in the "true" group and 52.7% in the sham group (P=0.353). The chemical PR was 7% in the true arm and 8.1% in the sham arm (P=0.786). There was no statistically significant difference in the clinical or chemical PRs between both groups. There was also no significant difference in the number of multiple pregnancies observed in the two groups.

Is it necessary to include a sham acupuncture control for a clinical trial on IVF? Is the sham acupuncture really a "sham"? What are the theoretical and methodological rationales for the use of sham acupuncture controls in trials of adjuvant acupuncture for *in vitro* fertilization (IVF)? Are there any drawbacks of using a sham acupuncture control that may have its own effects on the pregnancy outcome? These questions have been raised by practitioners and researchers for a long time. Manheimer [28] attempted to answer these questions.

Following the tradition of acupuncture clinical trials for pain conditions, sham acupuncture controls became an essential component for acupuncture clinical trials on IVF. But Manheimer [27] argued that pain is a subjective, patient-reported outcome and ratings of pain and similar subjective states can be strongly influenced by respondents' prejudgments, preferences, and expectations about treatment benefits. Therefore, controlling for these expectations or "placebo effects" by using a sham acupuncture control group is critically important in trials of acupuncture for pain-related conditions. "This need for sham acupuncture controls in trials of acupuncture for pain-related conditions may have led to the belief that sham acupuncture is always the most "rigorous" control, and that it should therefore be used for all acupuncture trials, including trials of adjuvant acupuncture for IVF." Manheimer continued: "In trials of adjuvant acupuncture for IVF, the outcome is pregnancy, which is entirely objective and unlikely to be affected by a patient's expectations of a benefit of acupuncture. Because it seems unlikely that an IVF patient's knowledge of whether she was receiving adjuvant acupuncture would affect her ability to become pregnant from IVF, using sham acupuncture to control for expectation/placebo effects seems unnecessary in this context. Even if adjuvant acupuncture were to increase IVF success rates only through a psychosomatic effect mechanism, such as by reducing stress, this stress-reduction effect would be integral to the working mechanism by which adjuvant acupuncture increases IVF pregnancy rates; therefore, it seems inappropriate to control for and separate out any such stress-reduction effect by using a sham control." Furthermore, "The risk that the sham is not an inert placebo but rather an active treatment that may affect the pregnancy outcome, using sham acupuncture as the control may unnecessarily confuse rather than clarify the interpretation of the effects of IVF adjuvant acupuncture." These theoretical arguments and methodological concerns bring forward the issue of weighing the benefits and drawbacks of using sham acupuncture in adjuvant acupuncture for IVF trials and assessing the risk of bias in the clinical trial results.

For a certain group of women, conceiving a baby is a very difficult process. Infertility in this group of women is due to failure of embryo implantation. Does acupuncture help for this group of women? Brazilian physicians and researchers [29] investigated this issue seriously. A prospective, randomized controlled clinical trial to evaluate the effectiveness of acupuncture and moxibustion as an adjuvant treatment in women undergoing *in vitro* fertilization (IVF) when embryo implantation has previously failed was conducted at the Faculty of Medicine of ABC, Clinic for Human Reproduction, Santo André, São Paulo, Brazil.

Eighty-four infertile patients who had had at least two unsuccessful attempts of IVF participated in the study. The patients were randomly allocated into three groups: control (n=28); sham (n=28); and acupuncture (n=28). The sample size was calculated by assuming a pregnancy rate of 10% when embryo implantation had previously failed. Blood β human chorionic gonadotrophin (βhCG) and subsequent transvaginal ultrasound were used as measurement for the pregnancy rates of the current IVF cycle. Acupuncture was performed according to the following protocol: on the first and seventh day of ovulation induction; on the day before ovarian puncture; and on the day after embryo transfer. In the acupuncture group, moxibustion and acupuncture were combined and patients were treated with moxibustion at nine acupuncture points: Ganshu (BL18), Sanjiaoshu (BL22), Shenshu (BL23), Zhishi (BL52), Zhongji (RN3), Guanyuan (RN4), Shimen (RN5), Yinjiao (RN7), and Mingmen (DU4), for about five minutes. After moxibustion, 11 points – Neiguan (PC6), Taixi (KI 3), Zhaohai (KI6), Fuliu (KI7), Yingu (KI10), Taichong (LR3), Gongsun (SP4), Sanyinjiao (SP6), Xuehai (SP10), Fenglong (ST40), and Lieque (LU7) – were needled unilaterally, plus the extra point Zigong bilaterally. The needles were manually inserted and stimulated to obtain qi sensation, and the needles were retained for 20 minutes. For patients in the sham group, acupuncture was performed in the arm and thigh, which are known not to correspond with classically described acupuncture points, using a total of eight needles (two needles in each region bilaterally). The needles were inserted superficially, without eliciting qi sensation. The sham group's needles were also retained for 20 minutes. No moxibustion or any other stimulation technique was performed in the sham group. The result showed that the clinical pregnancy rate in the acupuncture group was significantly higher than that in the control and sham groups (35.7% vs 7.1% vs 10.7%; $p=0.0169$). The researchers concluded that acupuncture and moxibustion increased pregnancy rates when used as an adjuvant treatment in women undergoing IVF, when embryo implantation had previously failed.

The Second Wave of Systematic Reviews and Meta-analysis (2012-2014)

By 2012, increasing numbers of clinical trials provided a lot of raw material for systematic reviews and meta-analyses. Three systematic reviews and meta-analyses by Chinese researchers which evaluated the effect of acupuncture on *in vitro* fertilization (IVF) outcomes reached conflicting conclusions in 2012. Conflicting conclusions have been rife in this area of research since the first systematic review with meta-analysis was published in 2008.

One systematic review with meta-analysis of the randomized controlled trials (RCTs) was conducted by Zheng, *et al.* [30] to evaluate the effects of acupuncture on IVF outcomes. Clinical trials from Pubmed, Embase, the Cochrane Library, Clinical Trials Register, Wanfang Database, CNKI Database, and VIP database were searched. Techniques used for the acupuncture-intervention groups included manual, electrical, and laser acupuncture. The control groups were given no acupuncture, sham acupuncture, or placebo acupuncture. The clinical pregnancy rate (CPR) and live birth rate (LBR) were the major therapeutic outcomes considered. A forest-plot analysis was used to evaluate the heterogeneity of the therapeutic effect. A funnel plot analysis was used to assess publication bias. Twenty-four trials with a total of 5,807 participants were included in this review. There were no significant publication biases for most of the comparisons among these studies. The study found that the pooled CPR (23 studies) from all of the acupuncture groups was significantly greater than that from all of the control groups, whereas the LBR (6 studies) was not significantly different between the two groups. And furthermore, "the results were different when the type of control was examined in a sensitivity analysis. The CPR and LBR differences between the acupuncture and control groups were more obvious when the studies using the Streitberger control were ignored. Similarly, if the underlying effects of the Streitberger control were excluded, the LBR results tended to be significant when the acupuncture was performed around the time of oocyte aspiration or controlled ovarian hyperstimulation." The study indicated that acupuncture improves CPR and LBR among women undergoing IVF based on the results of studies that do not include the Streitberger control. One explanation is that the Streitberger control may not be an inactive control. The authors concluded that additional positive effects from using acupuncture in IVF can be expected if more reasonable acupuncture programs are used.

Another systematic review with meta-analysis of the trials of acupuncture use during *in vitro* fertilization (IVF) or intracytoplasmic sperm injection (ICSI) treatment, related to the outcomes of clinical pregnancy, biochemical pregnancy, ongoing pregnancy, implantation rate, live birth, and miscarriage was conducted by Qu, *et al.* [31] Clinical trials from MEDLINE, SCISEARCH, the Cochrane Menstrual Disorders and Subfertility Group trials register, AMED, Cumulative Index to Nursing and Allied Health Literature, EMBASE, Wanfang Database, China Academic Journal Electronic full text Database in China National Knowledge Infrastructure, Index to Chinese Periodical Literature, ISI Proceedings for conference abstracts, and ISRCTN Register and Meta-register for randomized controlled trials were searched. Meta-analysis techniques such as study selection, quality appraisal, and data extraction were performed independently and in duplicate. The pooled relative risks (RR) of achieving clinical pregnancy, biochemical pregnancy, ongoing pregnancy, implantation rate, live birth, or miscarriage for women in the acupuncture group compared with women in the control group were the measures of treatment effect. Using the random-effects model, pooling of the effect estimates from all of the seventeen trials showed no significant difference in the clinical pregnancy outcome between the acupuncture and the control groups (RR=1.09, 95% confidence interval (CI) 0.94-1.26, p=0.25). No significant differences in the biochemical pregnancy (RR=1.01, 95% CI 0.84-1.20, p=0.95), ongoing pregnancy (RR=1.20, 95% CI 0.93-1.56, p=0.16), implantation rate (RR=1.22, 95% CI 0.93-1.62, p=0.16), live birth (RR=1.42, 95% CI 0.92-2.20, p=0.11), or miscarriage outcomes (RR=0.94, 95% CI 0.67-1.33, p=0.74) were found between the acupuncture and the control groups. This study concluded that it seems that no significant benefits of acupuncture were found to improve the outcomes of IVF or ICSI.

Clearly, these two systematic reviews with meta-analysis produced inconsistent implications: supportive evidence for acupuncture application to IVF vs. non-supportive evidence for acupuncture application to IVF. Why did the same statistical techniques addressing the same question produce such different answers? In applying these statistical techniques, inclusion criteria and methods of searching the literature, data extraction, and data analysis were different. Heterogeneous trials have been pooled, without examining variables that might explain the heterogeneity. The inconclusiveness of these systematic reviews with meta-analysis of adjuvant acupuncture for IVF illustrated from the above two reviews provoked further explorations. Manheimer, *et al.* at the University of Maryland Center for Integrative Medicine continued their involvement in this area and took on the challenge of explaining the heterogeneity.

Manheimer *et al.* [32] attempted to quantify the overall pooled effects of adjuvant acupuncture on IVF clinical pregnancy success rates, and evaluate whether estimates of effectiveness are influenced by the factors of study design, treatment protocols, and population selection. Their study selected randomized controlled trials that compared needle acupuncture administered within one day of embryo transfer, versus sham acupuncture or no adjuvant treatment. Clinical pregnancy rate was the primary outcome measure. Sixteen trials (4021 participants) were included in this meta-analysis. The authors obtained additional methodological details and outcome data not included in their original publications from all investigators. Sham-controlled and no-adjuvant-treatment-controlled trials were analyzed separately. Since there were no large or significant differences between these two subsets, all trials were pooled for subgroup analyses. Eleven subgroup variables (5 clinical and 6 methodological) were specified to investigate sources of heterogeneity, using single covariate meta-regressions. The meta-analysis found that there was no statistically significant difference between acupuncture and controls when combining all trials [risk ratio (RR) 1.12, 95% confidence interval (CI), 0.96-1.31; I(2) = 68%; 16 trials; 4021 patients], or when restricting to sham-controlled (RR 1.02, 0.83-1.26; I(2) = 66%; 7 trials; 2044 patients) or no-adjuvant-treatment-controlled trials (RR 1.22, 0.97-1.52; I(2) = 67%; 9 trials; 1977 patients). The type of controls used did not significantly explain the statistical heterogeneity (interaction P = 0.27). They discovered that the baseline pregnancy rate, measured as the observed rate of clinical pregnancy in the control group of each trial, was a statistically significant effect modifier (interaction P < 0.001), and this covariate explained most of the heterogeneity of the effects of adjuvant acupuncture across all trials (adjusted R(2) = 93%; I(2) residual = 9%). Trials with lower baseline pregnancy rate showed larger effects of adjuvant acupuncture (RR 1.53, 1.28-1.84; 7 trials; 1732 patients). Trials with higher baseline pregnancy rate showed smaller effects of adjuvant acupuncture (RR 0.90, 0.80-1.01; 9 trials; 2289 patients). The asymmetric funnel plot showed a tendency for the intervention effects to be more beneficial in smaller trials.

This latest meta-analysis confirms a suspicion which has emerged over the last few years of research into the effect of acupuncture applied on the day of embryo transfer: that it confers an advantage only for those patients whose chance of success with IVF is low. Manheimer explained his team's findings: "For IVF clinics with baseline pregnancy rates higher than average (32 percent or greater) adding acupuncture had no benefit. However, at IVF clinics with baseline pregnancy rates lower than average (less than 32 percent) adding acupuncture seemed to increase IVF pregnancy success rates. A direct association between the baseline pregnancy success rate and the effects of adding acupuncture was discovered: the lower the baseline pregnancy rate at the clinic, the more adjuvant acupuncture seemed to increase the pregnancy rate." The study of Manheimer et al. [32] demonstrated that an accepted economics principle also applies to acupuncture for IVF: the law of diminishing marginal returns.

The most recent systematic review and meta-analysis to evaluate the impact of acupuncture during *in vitro* fertilization (IVF) treatment on the outcome of clinical pregnancy in published randomized studies was conducted by Shen, *et al.* [33] from four data sources: MEDLINE, Embase, Web of Knowledge and the Chinese Biomedical Database. Their analysis showed that there was no statistically significant difference between the acupuncture group and the no-acupuncture (intervention) control group in regard to the following factors: the time of embryo transfer (ET) (risk ratio, RR, 1.24, 95% confidence interval, CI, 1.02-1.50); unblinded trials (95% CI 1.26-1.88); trials blinded to physicians (95% CI 0.82-1.33); and double-blind trials (95% CI 0.89-1.25). There was also no statistically significant difference when comparing acupuncture groups with sham acupuncture controls in the same areas: the time of ET (RR, 1.03, 95% CI 0.87-1.22); restriction to unblinded trials (95% CI 0.80-2.02); trials blinded to physicians (95% CI 0.82-1.18); and double-blind trials (95% CI 0.77-1.17). However, statistically significant differences were noted in the following instances. A statistically significant difference was shown when acupuncture was performed at 30 minutes after the ET and implantation phase (RR 1.76, 95% CI 1.22-2.55), and also when acupuncture was performed at the follicle phase and 25 minutes before and after ET (RR 1.56, 95% CI 1.04-2.33). The authors concluded that acupuncture did not significantly improve the IVF clinical pregnancy rate when performed only at the time of ET, but the pooled benefit of acupuncture for IVF showed when performed at the follicle phase and 25 minutes before and after ET, as well as 30 minutes after ET and implantation phase. The timing of acupuncture intervention is an important factor.

The Mechanisms of Acupuncture for IVF

This literature review focuses on the clinical aspects of acupuncture application to IVF. A basic scientific explanation of the mechanisms of acupuncture application to IVF is not the emphasis of this paper. But scientists have conducted numerous studies in an attempt to scientifically explain the benefits of acupuncture. A brief summary of developments in this area may be beneficial to readers. Ho, *et al.* [34] demonstrated that acupuncture can increase blood flow to the reproductive organs such as the uterus and ovaries. This facilitation of the blood flow can improve the thickness of the endometrial lining, thus increasing the chances of embryo implantation. Anderson, *et al.* [17] found that acupuncture regulates fertility hormones. Because stress and other factors can disrupt the function of the hypothalamic pituitary-ovarian axis (HPOA), acupuncture can modulate neuroendocrinological factors. Acupuncture regulates the release of beta-endorphin in the brain, which regulates gonadotrophin-releasing hormone from the hypothalamus, follicle stimulating hormone from the pituitary gland, and ovarian estrogen and progesterone levels. Liu, *et al.* [35] showed that acupuncture can promote embryo implantation through mediating sexual hormone levels and receptor expression. Magarelli, *et al.* [20]

indicated that acupuncture can normalize cortisol and prolactin levels on IVF medication days. Jin, *et al.* [36] demonstrated that acupuncture can increase egg production, thus increasing the chance of fertilization, and also showed that acupuncture can regulate follicle stimulation hormone-receptor expression. A study by Chen, *et al.* [37] indicated that acupuncture can improve oocyte quality, thus increasing the chances of fertilization. Huang, *et al.* [38] demonstrated that acupuncture can enhance luteal function to improve embryo implantation. Scientific evidence indicates that acupuncture improves ovulation by modulating the central and peripheral nervous systems, the neuroendocrine and endocrine systems, ovarian blood flow, and metabolism. Taken as a whole, clinical studies show that acupuncture can improve the outcome of IVF-ET, and that the underlying mechanisms may be related to increased uterine blood flow, modulation of immune function, inhibited uterine motility, and the anesis of depression, anxiety and stress. Even though there have been many positive findings in regard to the beneficial effects of acupuncture on infertility, well-designed, multi-center, prospective, randomized, controlled studies, and more rigorous studies are still needed to provide more reliable and stronger scientific evidence [39].

Conclusion

Starting with the "relatively silent revolution" of Dr. Paulus' 2002 study [1], the application of acupuncture to fertility medicine has had truly revolutionary implications in two dramatically different medical fields: traditional Chinese medicine and contemporary reproductive medicine. This literature review has attempted to document the development of this emerging field from the birth of the Paulus protocol to the variety of protocols which are in use by reproductive clinics today. We have detailed the Paulus protocol, the first wave of systematic reviews with meta-analysis (2008-2010), advanced clinical trials, and the second wave of systematic reviews with meta-analysis (2012-2014) in this review paper. The volume of clinical research studies and publications in the area of TCM applications to fertility medicine continues to grow at a staggering rate, thus insuring an ever-expanding supply of material for future systematic reviews and meta-analyses. It is encouraging to see how successfully traditional Chinese medicine stands up to the protocols of rigorous scientific analysis and the challenge of evidence-based medicine. The ancient art of acupuncture and modern reproductive medicine have met at a crossroads of scientific research, and it seems certain that they will walk side-by-side into the future.

Chapter Four

Acupuncture for Nausea and Vomiting

Understanding the Clinical Problem

Nausea and vomiting are internal medicine conditions. This chapter focuses on nausea and vomiting resulted from the side-effects of chemotherapy. From mild to constant and severe, symptoms can impact the quality of life, the ability to take in nourishment and; if prolonged, may affect the mood and weaken the will. In addition to interfering with activities of daily living, nausea and vomiting may diminish the patient's ability to tolerate treatment, resulting in sub-therapeutic doses that do not effectively resolve the cancer. Additionally, as weight loss and malnourishment may lead to weakness and the inability to gather the strength to recover, resolving nausea and vomiting can be the essential determining factors in whether the patient survives chemotherapy.

Fortunately, with the evolution of cancer treatment, many forms of chemotherapy no longer cause nausea and vomiting. For those that do, many oncology departments are incorporating complementary treatments to assist with side effects of treatments; and many insurance companies will now cover acupuncture for chemotherapy-related nausea. The difficulty in treating cancer arises from the fact that, in contrast to an exogenously derived condition, such as a bacterial, viral or fungal infection; cancer reflects a dysfunction of the normal death process of one's own cells. While an accumulation of exogenous or endogenous toxins may create the conditions that eventually lead to interference with normal cellular processes; treatment is often focused on destroying the aberrant cancerous cells rather than removing the substances that most contribute to creating a noxious cellular environment. Chemotherapies are extraordinarily toxic to the cellular matter targeted; and although targeting mechanisms have improved, the poisonous nature of the drugs sets off the body's natural alarm system; nausea and vomiting then ensue in an attempt to expel the toxin. Serotonin and substance P, neurochemicals released in response to noxious stimuli, can be key initiators that activate the nausea and vomiting process.

The negative impact of cancer depends on several factors. If tumors are interfering, impinging- upon, putting pressure on tissues; or blocking the circulation of vital substances, tumors may need to be removed or destroyed via medical intervention. Some cancers do not drastically infringe on the activity of healthy tissues or processes, or may be slow to grow; in which instances, patients can live for a long time without risky medical intervention. In cases where the tumor is rapidly growing, depriving local tissues of oxygen and blood, draining the body's energy or invading the circulatory system and thus metastasizing in distal locations, treatment methods often need to be strong enough to quickly stop the cancer from taking over. In cases where cancerous cells are rapidly growing, chemotherapeutic agents are targeted to break-down rapidly dividing cells; unfortunately, healthy cells in those body tissues that naturally exhibit a rapid turnover often take a beating as well. The digestive tract is one such body area lined end to end with rapidly dividing cells. The cellular lining from the mouth to the esophagus and stomach may be quickly eroded by chemotherapeutic agents, resulting in nausea and vomiting. The reaction to certain chemotherapeutics may be immediate or delayed until a few hours or days after administration. Expectation and nerves also play a role; in which case anticipation, may induce nausea and vomiting preceding chemotherapy. In addition to chemotherapy-induced nausea, patients may experience radiation-induced nausea and vomiting. Although the negative impact of radiation treatment has been lessened via improved targeting methods that limit exposure as much as possible to the cancerous cells; many receiving radiotherapies still experience nausea and vomiting.

Certain medical procedures, such as stem-cell transplantation may involve the administration of whole-body radiation, which is associated with a greater incidence if nausea and vomiting. In addition, certain treatment interventions may pose a greater risk of inducing nausea and vomiting as they may include both chemotherapy and radiation. The likelihood of radiation-induced nausea and vomiting may also depend on which part of the body is being treated. Radiation directed at the digestive system, alimentary tract and elimination pathways often are associated with an increased risk of nausea and vomiting. Dosing is also a factor as patients often experience less nausea and vomiting with a series of smaller doses as opposed to one large dose.

In addition to experiencing nausea and vomiting while undergoing a treatment series, nausea and vomiting may become chronic when those with advanced cancer undergo radiation treatment. Depending on area of the body affected by cancerous tumors, chronic nausea and vomiting may be induced in reaction to the tumor itself. Brain and colon tumors, stomach ulcers, dehydration blood imbalances and pharmaceuticals such as antidepressants, anti-anxiety medications or pain killers may produce or contribute to nausea and vomiting as well.

Mental anguish as well as physical pain and suffering related to nausea and vomiting are compounded by the monetary cost of prolonged or severe symptoms. Supplementary treatment, extended hospital stays, additional care providers, provisions for lengthy periods of unemployment and mental and spiritual support may all be required. Thus, it is advisable to do what can be done to resolve the seemingly less important symptoms of nausea and vomiting, as this may immeasurably benefit the patient and improve the overall success of the treatment intervention.

Many chemotherapeutic agents initiate a cascade of reactions beginning with dry mouth, poor appetite, nausea and vomiting, stomach and abdominal pain, hemorrhage and irregular bowel movements. Additionally, alkalizing and anti-cancer antibiotics may instigate acute adverse reactions affecting the digestive and elimination systems.

Pathogenesis: In 1953, Dr. Borison proposed a chemoreceptor trigger zone (CTZ) behind the brain area associated with emesis which was also external to the blood-brain barrier. The CTZ is thought to act via nerve impulse to the emesis brain area. In the past, the dopamine receptor was thought to be responsible for initiating the vomiting reaction; metoclopramide was then found to quell the urge to vomit and restore homeostasis. More recent research has indicated that neurotransmitters, such as 5-hydroxytryptamine, histamine AI, and toxic alkaline substances are also involved in initiating a vomiting response. Pharmaceutical interventions that block these receptors may also be serve to be preventative. Emesis is thought to be regulated via a network within the medulla, in close proximity to those structures responsible for respiration, vasomotor control and the autonomic nervous system; nausea and vomiting may be accompanied with headache, weakness, changes in breathing, dizziness or vertigo, changes in complexion, salivation and puffiness or swelling; and thus, emesis may be affected by influences affecting these symptoms as well.

The Three Manifestations of Nausea and Vomiting Caused by Chemotherapy: Emesis related to chemotherapeutic agents may occur immediately following administration, as often occurs with nitrogen mustard and streptozotocin; most chemotherapy drugs may elicit a vomiting response one- or two-hours following administration. Delayed vomiting, as sometimes occurs with high doses of cisplatin, may commence 1-3 days after chemotherapy. Anticipatory vomiting may occur in those who expect that vomiting will occur, or those who have been conditioned from previous experience.

Differential Diagnosis: As the primary cause of nausea and vomiting in cancer patients may be something other than the chemotherapeutic agents, a differential diagnosis is needed to rule-out nausea and vomiting that is related to an internal condition or exogenous pathogen. Other conditions that commonly produce nausea and vomiting in chemotherapy patients encompass a wide range of conditions. Nausea and vomiting are common early signs of brain metastasis If attributed to chemotherapy, the metastasis may not be diagnosed until other signs and symptoms appear. Nausea and vomiting due to acute renal failure, or tumor lysis syndrome (TLS) resulting in impeded kidney function occurs when chemotherapy releases uric acid from the tumor; kidneys are further stressed by emesis-induced dehydration and electrolyte imbalance. The uremia itself may lead to nausea and vomiting. If the emesis in this case is assumed to be chemotherapeutically-induced, the toll on the kidneys may be overlooked, and if supportive action is not taken, further damage may ensue. In cases where gastrointestinal tract obstructions lead to emesis related to gastrointestinal cancers of the stomach, intestine or pancreas, these must also be distinguished from chemotherapy-induced nausea and vomiting. Additional prescribed pharmaceuticals, such as morphine, estrogen, erythrocin, digitalis, etc., often contribute to nausea and vomiting during the chemotherapeutic process. Metabolic imbalance and neuroendocrine system diseases may also compound symptoms of nausea and vomiting. Systemic influences may also instigate emesis, such as hypercalcemia and hyponatremia that must not be confused with nausea and vomiting from chemotherapeutic agents so that the imbalance may be corrected.

Chinese Medicine Understanding

In traditional Chinese medicine, each organ system moves energy in a certain direction. The stomach, when functioning properly, sends energy downward so that food, once digested, can continue down through the intestines and out of the body. When the stomach qi is disordered, or a noxious substance enters the stomach meridian, stomach qi rebels upward, leading to feelings of nausea, frontal headache, dizziness; and if the impulse is strong enough, vomiting.

Nausea and vomiting of any kind is thus possible to treat with acupuncture by eliminating the pathogen, harmonizing the organ systems, strengthening the body and correcting the direction of qi-flow. In patients suffering from chemotherapy-induced nausea and vomiting, a differential diagnosis may be obtained that takes into consideration the constitution of the patient, the underlying factors regarding the primary condition (how a cancerous condition is manifesting in a particular person), other factors that may be contributing to nausea and vomiting, the noxious substance and the body's reaction to chemotherapy. In truth, providing acupuncture prior to chemotherapy may help stabilize the patient so that treatment is more easily tolerated from the beginning. It is almost always much easier in Chinese medicine to prevent an imbalance than to correct one; and via the harmonizing nature by which acupuncture exerts its effect, a great deal of suffering may be avoided. Although some hospitals and western medical clinics try to bypass traditional Chinese medicine theory and differential diagnosis assessment by administering standardized acupuncture protocols known empirically to produce anti-emetic effects, this short-cut may circumvent the opportunity to reap the full benefits of traditional Chinese medicine. A differential diagnosis will lead practitioners to choose the best combination of points in each case, and also may reveal new medically relevant information.

To further illuminate the differentiation possibilities belonging to nausea and vomiting from a traditional Chinese medicine perspective, some patterns are described here. A patient presenting with mild nausea may have a stomach deficiency; the specific type may be revealed through further questioning and examination. If the nausea and vomiting are severe, the imbalance may be due to a form of excess. If the nausea and vomiting are severe, rebellious stomach qi may be the case. If one vomits after eating, this suggests one has a full or excessive stomach condition. If one vomits liquids, this may indicate a deficiency pattern of the stomach. Vomiting sour liquid often indicates the condition is likely due to a stagnant liver invading the stomach. When vomitus liquid is bitter, heat may be lodged in the liver and gall bladder; whereas, thin, watery fluids are often a sign of excess cold in the stomach. When vomiting occurs immediately after eating, stomach heat is likely; while if vomiting occurs hours after eating, the condition is likely cold in nature. Waves of nausea and vomiting that come and go may be more closely related to emotional upset, and rebellious liver qi may be invading the stomach.

Excess patterns tend to manifest suddenly with acute and strong symptoms, which may seem unrelenting; however, tend to quickly pass. They may be due to exterior invasion, irregular or excessive eating habits or an excessive liver invading the stomach. Deficient patterns tend to become chronic; often expressing symptoms gradually over time. Often, they are associated with a constitutional weakness; or a weakening of the stomach due to a combination of factors or specific illness. Deficiency patterns, although long-term, may be less severe, may come and go or recur under stress. In the treatment of chemotherapy-related nausea and vomiting, it is well to be aware that several other symptoms of rebellious stomach qi may present themselves in the absence of nausea or vomiting, such as gastric reflux and hiccough; and thus, may be treated with acupuncture as well.

Vomiting may ensue from an internal imbalance. In this case the imbalance is diagnosed from a traditional Chinese medical perspective, and can then be corrected. When vomiting is induced by the body's own defense mechanisms in response to the ingestion of harmful substances, the expulsion of the pathogen through emesis may be advised; in which case, the first action in treatment may not intend to stop the vomiting until the pathogen is fully expelled. In cases where the patient is undergoing medical interventions that trigger the body's innate defense system, as is such when undergoing chemotherapy, the role of acupuncture may best be directed at harmonizing the patient's body with the purpose of the therapeutic action of the chemotherapeutic agents. With less natural resistance, the ability of the agent to target specific cells with as little as possible damage to the healthy aspects of the body may be maximized.

As always, referrals need to be made accordingly. Dehydration is always a consideration when a patient has been losing fluids through vomit, sweat, urine or feces; if the patient presents with dehydration or becomes dehydrated, a referral is necessary. An ER visit may be required if vomiting is accompanied by other serious symptoms, such as projectile vomiting with blood, high fever, stubborn or severe headache, a high level of irritability, agitation, confusion or any other mood change, pale, greenish, listless or any peculiar complexion, lethargy, extreme weakness, loss of control of bodily functions, shallow or difficult breathing or loss of consciousness.

Acupuncture Treatment Protocol

Body Acupuncture: Commonly used acupuncture points in the treatment of chemotherapy-induced nausea and vomiting may include the front-mu point of the stomach, Zhongwan (RN12), as front-mu or back-shu points of the affected organ system are often selected to elicit the greatest influence over a particular channel. Neiguan (PC6), is one of the most common distal points selected for any kind of nausea or vomiting. Combined with Gongsun (SP4), it regulates the Chong channel which powerfully influences the direction of the stomach channel, regulates the flow of blood and has a balancing effect on hormonal influences. Zusanli (ST36) also may be selected to strengthen and ground the qi of the stomach.

In cases where differential diagnosis has detected excessive stomach-heat, Hegu (LI4), Jinjin (Extra8), and Yuye (Extra8) may be added to the above protocol to release excess heat. If the stomach upset is due to excessive cold pattern, Shangwan (RN13) may be selected for its influence over the upper gastric; while, Weishu (UB21) the back-shu point of the stomach, may be selected for its strong warming and tonifying effect on the stomach. If a patient is presenting with a full pattern, and symptoms consistent with food stagnation, Xiawan (RN10) may be added for its influence over the epigastrium, and Xuanji (RN21) may be added to strongly descend rebellious qi. Treatments may be needed daily to support a patient undergoing chemotherapy.

Auricular Acupuncture: Auricular point protocols may easily be administered on their own or in conjunction with body acupuncture points to strengthen treatment effect and mind-body connection. Auricular treatments may be provided daily or every other day to help patients maintain stability. Commonly selected acupuncture points may harmonize the liver and stomach while deactivating the sympathetic response. Shenmen may also be included to induce a calm state that promotes the restoration of homeostasis.

Differentiation and Treatment

Once the pattern has been identified, an appropriate treatment principle may be defined. In cases where excess is causing nausea and vomiting, one might expel the pathogenic factors, transform turbidity, harmonize the stomach and liver and descend the rebellious stomach qi. For deficient patterns, treatment principles may be adopted that warm the middle jiao while fortifying the stomach. If fluids are deficient, one may nourish fluids and replenish stomach yin.

Excess patterns

Exterior pathogens invading the stomach: Weakened immunity to externally contracted illness, presenting with a history of periodic invasions. Headache, fever or chills, sensitivity to wind, body aches, queasiness or stomach pains may precede a sudden attack of vomiting. A sense of fullness, pressure or distention of the diaphragm, hypochondria or chest may also be present. The pulse tends to be floating and full and the tongue may have a greasy or thick coat. The treatment principle in this case is to release the exterior, transform turbidity and harmonize the middle jiao. Depending on specific presentation, points such as Zhongwan (RN12), the front-mu of the stomach; Zusanli (ST36), the stomach He-Sea point where qi of the channel gathers; Neiguan (PC6) combined with Gongsun (SP4), to open the Chong meridian and facilitate the normal direction of qi flow, settle the stomach and stop vomiting; Fengchi (GB20) to expel exterior wind; and Hegu (LI4) to clear the head and reinforce the exterior.

Retention or Stagnation of Food in the Stomach: An accumulation of food in the stomach may result in a sour stomach with retching and odiferous vomit. The condition is worse with food intake and better after vomitus is expelled. The diaphragm, hypochondrium and epigastric regions may be full and distended. Sour belching may relieve some pressure, aversion to food and vomiting at the sight, smell or hearing about food may predominate. Constipation, pressure in the lower abdomen and puffiness of the limbs and face may occur; or the stool may be pasty or sticky with a strong noxious odor. The tongue coat may be thick and greasy or curdled. The pulse is generally slippery and forceful at the middle jiao position. The treatment will focus on expelling or eliminating food stagnation, strengthening digestion and harmonizing the stomach and intestines. Acupuncture may be provided at points such as: Zhongwan (RN12), the front-mu of the stomach; Zusanli (ST36), to rectify the stomach qi; Neiguan (PC6) and Gongsun (SP4) to open the Chong and stop nausea and vomiting; Xiawan (RNI0) to stabilize and reinforce the stomach and Xuanji (RN21) to descend the qi.

Accumulation of Fluids in the Stomach: Queasiness with vomiting of clear liquids. Vomiting often occurs with fluid intake. The lungs and upper sinuses may also be congested, resulting in the coughing up of white or yellow sputum along with watery eye exudate and nasal discharge. Dizziness, difficulty concentrating, palpitations, fullness of the epigastrium, chest and diaphragm, gurgling or swishing stomach sounds, lack of desire to eat with aversion to taking-in liquids. This condition may occur more frequently in obesity or those with a rich diet with excessive sweets. The tongue may be wet, puffy, swollen or have a thick slippery coating. The pulse is often slippery and full. The treatment principle may focus on dispersing and expelling excess fluids, clearing the lungs, harmonizing the middle jiao, supporting the kidneys and transforming and regulating water while descending rebellious qi. Acupuncture may be given at: Zhongwan

(RN12), Zusanli (ST36), Tianshu (ST25), Neiguan (PC6), Gongsun (SP4), Tanzhong (RN17) to open the chest and diaphragm, and Fenglong (ST40) and (SP9) to dissolve mucus.

Stagnant Liver Qi Invading the Stomach: Sour vomiting and frequent belching or hiccup. Fullness and pain in the epigastric region and hypochondrium, focal distention may also be notable in the epigastrium accompanied by suppressed appetite, worse with stress or strong emotions. Emotions such as anger, frustration or resentment may precipitate a vomiting spell. The tongue may be swollen on the sides with toothmarks and a thin and greasy coat. The liver pulse may be especially wiry and the spleen pulse may be deficient and/or slippery. The practitioner will harmonize the liver and stomach, and unblock and facilitate the smooth flow of qi with points that may include: Zhongwan (RN12), Zusanli (ST36), Neiguan (PC6) and Gongsun (SP4), Danzhong (RN17), Taichong (LR3) to harmonize the liver and Yanglingquan (GB34) to remove damp-heat and facilitate the smooth flow of qi.

Deficiency patterns

Yang Deficiency with Cold Accumulation in the Spleen and Stomach: When cold and yang-deficient signs predominate, one may vomit clear, odorless cold liquids with undigested food particles. The condition may develop in a person with a cold constitution, and is made worse with irregular eating habits or fatigue. The condition is aggravated by habitual consumption of cold food or drink and improves with regular consumption of warm fluids or food. Complexion may be pale, whitish; or sallow, especially if the deficiency has lead to anemia, and the extremities and back may be cold. Fatigue may predominate with weakness, rigid and tight muscles and severe dislike and avoidance of cold. The tongue may be pale or bluish with thin white coating; the pulse will be deep, slow and tight; or, possibly thready and weak. Recovery will be aided by warming the spleen, dispersing the accumulation of cold, harmonizing the stomach and descending rebellious qi. Acupuncture may be provided at: Zhongwan (RN12), Zusanli (ST36), Yinlingquan (SP9), Neiguan (PC6), Gongsun (SP4), Pishu (BL20) (the back-shu point of the spleen) and Zhangmen (LR13).

Stomach yin-deficiency: Stomach yin-deficiency tends to be chronic, with vomiting or dry heaves that recur. The condition is made worse with dehydration, habitual diet of dry, spicy or hot food and alcohol; and is less frequent with moderate, regular eating habits that include moist food and proper fluid intake. Low appetite or hunger for small snacks, dry mouth and throat and dry stool may predominate. The tongue may be dry with transverse cracks especially in the middle, and may have little coating. The pulse may be rapid, thin and deficient. This kind of nausea and vomiting may best be treated by nourishing the spleen, replenishing stomach yin, descending stomach qi. A protocol that includes nourishing as well as descending points may benefit the patient; a helpful protocol may include: Zhongwan (RN12), Zusanli (ST36), Neiguan (PC6) and Gongsun (SP4), Sanyinjiao (SP6), Pishu (BL20) and Weishu (BL21) (the back-shu of the stomach).

Neiguan (PC6): An Essential Point in the Treatment of Nausea

Acupuncture at Neiguan (PC6) opens the chest, regulates the heart and calms the mind. Its harmonizing influence over the stomach tends to alleviate nausea and vomiting. This point also helps clear heat from the channel and organ and opens the yin linking vessel. Indicated for many symptoms affecting the chest and heart, acupuncture at Neiguan (PC6) alleviates symptoms related to the heart, lungs, stomach, liver as well as many symptoms related to the blood, menstruation and gynecology. Commonly, acupuncture at Neiguan (PC6) is selected to treat dull or acute heart pain, stuffiness of the chest, agitation, palpitations, a sense of fright, pounding sensations, irregular heart rate and rhythm, hypochondrial pain, cough, asthma and irregular menstruation and heat syndromes.

Conditions related to the heart and mind, such as insomnia and anxiety are effectively treated with acupuncture at Neiguan (PC6), as are many spastic conditions such as epilepsy. Its influence over mania, poor memory, insecurity, sadness, disorders of speech and high blood pressure reflect the range of influence Neiguan (PC6) has. Conditions related to blockage of qi or blood between the chest and epigastrium may also be regulated via acupuncture at Neiguan (PC6). Some symptoms positively affected include those related to digestion; such as nausea, vomiting, hiccup and belching. According to traditional Chinese medicine, conditions such as qi and yang deficiency of the spleen and stomach with relentless vomiting; spleen and stomach qi deficiency leading to indigestion, distention and fullness; disharmony of the spleen and stomach, resulting in stomach pain, stabbing epigastric pain and dull abdominal pain are all indications of Neiguan (PC6).

The ability of Neiguan (PC6) to open the diaphragm and move blockages is reflected in the successful treatment of food stagnation, masses and blood stasis. Lower GI symptoms such as borborygmus, diarrhea, blood in the stool and rectal prolapse may be positively influenced by acupuncture at Neiguan (PC6) as well. Via influence on the Yin Wei linking vessel, externally contracted fever with lack of sweat, frontal or headache, stiffness and pain of the head and neck may also be treated with Neiguan (PC6). While, influence over heat in the liver and diaphragm is reflected in the ability of Neiguan (PC6) to treat jaundice, red eyes, red face with hot skin, symptoms of febrile disease such as those exhibited in malarial disease, severe internal heat exhibited as a cracked and bleeding tongue and dizziness. Via influence over the Chong meridian, Neiguan (PC6) regulates many aspects of menstruation and gynecology. Dizziness related to blood loss after menstruation or childbirth, irregular menstruation and urinary tract infection and irritation.

Neiguan (PC6) may be the most influential distal point for any condition affecting the chest. So powerful in action, it may be selected during heart surgery for its analgesic effects. Almost any condition related to the heart or lung may also be treated with Neiguan (PC6). Although PC has a wide range of applications, angina pectoris, may be better resolved with Ximen (PC4, the xi-cleft point). Asthma and cough are commonly relieved via acupuncture at Neiguan (PC6).

Clinical Studies on Anti-Emetic Effects of Acupuncture at Neiguan (PC6)

Although many undergoing chemotherapies receive anti-emetic pharmaceuticals to lessen the severity of chemotherapy-related nausea and vomiting, some patients still feel nauseous or tend to vomit frequently. Corticosteroids, antidopaminergic agents and 5-HT3 antagonists are commonly prescribed for their ability to influence key factors involved in the nausea and vomiting reflex. It may be presumed that acupuncture mediates this reflex by other means as it may quell nausea and vomiting in cases where pharmaceuticals have been unsuccessful. To assess the effect of acupressure in patients that have not responded well to anti-emetic drug therapy, 40 patients with various kinds of advanced cancers participated; colorectal, lung and breast cancer being most prevalent. Patients received chemotherapy with those agents that tend to elicit the nausea and vomiting response, such as cisplatin and anthracyclines. Each also received acupressure at PC6 for a minimum of six hours per day throughout treatment.

Researchers [1] found that 70% of patients experienced less nausea and vomiting regardless of chemotherapeutic agent or cancer type. These findings are hopeful, as the relief from the body's emetic response to chemotherapeutic agents is of great benefit to the patient in terms of limiting the amount of suffering during a course of treatment, and may improve the ability of chemotherapeutic agents to more effectively producc results. According to these findings, it may be worth further examining the ability of acupressure at Neiguan (PC6) to reduce the chemotherapy-induced nausea and vomiting when pharmaceutical anti-emetics have not helped. These results seem to indicate that patients with nausea and vomiting related to other medical conditions may also benefit by the anti-emetic action of acupressure at Neiguan (PC6), such as morning-sickness during pregnancy.

Studies [2] have revealed that acupuncture relieves nausea and vomiting induced by medically-related conditions such as sickness following an operation and morning-sickness, in addition to chemotherapy-induced nausea and vomiting. Randomized trials have also attested to the benefits of acupoint stimulation in cases of motion sickness. Specifically, 26 trials have confirmed a reduction in nausea and vomiting in patients recovering from surgery. While 11 trials revealed different effects depending on the particular type of acupuncture application, acupressure was found to improve nausea on the first-day of chemotherapy, electroacupuncture lessened vomiting on the first-day, and noninvasive electrostimulation was equal in effect to placebo in influencing outcomes. No clear effects were noted in morning-sickness. Functional magnetic resonance imaging (fMRI) revealed that Pc6-stimulation influenced activations affecting the gastric myoelectrical system, vagal modulation and vestibular influences within the cerebellum. These highlights provide a glimpse of the anti-emetic influence of Neiguan (PC6) that have been revealed in over 40 randomized controlled trials. Studies continue to illuminate the mechanisms behind the anti-emetic effects of acupuncture as well.

Nausea and vomiting can be of exceptional concern in children receiving chemotherapy. To assess the potential for acupuncture to reduce the need for antiemetic rescue medication, researchers [3] conducted a crossover study, including 23 children (10-17 years in age) from 5 tertiary hospitals in Germany. Each patient was undergoing a chemotherapeutic regimen for solid and malignant tumors known to elicit a strong emetic response. Acupuncture was administered after the second or third chemotherapy course along with standard anti-emetic pharmaceutical intervention. After assessing a total of forty-six courses of chemotherapy, researchers found a significantly reduced need for rescue anti-emetic medication when acupuncture was applied. Significantly less chemotherapeutically-induced vomiting occurred when acupuncture was included. Researchers also noted that acupuncture reached a high rate of acceptance among patients. Researchers concluded that acupuncture significantly reduced the emetic response to chemotherapy in children receiving chemotherapeutic agents associated with a high rate of emesis.

Acupuncture at Neiguan (PC6) is known to be effective in reducing the occurrence or severity of those recovering from surgery or experiencing morning-sickness. While many have reported benefits from receiving acupuncture during a course of chemotherapy; many cancer patients suffer tremendously at the end of an unsuccessful course of treatment and are prescribed therapeutics to make the last stages of life more comfortable. As some survive for many months or even years in continuous, unrelenting, severe pain, debility, weakness and mental disturbance; effective means of alleviating distress during this time may be of immense benefit. To determine the effects of acupuncture at Neiguan (PC6), researchers [4] administered acupuncture between courses of chemotherapy in those who were experiencing nausea and those who were not nauseous; although, had become nauseous with previous courses of chemotherapy. Sixteen patients received a four-week course of 10 acupuncture treatments at Neiguan (PC6). Of the 15 patients who completed the study, researchers found that severity of nausea was significantly lower after the course of acupuncture than at the start. Additionally, of those who started acupuncture while not nauseous, remained free of nausea throughout the course of acupuncture treatment. Researchers did not find any connection between nausea, pain or constipation. These findings showed that acupuncture at Neiguan (PC6) may reduce the intensity of nausea during late-stage chemotherapy treatment.

The potential therapeutic benefit of administering injections at specific acupuncture points has not been well-researched. To supplement scientific knowledge in this area, effects of injecting B6, an important co-factor in many biochemical processes, was assessed for its ability to reduce nausea and vomiting in women undergoing chemotherapy for ovarian cancer. Patients (n=142) received either acupuncture and vitamin B6 at Neiguan (PC6), acupuncture alone or vitamin B6 injection at Neiguan (PC6) in conjunction with a highly toxic course of chemotherapy and anti-emetic pharmaceutical intervention. Researchers [5] found that the greatest significant improvements occurred when acupuncture was provided and vitamin B6 was injected at Neiguan (PC6), both in terms of number of emetic episodes and days free from nausea and vomiting. Therefore, tolerance to highly emetogenic chemotherapy may be positively impacted by receiving both acupuncture and B6 injections at Neiguan (PC6).

Wristbands (sea-bands) can be worn to extend the effect of pressing on acupuncture at Neiguan (PC6). A convenient method of easing pain or nausea in those with continuous symptoms, wristbands are often given to those undergoing chemotherapy. To understand the impact of this treatment method, researchers gathered data on the anti-emetic effects of therapeutic wristbands on women undergoing chemotherapy for gynecological concerns. Findings [6] showed a significant reduction in nausea as well as a reduction in need for anti-emetic pharmaceuticals. Additionally, retching and vomiting were reduced to a less than significant degree. Researchers suggested more studies be conducted to further assess the applicability of wristbands as an anti-emetic device in patients undergoing chemotherapy.

Wristbands administering continuous acupressure at Neiguan (PC6) were further assessed for their ability to limit nausea and vomiting in 32 patients undergoing chemotherapy for early stage (stages 1-3) breast cancer. When researchers [7] compiled data according to the Patient Information Form, Beck's Anxiety Inventory, and the Index of Nausea, Vomiting and Retching; they found, compared with controls, patients who received continuous acupuncture at Neiguan (PC6) via wristband, experienced significantly reduced nausea, vomiting and retching. Patients receiving the acupressure intervention also exhibited improved overall scores reflecting experience, occurrence, and level of distress. Statistically significant reductions in anxiety scores were observed as well in those who wore wristbands throughout the course of chemotherapy treatment compared with those who did not. Researchers concluded that this study showed that wristbands applying acupressure to Neiguan (PC6) while undergoing chemotherapy for breast cancer reduced anxiety, nausea, vomiting and retching. More research is needed to fully determine the role of wristbands in chemotherapy treatment.

A randomized controlled trial [8] was conducted on the impact of wristbands, applying acupressure at Neiguan (PC6), on patients undergoing chemotherapy for acute myeloblastic leukemia. Compared with 30 patients who received finger acupressure for four days and controls, those who wore wristbands for four days experienced less frequent and less intense nausea and vomiting. Thus, wristband acupressure at Neiguan (PC6) was shown to be effective at limiting chemotherapeutically-induced nausea and vomiting in those with acute myeloblastic leukemia.

Clinical Evidence: Individual Clinical Trials

With the expanse of interest in acupuncture as a form of complementary medicine and adjunctive intervention in many conditions, including various forms of cancer; research on the topic continues to grow, especially in the area of pain, nausea/vomiting and anxiety. Although the best methods for researching the topic have yet to be developed; the consensus is that acupuncture is a safe and effective form of adjunctive care with which to help limit the negative impact of various forms of cancer treatments. The collective literature suggests that pain, nausea, vomiting and xerostomia all may be improved with acupuncture. In acknowledgment of these findings, The International Society of Integrative Oncology has set forth guidelines by which acupuncture recommendations may be given in the oncology setting.

To gather more clinical evidence regarding the potential benefit of adjunctive acupuncture care, researchers examined the effects of electroacupuncture at Zusanli (ST36) on chemotherapy-induced nausea and vomiting. A multicentered, randomized controlled trial was conducted among 127 patients undergoing chemotherapy for malignant tumor in patients also receiving an intravenously administered anti-emetic, granisetron. Researchers noted, in terms of preventing and quelling chemotherapy-induced nausea and vomiting, a significantly greater efficacy was seen with acupuncture and anti-emetic IV, compared with anti-emetic IV alone. Findings [9] revealed a 90.5% rate of effectiveness was achieved when electroacupuncture at Zusanli (ST36) was administered with granisetron IV; compared with an 84% rate of effectiveness in those receiving anti-emetic IV without electroacupuncture.

The human mind may influence the outcome of medical treatments to varying degrees depending on the individual. Just as a stubborn mind is often associated with lack of ability to overcome an illness no matter what kind of treatment one undergoes, positive expectation is often associated with improvement or resolution of a condition whether a proven curative intervention is applied or not. Although the placebo effect is not easily measured in acupuncture studies, researchers attempted to assess the potential placebo effects involved in anti-emetic acupuncture via sham non-penetrating acupuncture placebo. Researchers [10] administered true acupuncture or sham acupuncture two-three times per week at Neiguan (PC6) to patients undergoing anti-cancer abdominal/pelvic radiotherapy. Researchers found that those who received true or sham acupuncture experienced less nausea than those who received only standard treatment,

37% versus 63%, respectively. A lessening of intensity of nausea was also observed in those who received acupuncture or sham compared with those who did not. Notably, 95% of those receiving acupuncture or sham acupuncture expected an anti-emetic effect; while patients who anticipated nausea experienced nausea more often than those who had a low expectation of nausea. To summarize, less nausea and vomiting was seen in those who received either true or sham acupuncture throughout a course of anti-cancer radiation therapy than those who did not. Expectation and effect of care was also considered to play an influential role in observed outcomes.

Researchers attempted to improve methodology of acupuncture studies through a pilot study. Feasibility, compliance, method of data collection, blinding and expectation were attended to during a modified single subject experiment. Researchers administered two or three weekly acupuncture or non-insertion sham acupuncture treatments to 10 cancer patients for a duration of 30 minutes per session. Patients received radiotherapy over abdomen/pelvis simultaneously.

Patients noticed a variety of effects. All patients noticed anti-emetic effects, most experienced a sense of relaxation, half reported an analgesic effect and half found they slept better. Only one of five patients who received true acupuncture became nauseous; while all except for one of those who received sham acupuncture experienced nausea. Nausea was found to coincide with a lowered sense of well-being and diminished ability to adequately complete daily activities. All patients were blinded, complied with treatments and willingly provided data. Researchers [11] concluded that the design of this study could be applied to randomized controlled studies to determine the impact of acupuncture on radiotherapy-induced emesis in the treatment of cancer.

To further examine the effect of acupuncture on radiotherapy-induced nausea and vomiting, 215 blinded cancer patients were administered either true acupuncture with deqi or non-penetrating sham acupuncture, two or three times per week. Among patients who all were experiencing daily nausea, 70% of those who received true and 62% of those who received sham acupuncture experienced nausea at least once during the course of radiotherapy treatment. Vomiting occurred in 25% of those who received acupuncture and 28% of those who received sham treatment. While 42% of those who received acupuncture needed anti-emetic pharmaceuticals, 37% of those who received sham needed medication. An overwhelming agreement of 95% in those who received true acupuncture and 96% in those who received sham expressed the belief that acupuncture had reduced nausea and vomiting. Most of those who received either treatment also noticed improvements in perceived level of stress, mood, sleep or pain and 89% reported they would like to receive more treatment. Researchers [12] concluded equal benefits from acupuncture with deqi and sham in reducing radiotherapy-induced nausea.

Among 40% of children receiving cancer treatment with or without anti-emetics, nausea and vomiting are more distressing than any other side-effects of chemotherapy. To address this common complaint, a pilot study was conducted on the effects of auricular acupressure in Taiwanese children. A crossover randomized study design was adopted in which baseline assessments were made during the seven days following the first round of chemotherapy. Each group then received either auricular acupressure at a real or sham point during the second course of chemotherapy; during the third round, those who had received real acupressure received sham and vice versa. Findings showed that real auricular acupressure significantly reduced the frequency and intensity of emesis compared to sham acupressure. Significant differences in emetic response were not noted between groups. Although all patients received anti-emetic pharmaceuticals on each day chemotherapy was administered, 80% reported no alleviation of symptoms from the medication.

As auricular points can produce an intense and lasting alleviation of symptoms and may even break a patterned response via more direct action on mechanisms affecting brain networks, the difference between real and sham point effects may be difficult to determine and isolate as both groups received acupressure at the active point. Researchers [13] posed that in future studies, a larger sample size be assessed, and psychosocial benefits related to attention and presence of the practitioner be considered.

Integrative medical centers are becoming more popular as demand for complementary medical treatment rises. The State of Sao Paulo Cancer Institute emulates the model and vision of many oncology care centers in the United States in their efforts to include acupuncture for the purpose of reducing life-depleting aspects of cancer or negative side-effects of cancer treatment such as post-surgical pain, cancer-related pain, treatment-induced pain, nausea, vomiting, xerostomia and fatigue. To gather data on potential benefits of acupuncture in integrative oncology, 183 patients either in remission or receiving radiotherapy, chemotherapy or hormone therapy, were assessed for baseline readings of current symptoms. After acupuncture, researchers [14] noted a 64% reduction in symptoms. As quality of life can be a major factor during cancer care and treatment, such an improvement in symptomology overall indicates that acupuncture in an integrative oncology center may be highly beneficial for patients experiencing a range of discomforts.

Many routes may be taken to prevent or alleviate nausea and vomiting in cancer patients. As specific biochemicals have been implicated in the intrinsic reaction leading to emesis, mediating the release of these biochemicals may lead to a greater ability to control emetic symptoms. Researchers attempted to determine the influence of electroacupuncture at Neiguan (PC6) and Jianshi (PC5) combined with pharmaceutical anti-emetic, granisetron on chemotherapy-induced nausea and vomiting and these crucial biochemicals. Serum levels of 5-hydroxy-tryptamine (5-HT) and dopamine (DA) were selected as measures for comparison. Seventy-two patients received granisetron injection with electroacupuncture at PC6 and PC5 or granisetron and sham electroacupuncture. Findings showed that during the acute stage, within 24-hours after administration of chemotherapy, frequency of vomiting did not significantly vary between groups. After 24-hours, nausea severity was significantly greater in those who had received sham electroacupuncture. Efficacy was similar between both groups during the acute stage; however, vomiting was reduced to a greater degree in those who received true electroacupuncture compared to controls. Electroacupuncture also reduced serum levels of 5-HT and DA; while no significant difference was seen in these levels among controls. Researchers [15] concluded that the combination of anti-emetic pharmaceutical, granisetron, along with electroacupuncture at Neiguan (PC6) and Jianshi (PC5) alleviated the delayed effect of chemotherapy-related nausea. A concordant reduction of serum 5-HIT and DA may be key factors in the underlying mechanism of action.

Acupuncture has become an acceptable form of complementary care when anti-emetics are ineffective during chemotherapy treatment. As acupuncture influences diverse aspects of health, its use in complementary cancer care may reduce a number of unpleasant side-effects of chemotherapy. The effect of adjunctive acupuncture care on nausea, vomiting, pain, insomnia and anxiety was assessed in 45 inpatients at Numune Hospital. Patients received acupuncture for three consecutive days, the initial session on the day before start of chemotherapy, the second session on the first day of chemotherapy treatment, and the third on the day following chemotherapy. Most of the 45 patients, 71%, had advanced cancers and were receiving palliative chemotherapy. Acupuncture was found to diminish all symptoms assessed to a statistically significant degree [16]. Thus, chemotherapeutically-induced nausea, vomiting, pain, sleep and anxiety improved with acupuncture given in conjunction with each chemotherapy treatment.

The prevalence of chemotherapy-induced nausea and vomiting profoundly affects cancer patients, loved-ones and care-givers. As cancer and medical interventions tend to dominate life for months to years, the consequences of unresolved chemotherapy-related side-effects may take a devastating toll on quality of life, mental state, endurance and will to live. As Yongquan (KI1), an acupuncture point on the sole of the foot, associated with having a strongly grounding or descending effect on the qi, is thought to be effective in reducing nausea and vomiting. To compare the effect of electrostimulation at Yongquan (KI1) with a sham point on the sole, a trial with 103 patients receiving transcatheter arterial infusion (TAI) of cisplatin or oxaliplatin was conducted. An anti-emetic, tropisetron, was also administered in each case. Electrostimulation was provided at Yongquan (KI1) or a sham point for 20 minutes, one to two hours prior to infusion on each day for six days. According to quality-of-life assessment measures documented daily during the course, those who received Yongquan (KI1) electrostimulation expressed some higher quality of life scores on day four than those in the sham group. Researchers [17] concluded that electrostimulation at Yongquan (KI1) had no effect on prevention of chemotherapy-induced nausea or vomiting.

The anti-emetic effects of acupuncture at Neiguan (PC6) were compared to the impact of anti-emetic pharmaceutical, ondansetron. Delayed chemotherapy-induced nausea and vomiting (CINV) in 70 patients was assessed in a randomized cross-over study. All patients underwent treatment consisting of two daily five mg doses of oral dexamethasone for three consecutive days. Additional ondansetron was provided every 12 hours as needed.

Researchers [18] discovered that acupuncture produced a significantly higher cure rate in the total prevention of delayed chemotherapy-induced nausea and vomiting. Additionally, acupuncture significantly diminished delayed nausea and severity of nausea. Acupuncture at Neiguan (PC6) also reduced the need for additional anti-emetic medication. A significant reduction in side-effects was also observed in those who received acupuncture, including constipation and insomnia. Quality of life ratings were also significantly higher in those who received acupuncture. Overall, acupuncture at Neiguan (PC6) was found to be effective in improving side-effects of chemotherapy including the prevention of delayed nausea, constipation and sleep quality, while raising the quality of life for cancer patients.

Chemotherapeutic agents targeting rapidly dividing cells are a source of continuous irritation to the lining of the gastrointestinal tract, causing nausea and vomiting which may last long after the chemotherapeutic agent has been administered. Wristbands that provide continuous pressure to an acupuncture point help alleviate symptoms of an unrelenting nature, such as those associated with the treatment of cancer. Acupuncture protocols that combine wrist and ankle points are also known to be extraordinarily effective in preventing or alleviating nausea and vomiting. Moxibustion with ginger is often used when cold accumulates in the digestive organs or stagnates in the intestines, or when chronic deficiency leads to impaired ability to warm the body. To address the need for adjunct agents that protect or restore the GI tract, researchers gathered data on the efficacy of wrist and ankle acupuncture with ginger moxibustion on chemotherapy-induced nausea, vomiting, and constipation.

During a course of chemotherapy for gynecological tumors, 60 women received either wrist and ankle acupuncture combined with ginger moxibustion or served as controls, receiving tropisetron hydrochloride and dexamethasone intravenously. Findings showed that fewer nausea episodes occurred in those who received acupuncture and moxibustion than those who received standard anti-emetic pharmaceuticals; the difference between the experimental group and controls reached significance on the 2nd day of chemotherapy which continued through the 5th day of chemotherapy. Acupuncture and moxibustion displayed a significantly greater anti-emetic effect than standard treatment on the 3rd day of chemotherapy. Those receiving acupuncture and moxibustion also experienced significantly less constipation than controls. An additional benefit, the cost of anti-emetic acupuncture and moxibustion was significantly lower than the anti-emetic pharmaceuticals. Researchers [19] surmised that the combination of wrist and ankle acupuncture with ginger may be safe, effective and economical in preventing or treating the adverse impact of chemotherapy on the gastrointestinal tract.

High-quality randomized controlled studies offer a means of validating the millennia-old practice of acupuncture, results obtained in the clinic and outcomes seen in preliminary trials. The feasibility of such a study was assessed with the purpose of comparing the effects of electroacupuncture on delayed chemotherapy-induced nausea and vomiting with sham electroacupuncture or standard anti-emetic drug therapy. Patients undergoing chemotherapeutic treatment with a moderately-high potential of inducing nausea and vomiting received either electroacupuncture or sham electroacupuncture with anti-emetics. Standard electroacupuncture or sham electroacupuncture was administered during chemotherapy on the first and third day. Functional Living Index Emesis (FLIE) was used to assess outcomes of 60 patients. Of those who completed the study, nausea and vomiting scores were low regardless of anti-emetic approach. Researchers determined a randomized controlled study would be feasible in a busy oncology department. The results [20] were unclear in this study as few patients experienced nausea during the initial round of chemotherapy and differences between electroacupuncture and standard emetics were not observed. Researchers also noted that a numerical rating scale may be a better measure of nausea than FLIE.

Researchers assessed the efficacy of auricular acupressure as an adjunct treatment for chemotherapy-induced nausea and vomiting among breast cancer patients. During the initial course of chemotherapy, 48 patients received either standard anti-emetics and auricular acupressure for five consecutive days; or served as controls, receiving pharmaceutical anti-emetic therapy. Researchers discovered that auricular acupressure significantly reduced frequency and intensity of initial and delayed nausea and vomiting compared to those receiving drug therapy without acupressure. The results [21] suggest that this method may be applicable as safe, effective and inexpensive means of reducing the negative side-effects of chemotherapy.

Clinical Evidence: Systematic Reviews and Meta-analysis

Since 1998, the National Institutes of Health (NIH) has supported the use of acupuncture in adult post-surgical and chemotherapy-induced nausea and vomiting. This has led to its inclusion in many health insurance coverage policies. Acupuncture at Neiguan (PC6), the most common point explored for this use among trials has shown to be effective in many kinds of cancers with diverse chemotherapy protocols. Many of these assessments of Neiguan (PC6) have been described in Cochrane systematic reviews, especially those concerning post-surgical nausea and vomiting, chemotherapy-induced nausea and vomiting, and morning-sickness. Consistent positive data on the efficacy of PC6 over sham in children and adults has been collected from 26 trials including an excess of 3000 post-operative sickness cases. Compared with many different pharmacologic anti-emetics, Neiguan (PC6) has more effectively reduced nausea and shown equal efficacy as an anti-emetic. Effects of Neiguan (PC6) were equal whether insertion or non-invasive methods were applied.

Compiled evidence on chemotherapy-induced nausea and vomiting encompassed 11 trials, including 1200 patients. Interestingly, different methods and modalities were more or less effective at different stages during chemotherapy. Electroacupuncture was found to be effective in treating vomiting associated with the initial chemotherapy treatment, whereas manual acupuncture was not. Acupressure lessened queasiness, but had no effect on vomiting during the initial chemotherapy session. Wristbands emitting electrical frequencies were not found to be effective at reducing any chemotherapy-related symptoms.

Collective morning-sickness research of six trials with nearly 1150 patients produced inconsistent results. In studies of nausea and vomiting related to a range of conditions, Neiguan (PC6) was found to positively influence some kinds of nausea and vomiting. Researchers [22] suggested that future studies might best be focused on chemotherapy patients with refractory nausea and vomiting. Combining Neiguan (PC6) with other potentially effective points; or, selecting protocols according to differential diagnosis was also suggested in order to build on current knowledge and improve outcomes.

Collective information on the use of acupuncture modalities in mitigating negative side-effects of breast cancer treatment was gathered from eight English and Chinese databanks. The effects of acupuncture techniques on cancer treatment-related vasomotor syndrome, chemotherapy-induced nausea and vomiting, lymphedema, post-surgical pain, joint pain due to aromatase inhibitors and leukopenia were compiled and presented to provide a meaningful understanding of the overall impact of acupuncture modalities. Among the 26 trials, 88% showed some benefit related to at least one side-effect. Overall quality of studies was not exceptional; with only 35% reflecting a high degree of quality, improvement in this area may provide more telling results in future studies. Neiguan (PC6) was found to improve chemotherapy-induced nausea and vomiting in three high quality studies. As results on other side-effects were obtained via low quality trials, the evidence remains equivocal. Acupuncture modalities did appear safe as only a few minor adverse effects were reported. Researchers concluded that acupressure at Neiguan (PC6) showed promise in treating chemotherapy-induced nausea and vomiting; with greater benefit during the initial administration of chemotherapeutic agents. An important finding was that patients often become conditioned to the initial response to chemotherapy; if nausea and vomiting become associated with chemotherapy in the beginning, the emetic response may be triggered throughout the course of treatment and even after by associated stimuli. Researchers [23] suggested improving methodology and design to gather more accurate and applicable data on the role of adjunctive acupuncture care in treating side-effects of cancer treatment.

Many seek the clinical benefits of complimentary acupuncture care while undergoing cancer treatment based on perceivable external effects on pain, nausea and vomiting. A desire for scientific validation of these external observations has inspired the exploration into various mechanisms by which acupuncture exerts such effects. Through imaging technologies, convincing studies describing a neurological basis for acupuncture effects are accumulating. Although, especially in the advent of acupuncture research, low quality studies have aroused critical skepticism of acupuncture as a whole; improved study design and attempts to meet scientific standards have reversed the negative impact to some degree.

Subjective factors, mentioned in some early studies, make assessment of benefits difficult, such as the practitioner-patient relationship or the effects of a particular practitioner's level of empathy. In response, randomized control trials (RCTs) have been conducted; although outcomes are not clear. Collective RCTs on acupuncture and cancer suggest acupuncture poses some benefit in terms of pain, nausea and vomiting, xerostomia, hot flashes, fatigue, anxiety, depression and insomnia. Although acupuncture is considered safe and effective, further high-quality studies are needed to assess the full benefit and most efficacious applications for use among those under-going cancer treatment. Researchers [24] further suggested clinicians weigh potential benefits and, considering the low risk, include appropriate acupuncture modalities to mitigate negative symptoms associated with cancer care.

With the growing popularity of acupuncture and its inclusion in integrative cancer centers, more information of the true effects of acupuncture modalities is now available. A systematic review was conducted to assess the influence of acupuncture on cancer treatment-related symptom reduction. Researchers pulled 41 Randomized Controlled Trials (RCTs) from reputable scientific databases through the year 2011, including those on pain, nausea, hot flashes, fatigue, xerostomia, prolonged post-surgical ileus, anxiety and other mood disorders, and insomnia. Most of the studies reported positive findings leading researchers to consider the validity of acupuncture for treating chemotherapy-induced nausea/vomiting, although more research in this area is called for. Researchers found conflicting information regarding efficacy of acupuncture in treating other negative side-effects of cancer treatment. Standardizing groups and treatment were suggested to improve future studies. Blindness and larger sample sizes may be key factors in increasing objectivity and generalizability of results. Studies [25] revealing the mechanisms underlying the acupuncture response are crucial to determine potential clinical effects in specific medical applications. As styles, technique and skill of practitioner varies greatly between acupuncturists, involving a greater number of acupuncturists in research may also produce results more representative of clinical reality.

In search of valid results regarding the role of acupuncture in complementary and palliative cancer care, researchers conducted a systemic review. In seventeen reviews, acupuncture was affirmed as a valid modality with which to mitigate cancer treatment-induced nausea and vomiting. Pain, fatigue, hot flashes, radiation-induced xerostomia, dyspnea and anxiety were also positively impacted by acupuncture. Although inadequate rigor and lack of heterogeneity limited the ability of researchers to fully assess results; conditional recommendation was made for cases in which limited patient options are available, or potential benefit deems appropriate. Researchers acknowledged the need for sufficient study that suits the level of complexity innate to acupuncture. They [26] suggested developing research approaches that apply a sufficient level of treatment, select relevant outcome measures regarding the patient and modality and comply with standard reporting methods in order to gain confidence in validating the extent of efficacy of acupuncture in complementary and palliative cancer care.

Patient interest in complementary medicine continues to drive research efforts in that direction. While mechanisms may involve the brain and nervous system, the endocrine system, cytokine regulation or immune system, the role of acupuncture has shown profound promise within the field of oncology; specifically, in the alleviation of negative side-effects of both chemotherapy and radiotherapy. To consolidate the existing knowledge basis on acupuncture mechanisms and applications as they relate to cancer patients, systemic reviews and RTCs were analyzed. Of 25 articles on hot flashes in breast cancer, xerostomia induced by radiotherapy in head and neck cancer, post-chemotherapy nausea and vomiting, pain, fatigue and insomnia, researchers reported mixed results. Overall; however, researchers found acupuncture modalities to reduce negative symptoms associated with cancer treatment. Researchers [27] suggested creating effective strategies that maximize benefits of acupuncture in specific applications.

Pharmacopuncture, the injection of medication or herbal remedies at specific acupoints for a specific intention is currently being utilized to quell side-effects of cancer treatment in Korea and China. To gather the collective data on this relatively isolated intervention, twenty-two studies including 2,459 patients were reviewed. The total findings [28] revealed that, compared with controls, pharmacopuncture significantly diminished the frequency and intensity of chemotherapy-induced nausea and vomiting. According to 17 trials which gathered information regarding various symptoms, and as revealed in most studies; pain, ileus, hiccup, fever, and gastrointestinal symptoms all tended to improve with pharmacopuncture. Overall, quality of life was positively influenced. Pharmacopuncture, thus, may provide relief concerning multiple treatment-related symptoms in cancer patients; however, clinical heterogeneity and ROB need to be improved in future studies to confirm these preliminary findings.

Acupuncture, moxibustion and transcutaneous electrical nerve stimulation are thought to offer some benefit in complementary cancer care. To provide a summary of the scientific findings on acupuncture in palliative cancer care, a systematic review was conducted of clinical cancer trials. After determining satisfactory methodological quality of 23 systematic reviews, researchers found substantial support for use of acupuncture in treating cancer-related fatigue, chemotherapy-induced nausea and vomiting and cancer-related leucopenia. They found inconsistent support for cancer-related pain, hot flashes and hiccups. The benefits concerning quality of life and xerostomia, dyspnea, lymphedema and mental health were also unclear. As acupuncture was regarded as safe, and may provide some benefit in palliative cancer care, researchers [29] recommended its use especially when options are limited.

CHAPTER FIVE

ACUPUNCTURE FOR PARKINSON'S DISEASE

Introduction

The ability of acupuncture to mitigate some of the most debilitating aspects of Parkinson's disease has attracted much attention from both clinicians and researchers. In order to provide greater understanding of the rational basis for the application of acupuncture in these cases, the following paper provides some explanation of how traditional Chinese medicine theory addresses different types of Parkinson's disease manifestations. Current scientific research is also shared to give credence to subjective improvements seen in patients who have received acupuncture for Parkinson's disease, tremors and related symptoms. This chapter begins with a patient history and proceeds to a summary of Western and Eastern medicine theory and treatment. A few classical cases from leading acupuncturists are selected to demonstrate the diversity of treatment protocols; scientific research is also included that provides evidences and proposes potential mechanisms of action by which acupuncture influences Parkinson's disease.

A Patient History

A 71-year-old male patient suffering from Parkinson's disease for seven years sought out acupuncture to manage related symptoms and debility. He presented with difficulty getting up in the mornings, constant, continuous trembling hands, weak grip, ambulatory slowness, bradykinesia, and low energy. He graded the intensity of overall symptoms at 9/10, frequency at 8/10 and duration at 8/10 on an increasing scale from asymptomatic to the most extreme. The levodopa and physical therapy his neurologist had prescribed did not seem to be helping.

Upon initial exam, the patient's (tongue was red and his pulse wiry), he was initially diagnosed with qi and blood deficiency with wind according to traditional Chinese Medicine theory. He received one session of three sequential 15-minute units of daily electro-acupuncture to tonify qi and blood, sedate liver wind, descend liver yang at points: Baihui (DU20),

Fengchi (GB20), Taichong (LR3), Neiguan (PC6), Waiguan (TB5), Tianshu (ST25), Sanyinjiao (SP6), Zusanli (ST36) and Hegu (LI4). Scalp motor point was used. Infrared heat lamp was provided as well. Chinese herbal formula to tonify yin and quell wind was prescribed: Tian Ma Gou Teng Yin (*Gastrodia-Uncaria Decoction*). Having achieved significant improvements after a course of twenty-one treatments, the patient was happy, noting remarkable progress. He also noted that he received greater benefit from electro-acupuncture than any other modality he had thus tried and regretted not having tried acupuncture before. The overall intensity of symptoms had decreased from 9/10 to 5/10; frequency had abated from 8/10 to 5/10; and duration had lessened from 8/10 to 4/10. Mental clarity and concentration had improved. Trembling was reduced by 40% and he was able to lift light objects. He even regained the ability to drive himself for a few minutes at a time. Range of motion increased 30%. Remainder of symptoms at treatment conclusion included (in addition to those listed above): low energy level and insomnia, with symptoms getting worse with physical activity, noise, stress, and fatigue. Continued weekly acupuncture was recommended to maintain and increase improvements, while addressing the remainder of symptoms.

The Clinical Problem

Parkinson's disease (PD) is a motor system disorder, resulting from the loss of dopamine-producing brain cells. Four symptoms primarily tend to predominate among those afflicted: tremor or trembling hands, arms, legs, jaw, and face; a rigid or stiff body; bradykinesia and lack of postural stability, balance and coordination. With greater prevalence in those over fifty years of age, progression of disease may create pronounced difficulty in walking, talking, or completing other simple tasks. Although onset may be subtle, producing a gradual manifestation of symptoms, rate of progression varies. Shaking or tremors create the greatest interference to daily activities for the majority of Parkinson's patients. Other symptoms commonly experienced consist of: depression and other emotional changes; difficulty in swallowing, chewing, and speaking; urinary symptoms or constipation; skin issues and disrupted sleep. In cases of intermittent Parkinson's, diagnostic measures are limited. Blood and laboratory tests are insufficient, although brain scans or laboratory tests may rule out other diseases. Accuracy and certainty of diagnosis remains difficult, relying on medical history and neurological examination.

No cure exists for Parkinson's disease; however, medication may produce an extraordinary reduction in symptoms. Levodopa combined with carbidopa is a commonly prescribed remedy. Carbidopa acts by creating a delay in the conversion of levodopa into dopamine until reaching the brain. Nerve cells then convert levodopa into dopamine and replenish depleted stores in the brain. Seventy-five percent of those with Parkinson's receive some benefit from medication, with some symptoms improving more than others. Bradykinesia and rigidity are among the most responsive symptoms, while tremor (the disease's main component) may be only marginally affected; and medication may not improve balance and other symptoms at all. Anti-cholinergics may serve to diminish tremor and rigidity. Bromocriptine, pramipexole, and ropinirole mimic the role of dopamine in the brain, causing a similar response. The anti-viral, amantadine, also seems to alleviate symptoms. In May of 2006, the FDA approved rasagiline to be administered in conjunction with levodopa for advanced Parkinson's, and to be given alone during the early phase of the disease.

Periodically, surgery may be advised when medications are unsuccessful. In deep-brain-stimulation (DBS) therapy, electrodes are implanted into the brain and connected to a small, programmable, electrical pulse generator. DBS can reduce the need for medications that produce negative side-effects, such as involuntary movement or dyskinesias, and may alleviate other mood-related symptoms, reduce tremors and improve movement and gait issues.

The National Institute of Neurological Disorders and Stroke (NINDS) engages in Parkinson's disease research at the National Institutes of Health (NIH) and also funds research via grants to major US medical institutions in hope of deepening the understanding as to the etiology and mechanisms underlying the disorder. Available current medical treatments for Parkinson's patients provide only symptomatic abatement. Acupuncture, through its 2000-plus years history, has provided effective relief from many of the symptoms seen in Parkinson's patients; subjective clinical experience is supported by recent laboratory findings confirming the biochemical benefits of acupuncture in those diagnosed. Recent research conducted at Cornell University showed that acupuncture is neuroprotective, as it increases the release of brain-derived neurotrophic and glial cell line-derived neurotrophic factor as well as cyclophilin A. They also found that acupuncture slows cellular death and moderates oxidative stress effects on dopaminergic neurons in the substantia nigra. Acupuncture was also seen to affect neuronal activity within the basal ganglia. Researchers assessed that acupuncture provided at the early onset of disease may produce the greatest benefits and suggested that the translation of Parkinson's acupuncture research will help optimize benefit of acupuncture treatment.

Chinese Medicine Approach to Parkinson's Disease

In terms of traditional Chinese medicine, Parkinson's disease is always characterized by internal wind as tremors always signify wind. In terms of affected organ systems, the actual wind is always a pathology of the liver, however the root cause of the wind may arise from pathologies within other organ systems. The main clinical manifestations of interior wind are: tremors, tics, dizziness, vertigo, unsteady gait, loss of balance, ringing in the ears, scattered thought, confusion and numbness. In severe cases, wind may take the form of convulsions, unconsciousness, deafness, opisthotonos, hemiplegia and deviation of the tongue and mouth. In cases of Parkinson's, interior wind is always related to a liver disharmony as convulsions and tremors are explained in Chinese medicine as "shaking of the sinews." The quality of the sinews, tendons, ligaments and fluidity of movement are controlled by the liver system in traditional Chinese medicine theory.

Liver wind arises from any one of four conditions: heat, liver yang rising, liver blood deficiency, liver yin deficiency or liver fire. The first of these conditions, heat, can give rise to liver wind. The more extreme the heat, the greater the potential for producing extreme cases of liver wind. Much like a dust storm in the desert, where a combination of intense heat and lack of moisture generate strong winds that obscure vision and toss objects about, intense heat affecting the body can dry up fluids, and deplete the yin and blood. Wind then arises in the empty channels which have been left vacant by lack of blood, yin or fluids; if severe, wind courses through the meridians, creating a wind-storm that may cause erratic or uncontrollable movement, potentially knocking the patient out. The range of clinical manifestations that heat-generated internal wind create include: high fever, lack of sweat, hot/dry skin, nausea, dry-heaves, delirium, weakness (from depletion of blood), dehydration, incoherent speech, red chest and face, red/dry/cracked lips and mouth, severe thirst or thirst with inability to drink, dry sore throat, red/dry eyes, dry/red skin sores, hot/burning scanty urine, constipation, opisthotonos, high-pitched ringing or whistling in the ears, mania, convulsion, dizziness, vertigo, seizure, fainting, heat-stroke and coma.

Liver yang rising can also produce liver wind. When the yin is not sufficient in relation to the yang, or the yang is excessive in relation to the yin, the Yang energy of the body can rise upward with internal wind, affecting the heart and head. The outward expressions of liver yang rising include fullness in the chest, palpitations, anxiety, mania, extreme dizziness, vertigo, earache or high-pitched ringing in the ears, bulging veins, yelling or loud voice, high blood pressure, headache at the vertex or migraine, tremors, tics, deviated mouth or tongue, and irritability, agitation, intense frustration or anger. Extreme cases may provoke a heart attack, seizure, spasms or stroke.

As was mentioned in cases of heat, where heat has burned up fluids and blood, resultant deficiency of liver blood and/or liver yin readily give rise to liver wind. Liver blood and/or liver yin may also manifest from etiologies other than pathogenic heat. Liver wind is created when any deficiency of blood or yin creates an empty space within the blood vessels. The empty space provides a tunnel which internal wind fills. The clinical manifestations are numbness, dizziness, blurred vision, dry eyes, floaters, tics, pale tongue, or peeled sides of tongue, weakness, dehydration, dry skin, dry nose, dry throat, thirst with little desire to drink, scant urine, poor memory, empty sensation in the head, lack of concentration, scattered mind, anxiety, insomnia, anemia, amenorrhea or light periods, menses blood may be scant or thick, shakiness, slight tremors.

Liver fire can give rise to liver wind. As a raging forest fire generates gale-force winds, liver fire can stir up liver wind. Phlegm easily combines with fire, especially when the person consumes alcohol, leading to phlegm fire manifesting with greater signs of confusion. Phlegm fire alone would not cause Parkinson's disease but it creates tremors and other related symptoms when the phlegm fire stirs up liver wind; this is common in the elderly. Phlegm can obstruct the channels, preventing normal fluids and blood from nourishing them, wind then gives rise to tremor.

Thus, liver wind, manifesting as tremor in Parkinson's disease may arise from an empty or a full condition. The most common empty causes of liver wind are liver blood, liver yin or kidney yin deficiency or a combination of these. When deficient liver blood fails to nourish and moisten the sinews; the empty space in the vessels is taken up by wind, which shakes the empty sinews, causing tremors. In more prolonged or severe cases, a deficient kidney yin fails to nourish liver yin and, in time, this may lead to the development of liver wind, with resultant tremor. As mentioned above, the deficiency of liver yin fails to nourish and moisten the sinews: this dryness of the sinews, combined with liver wind, leads to tremors.

The above-mentioned pathological liver wind conditions can be observed in Parkinson's patients. According to traditional Chinese medicine pattern differentiation, tremors in Parkinson's liver wind manifests when there is insufficient fluid, yin or blood to nourish the channels and sinews. Parkinson's disease must then always be related to a liver disharmony. In professional practice it can be observed that the heart is also often involved, especially in empty conditions. Liver blood or liver yin deficiency often manifests with heart blood and heart yin deficiency. An empirical point for tremors, Xiaochanxue (*Stopping Tremor Point*) located 1.5 cun below Shaohai (HT3) on the heart channel validates this clinical observation.

Pattern Differentiation and Treatment

According to Giovanni Maciocia [1], Parkinson's disease may be differentiated into the following five traditional Chinese medicine patterns: liver blood deficiency generating wind; liver yang rising, generating wind; liver fire generating wind; phlegm heat agitating wind; and liver and kidney yin deficiency, giving rise to wind. The following summarizes his pattern descriptions, acupuncture prescriptions and herbal medicine treatment.

Liver-Blood deficiency Generating Wind Specific indicators differentiate this pattern from other wind disharmonies. Parkinson's-related wind signs generated from liver blood deficiency include long-standing (as a blood deficiency persists over time), pronounced tremor of a limb (as there is insufficient blood to stabilize the channels), sallow complexion, staring look, dislike of speaking, occipital stiffness, cramps in the limbs (due to blood not nourishing the tendons and muscles), difficulty in moving, unsteady gait, lack of coordination, dizziness, blurred vision and spontaneous sweating; with symptoms generally worse with movement.

Patients exhibiting liver blood deficiency wind tend to have a pale (especially on the sides), thin, dry, quivering tongue and a fine or choppy pulse. This pattern can be treated by fortifying the blood, invigorating the connecting channels and extinguishing wind. An effective acupuncture protocol may include: Taichong (LR3), Fengchi (GB20), Hegu (LI4), Waiguan (TB5), Houding (DU19), Sanyinjiao (SP6), Zusanli (ST36), Ququan (LR8), Taixi (KI3), Geshu (BL17) and Guanyuan (RN4). Points that extinguish wind are reduced; points that nourish liver blood are tonified. Taichong (LR3) combined with Fengchi (GB20) extinguishes wind, Hegu (LI4) quells wind by harmonizing, Waiguan (TB5) and Houding (DU19) extinguish liver wind; while Sanyinjiao (SP6), Zusanli (ST36), Ququan (LR8) and Taixi (KI3) nourish liver blood, yin and tonify qi, and Guanyuan

(RN4) with Geshu (BL17) nourishes blood. Beneficial herbal prescriptions for patients with Parkinson's disease due to liver blood deficiency wind may be selected from: E Jiao Ji Zi Huang Tang (*Colla Corii Asini-Egg Yolk Decoction)* as it nourishes liver blood and extinguishes wind; or Ba Zhen Tang plus Tian Ma Gou Teng Yin (*Eight Precious Decoction* plus *Gastrodia-Uncaria Decoction)* for nourishing the blood, sedating liver yang and extinguishing wind.

Liver-Yang rising generating Wind Persistent liver yang rising may generate wind. This happens more commonly in the elderly, those with a naturally weak constitution or those recovering from a debilitating illness. The clinical manifestations are distinguished according to the precipitating pattern leading up to liver yang rising: liver yin deficiency, liver and kidney yin deficiency, or liver blood deficiency.

When liver yang rising coincides with liver yin deficiency, the combination of underlying deficiency producing signs of relative excess may bring about symptoms such as: tremor, facial tics, severe dizziness, high-pitched tinnitus, vertex headache (with or without pressure behind the eyes), hypertension, dry throat, dry eyes, blurred vision, numbness or tingling in the limbs and poor concentration. The patient may have a normal-colored tongue, although it may be peeled on the sides or all over, or may have no coat or dirty/dry coat from materials brought up by the liver yang rising. The pulse will most likely be wiry-fine, which may be felt more strongly on the surface (floating).

Consistent with diagnosis, the treatment principle in these cases focus on subduing liver yang, extinguishing liver wind and replenishing liver yin. An effective acupuncture protocol may include Taichong (LR3), Fengchi (GB20), Hegu (LI4), Waiguan (TB5), Houding (DU19), Sanyinjiao (SP6), Ququan (LR8), Taixi (KI3). Taichong (LR3) helps settle liver yang, combined with sedation at Fengchi (GB20), wind (especially from the head and marrow) is extinguished; sedating Hegu (LI4) assists in balancing yin and yang; sedating Waiguan (TB5) and Houding (DU19) subdues liver yang and extinguishes wind; tonifying Sanyinjiao (SP6), Ququan (LR8) and Taixi (KI3) nourish the liver yin and blood. A synergistic formula in this case is San Jia Fu Mai Tang *(Three Carapaces Restoring the Pulse Decoction),* which nourishes the liver blood and liver yin, while descending the liver yang and subduing wind.

A similar but more severe pattern, liver yang rising as a consequence of liver and kidney yin deficiency, may manifest with tremor, facial tics, severe dizziness, high- or low-pitched ringing in the ears, headache, hypertension, dry throat, dry eyes, blurred vision, numbness or tingling of limbs, poor memory, backache or weakness, knee pain or weakness, exhaustion, scanty urination, night sweating, dry nails/hair/skin. Upon examination, the tongue may be normal-colored, thin, peeled on the sides or all over, dry or lacking coat. The pulse may be wiry-fine or floating-fine.

According to traditional Chinese medicine theory, the recommended treatment principle for this condition would be: descend the liver yang and subdue wind while replenishing liver and kidney yin. An effective acupuncture prescription for this condition may be based on: Taichong (LR3), Fengchi (GB20), Hegu (LI4), Waiguan (TB5), Houding (DU19), Sanyinjiao (SP6), Ququan (LR8), Taixi (KI3), Zhaohai (KI6) and Guanyuan (RN4). Sedation is used on Taichong (LR3), Fengchi (GB20), Hegu (LI4), Waiguan (TB5) and Houding (DU19). Reinforcing method is applied to Sanyinjiao (SP6), Ququan (LR8), Taixi (KI3), Zhaohai (KI6) and Guanyuan (RN4); Zhaohai (KI6) and Guanyuan (RN4) are included to replenish kidney yin. A good Chinese herbal prescription that might be selected for this case may be Zhen Gan Xi Feng Tang (*Pacifying the Liver and Extinguishing Wind Decoction),* which replenishes liver and kidney yin, subdues yang and extinguishes wind; or Jian Ling Tang (*Constructing Roof Tiles Decoction)*, which nourishes liver blood and liver yin, settles liver yang and subdues the wind.

When liver yang rising is a consequence of liver blood deficiency, the patient may present with tremor, dizziness, weakness, lack of concentration, insomnia, high-pitched tinnitus, headache, hypertension, dry throat, blurred vision, numbness or tingling of limbs, poor memory and insomnia. The tongue may be pale and thin; pulse may be wiry-fine, choppy and/or weak. The treatment principle consistent with this case advises to subdue liver yang, extinguish wind and nourish the liver blood. A good choice of points for this patient may include Taichong (LR3), Fengchi (GB20), Hegu (LI4), Waiguan (TB5), Houding (DU19), Sanyinjiao (SP6), Ququan (LR8), Taixi (KI3), Geshu (BL17), Guanyuan (RN4). Tonifying Geshu (BL17) and Guanyuan (RN4) nourish blood in this prescription; tonification can also be applied to Sanyinjiao (SP6) and Ququan (LR8) while applying sedation to the other points. A complimentary herbal prescription for this condition would be E Jiao Ji Zi Huang Tang *(Colla Corii Asini-Egg Yolk Decoction),* as its function is to nourish liver blood and quell the wind.

In cases of Liver-Fire generating Wind, the wind takes on qualities similar to wind gusts that occur during a forest fire. A patient with wind derived from liver fire will tend to present with a more outward manifestation of symptoms such as tremor, irritability, propensity to outbursts of anger, shouting, tinnitus and/or deafness (with sudden onset), temporal or vertex headache, dizziness, red face and eyes, thirst, bitter taste, dream-disturbed sleep with tossing and turning, constipation with dry or hot-burning stools, dark-yellow or burning urination, epistaxis, haematemesis, haemoptysis, feeling overheated and sensitivity to heat; in addition to anger, mental disturbances may include mania, delirium or loss of consciousness. Red tongue with redder sides and dry yellow coating are typical of this pattern. The pulse is likely to be wiry, forceful, full and rapid. The treatment principle needed to resolve this condition includes clearing heat from the liver, draining the fire and calming the wind.

An effective acupuncture prescription to start with likely includes reducing method on: Xingjian (LR2), Taichong (LR3), Fengchi (GB20), Quchi (LI11), Tongziliao (GB1), Sanyinjiao (SP6), Dadun (LR1) and Jinsuo (DU8). Fire-point LR2 is the primary point responsible for draining the liver fire, while the harmonizing function of Taichong (LR3) calms the liver wind, Fengchi (GB20) drives out wind, especially from the head and marrow. Quchi (LI11) drains fire and cools heat, Tongziliao (GB1) is uses to quell liver wind. Sanyinjiao (SP6) is the only tonifying point; it assists in discouraging and draining fire by nourishing the yin. Taichong (LR1) provides an exit by which liver wind can be expelled. Needling Jinsuo (DU8) relieves spasms and tremors. An appropriate Chinese herbal prescription in this case is Ling Jiao Gou Teng Tang (*Cornu Antelopis-Uncaria Decoction),* which drains heat and liver fire, anchors the yang, stops tremors, controls convulsions and extinguishes wind.

For tremors due to Phlegm-Heat agitating the Wind, co-occurring symptoms may include: phlegmy appearance or obesity, staring or blank eyes, dislike of or low motivation for exercise, oppressed sensation in the chest, dry mouth, excessive sweating, dizziness, spitting of yellow phlegm, stiff neck and back and limb-tremor which can be stopped. There is also more confusion when Phlegm combines with Wind and diminished clarity of thought. The patient may also present with a red tongue with yellow-sticky coating. A wiry-fine-rapid pulse is common in patients with tremor due to Wind agitated by phlegm heat.

The treatment principle most helpful in this case resolves phlegm, clears heat, subdues wind and resolves congestion by invigorating the luo-connecting channels; this may be accomplished by combining the acupuncture points: Fenglong (ST40), Zhongwan (RN12), Pishu (BL20),

Sanyinjiao (SP6), Yinlingquan (SP9), Taichong (LR3), with even method, while tonifying Zhongwan (RN12) and Pishu (BL20). Fenglong (ST40) resolves phlegm directly, Zhongwan (RN12) and Pishu (BL20) tonify the spleen to resolve phlegm, Sanyinjiao (SP6) and Yinlingquan (SP9) also help to resolve phlegm and tonify yin while Taichong (LR3) subdues wind. Herbal prescription Dao Tan Tang plus Tian Ma Gou Teng Yin *(Conducting Phlegm Decoction* plus *Gastrodia-Uncaria Decoctio)* further supports the patient by resolving phlegm, anchoring liver yang and settling the wind.

Tremors resulting from qi and blood stagnation are often chronic; they coincide with agitation, insomnia, a dark complexion, muscle rigidity, a staring gaze or eyes that appear to bore into the foreground, numb sensations in the limbs, slurred stuttered speech, agonizing headache, dark nails and lips. The tongue is commonly enlarged and purple or dusky with toothmarks around the edges. The pulse may be wiry, firm, or choppy.

A successful approach in this case would invigorate and move the qi and blood, break-up or dissolve the stasis, open up the Blood connecting channels and quiet the tremor. An effective acupuncture protocol might be to apply even-method on: Taichong (LR3), Xuehai (SP10), Geshu (BL17), Gongsun (SP4) and Neiguan (PC6). The combination of Taichong (LR3), Xuehai (SP10), Geshu (BL17) and Neiguan (PC6) invigorates the blood; Gongsun (SP4) with Neiguan (PC6) powerfully influences the blood by opening the Chong Mai. Adding herbal formula: Tong Qiao Huo Xue Tang *(Opening the Orifices and Invigorating Blood Decoction)* further invigorates the blood, eliminates stasis and dissipates the wind.

Tremors that occur within Liver- and Kidney-Yin deficiency Wind patterns may present with a thin body, dizziness or vertigo, tinnitus, insomnia, dream disturbed sleep, headache or migraine, night sweating, mental restlessness, poor vision, diminished night vision, dry eyes, dry throat, sore back and knees, numbness of the limbs, stiff neck and back, tremor of head, clenched teeth, TMJ, and tremor of jaw, long-standing tremor of a limb with marked amplitude, cramps in the limbs, difficulty walking, unsteady gait, staring gaze and poor memory. A patient with this condition may have a thin, quivering or deviated tongue, peeled with no coat on the sides or all over, and a fine, rapid and/or floating pulse.

A treatment principle that counteracts tremors related to liver and kidney yin deficiency nourishes liver and kidney yin, settles the wind, opens the luo-connecting channels and stops tremors. A beneficial acupuncture prescription for a patient with this condition may consist of reinforcing

Guanyuan (RN4), Shenshu (BL23), Taixi (KI3), Sanyinjiao (SP6), Ganshu (BL18), and Ququan (LR8) while also needling Fengchi (GB20) and harmonizing Taichong (LR3). Guanyuan (RN4), Shenshu (BL23), Taixi (KI3) and Sanyinjiao (SP6) all replenish kidney yin; Ganshu (BL18) and Ququan (LR8) tonify liver yin and blood; Taichong (LR3) and Fengchi (GB20) subdue liver wind. A formula with like action could be chosen to reinforce the acupuncture treatment. Da Ding Feng Zhu (*Great Extinguishing Wind Pearl* Variation) is a good choice for nourishing liver yin, replenishing kidney yin, descending liver yang and quelling wind, for this formula, there would have to be some excess leading to liver yang rising.

Case Histories from Leading Acupuncture Doctors

Five cases histories are presented that illustrate the relevance of acupuncture in the treatment of Parkinson's disease and elucidate the diversity that exists among acupuncture protocols.

1. Zhu Rugong's Case [2]

A fifty-two-year-old male patient presented with tremors in both hands; with shaking in the right hand more pronounced than in the left. The tremors had started over six years ago when the patient noticed a slight trembling of the right hand. Two years later, the tremor had increased to the degree that it became difficult to hold objects and write. Chest congestion was noticed one year later. Tremors had first appeared on the left hand two years ago. Over the past year, both hands had been trembling incessantly; however, the trembling would stop when the patient goes to bed. The patient sought medical attention and was admitted into two hospitals where he was diagnosed with Parkinson's disease. He received over one hundred acupuncture treatments as part of his care. A combination of acupuncture and Chinese herbal medicine was offered afterwards. Chest congestion was relieved, but no improvement was observed for the trembling.

On his first visit with Zhu Rugong, both hands were trembling, with tremors in the right hand worse than those in the left hand. The patient had a pale and dark complexion, murky vision and occasional chest congestion. His pulse was thin and wiry. His tongue had a white and greasy coating. After traditional Chinese medicinal examination, the patient was diagnosed with liver and kidney deficiency, with tremors resulting from internally generated wind. Scalp electroacupuncture was performed in the first treatment session at the Area of Chorea and Tremor, Visual Area, and the Thoracic Cavity Area. The needles were retained for twenty minutes after manual stimulation by twisting and rotating.

Two days later, the patient reported that trembling of the right arm had stopped after the first treatment; although trembling resumed every two hours. The same acupuncture protocol was applied again, with the addition of auricular acupuncture points needled at the Brain, Shenmen, and the Occipital Point. Four days later, improvements were noticed in right-hand trembling. It was also noticed that just pressing the auricular points ceased tremor. The previous acupuncture protocol was repeated.

In the fourth visit, the eighth day after the initial visit, the patient reported that the left arm was trembling; in this case, the tremors were not alleviated by pressing the auricular points. The same scalp acupuncture protocol was provided; however auricular treatment was changed to embedded needles at the brainstem, sympathetic and heart points. Three days later, no remarkable changes were seen. Body acupuncture was provided at points on du meridian, bladder meridian and gallbladder meridian. Warming needles with moxa was applied to Fengfu (DU16), Tianzhu (BL10), and Fengchi (GB20); while Baihui (DU20), Houding (DU19), Qiangjian (DU18), Yuzhen (BL9), and Dazhu (BL11) were stimulated with rotating technique. Once de qi was achieved, the needles were retained for twenty minutes; manipulation with rotating technique was administered once during needle-retention time. Additionally, embedding needles were inserted at the subcutaneous, kidney and shenmen auricular points.

In the sixth visit, two days later, right-handed trembling ceased immediately with stimulation of Baihui (DU20), Houding (DU19), and Qiangjian (DU18); however, trembling recurred four to five hours post-stimulation. Trembling stopped after pressing the auricular points, and the time interval between recurrence increased. The same protocol as in the previous visit was followed on this day and for seven subsequent visits, after which, the patient's symptoms improved substantially; trembling decreased in both hands, his pulse normalized and his tongue coating became thin and white. Moreover, his symptoms became stable, and he could eat with his right hand. The following prescription was applied to address change in symptoms: acupuncture and moxibustion on Fengfu (DU16), Tianzhu (UB10) and Fengchi (GB20), with five moxa cones on each point; needling Baihui (DU20), Houding (DU19), Qiangjian (DU18), Naohu (DU17), Yuzhen (BL9), and Dazhu (BL11) with the same technique as above; and auricular acupuncture at the heart, brainstem and sympathetic points.

After completion of the fourteen treatments, the patient's symptoms were under control, and he went back to his hometown for two months during Spring Festival. The patient noticed a recurrence of symptoms when he was tired; but they only lasted for a few minutes. The patient also maintained a healthy appetite and was in good spirits. He continued treatment, and at the twentieth visit, no tremors were observed in the right hand. In order to maintain the effect, treatment was recommended once every other day. In total the patient received twenty-eight sessions. No attacks occurred during the follow-up visit.

Although no specific records about tremors are found in classical literature, tremor is often caused by deficiency of liver and kidney which coincides with malnutrition of tendons and vessels. Suboptimal levels of fluid and blood in the tendons leads to liver-wind stirring in the meridians and disturbing the limbs. The patient in this case, had resided in a damp area during war, which allowed for the exogenous pathogen to invade the collaterals. Compounding this, the patient was stressed out by his work, which over time leads to the manifestation of internal liver wind. The external pathogenic invasion combined with the internal disharmony exhausted the blood, which allowed for an uprising of internal wind. The condition persisted over time, and finally caused the disease.

In traditional Chinese medicine, there are many possible solutions to one problem or one disease. In this case, Dr. Zhu followed his first instinct by applying scalp acupuncture first. When he did not see any change in the patient's condition, he then chose to needle influential points along the bladder, gallbladder and du meridians: Fengfu (DU16), Fengchi (GB20), Tianzhu (UB10), Baihui (DU20), Houding (DU19), Qiangjian (DU18) and Naohu (DU17). Combining these with auricular acupoints proved to be an effective strategy as the symptoms were well controlled. The patient continued to improve over the next few consecutive treatments.

Dr. Zhu is adept at applying comprehensive treatment, considering it to be effective in treating diseases with mixed interior-exterior patterns. In this case, selecting the du meridian, gallbladder meridian and bladder meridian addresses the interior-exterior relation of shaoyang and jueyin and the interior-exterior relation of taiyang and shaoyin; this approach is common in clinical practice. Moreover, the du meridian dominates the whole body's yang, connecting with the kidney meridian at the coccyx and meeting the liver meridian at the vertex. Additionally, the du meridian has a close relationship with the liver and kidney; therefore, selecting the du meridian for tonifying the liver and kidney can achieve equally satisfactory results.

2. Shi Xuemin's Case [3]

A sixty-year-old male patient was admitted to the hospital. He had been experiencing tremors in the right arm for over one year. The patient had high blood pressure, 150/80mmHg, and he was over-occupied with excessive physical work. The tremors started over a year ago and were involuntary, limiting his ability to hold objects firmly. The symptoms worsened with emotional disturbance. The patient initially ignored symptoms until an occurrence of involuntary tremors of the head started, two months ago. He went to the hospital for acupuncture treatments then. Symptoms improved somewhat, but the patient did not continue receiving treatments.

He then returned to the Acupuncture Department. On examination, his mind seemed clear, although his reactions were slow and his face reflected feelings of apathy. His head was positioned at a forward incline. His body also leaned forward and was tense, with stiff muscles of the arms and legs. Constant contraction forced his waist to be curved when he stood up. Fingers curved inward as well. Involuntary tremors were observed on the upper limbs and his head was shaking slightly. Examination showed that the cranial nerves did not respond positively and he was slow to talk. Overall, his movements were slow, although his four limbs were fine, and his gait was unsteady. The patient's blood pressure was 140/80mmHg, heart beat was 75 bpm. His pupils were dilated 2.5:2.5mm and were responsive to light. No abnormalities with heart and lungs were detected. The patient's physiological reflexes were normal, and muscles were not atrophied. The patient's tongue had a white coating, and his pulse was wiry and slippery. After examination, the hospital diagnosed him with Parkinson's disease.

The patient was over sixty-year-old. According to traditional Chinese medicine theory, both essence and blood were deficient. Insufficient nourishment of the tendons and collaterals over time led to wind collecting in the channels, which then stirred uncontrollably. The Spleen's ability to control the four limbs, was impaired, and unable to root the yang. Liver wind swept unchecked through the body, resulting in tremors. Acupuncture points were selected to nourish the kidney and liver yin, while extinguishing wind, tonifying blood and improving smooth circulation of qi, yin and blood in the collaterals. Fengchi (GB20), Hegu (LI4), Taichong (LR3), Baihui (DU20), Ganshu (BL18), Geshu (BL17), and Shenshu (BL23) was the protocol selected in this case. Baihui (DU20) was needled to 0.5 cun and the needle was twisted with tonification. Fengchi (GB20) was needled in the direction of Adam's apple to a depth of 2 cun and the needles were rotated with high frequency for one minute. Ganshu (BL18), Geshu (BL17) and Shenshu (BL23) were needled to 1.5 cuns with rotation for one minute. Hegu (LI4) and Taichong (LR3) were needled to one cun vertically, while a breathing method for reducing was applied for one minute.

After five sessions the symptoms improved, although less severe tremors persisted. After fifteen sessions symptoms had almost disappeared. Tremors still occurred, especially during emotional upset.

Tremors, stiffness and reduction of movements are the three essential symptoms of Parkinson's disease. Chinese medicine sees a strong connection between this condition and impairment of the liver and kidneys, especially the liver. *Yellow Emperor's Classic of Medicine* states that all wind disorders are related to the liver. Deficiency of essence, blood and liver yin and lack of nutrition results in stiffness of the body and slowness of body movements. Deficiency of yin blood leads to the arising of wind, excess of wind in the channels and collaterals leads to movement, manifesting as tremors. The appropriate treatment principle, nourishing the kidneys and liver, extinguishing wind and invigorating collaterals is effective in treating this condition. For patients with a long history, purple tongue, body aching and numbness and both kidney and liver deficiency, invigorating the blood and dissolving stasis are also needed. This approach reflects the Chinese medicine principle to treat the blood first when eliminating wind; the circulating blood will then help extinguishing the wind.

3. Chen Quanxin's Case [4]

A 58-year-old male patient was diagnosed with Parkinson's disease and hospitalized for a few years. While hospitalized, he was treated with trihexyphenidyl and amantadine, with no improvement. Intervention was discontinued and he was referred to acupuncture. Upon examination, the patient presented with a dull expression, mask-like face, neck stiffness, trembling hands, unstable footing, uncoordinated limbs, normal appetite, unobstructed stool and interrupted urine. His tongue was dark red with a thin, white coat; his pulse was deep and thin.

From a Chinese medicine pathogenesis viewpoint, the patient had suffered from mental overload and excessive thinking. The mental strain consumed qi and blood of both the heart and spleen. The resulting deficiency of qi and blood was unable to fully nourish the tendons and fill the vessels, allowing for internally-generated liver-wind to course through the channels and collaterals, causing the lack of coordination in the limbs, frequently manifesting as tremor. The patient was diagnosed with tremor in Chinese medicine and diagnosed with Parkinson's disease in Western medicine. The patient was treated with acupuncture for tonifying the liver and kidneys while nourishing the yin and eliminating wind.

The following acupoints were manipulated with even reinforcing and reducing method: Dance tremor area, Baihui (DU20), Fengchi (GB20), Benshen (GB30), Ganshu (UB18), Shenshu (UB23), Taichong (LR3), and Hegu (LI14). Auricular acupoints were also pressed alternately with magnetic beads, on the liver, kidney, spleen, shenmen, heart and endocrine points. Additionally, the patient was needled at Dazhui (DU14), Shaohai (HT3) and Houxi (SI3) when he suffered from excessive shaking; with Dabao (SP21) and Qimen (LR14) with moxibustion and bloodletting if he had severe stiffness; with Feishu (BL13) and Pishu (BL20) when he had severe sweating; with Liangmen (ST21), Zhongwan (RN12), and Qihai (RN6) when the patient had fullness of stomach and abdomen; with Tianshu (ST25) and Qihai (RN6) when the patient had constipation; and with Chengjiang (RN24), Lianquan (RN23) and Fuliu (KI7) when the patient had a dry mouth.

While needling acupoints on the head, all needles were manipulated obliquely with a thirty-degree angle first, and then transversely with a fifteen-degree angle. Once the needle was inserted at two-thirds the full insertion depth, the needle was rotated quickly, two to three times per second; after achieving the hot, sore and heavy sensation, the needle was manipulated with the same technique once every five to ten minutes. When applying electric needles, all needles were retained for thirty to forty minutes, and the patient was treated once every other day. The patient had significant improvement after sixty treatments, and in order to reinforce the effect, the patient was treated with auricular acupuncture intermittently. The follow-up after two years showed no relapse, and the patient was able to take care of himself.

In this case, Dr. Chen selected acupuncture points based on the main symptom and then choosing adjunct points according to pattern differentiation. Generally, the clinical effects of treating Parkinson's disease with acupuncture includes: symptoms improvement; decreased use of Western medicine; delaying the progression of disease; and strengthening physique and improving disease resistance. Acupuncture has shown efficacy in cases of Parkinson's disease, especially in terms of symptom reduction and delaying disease progression.

4. Yang Jiasan's Case [5]

A 62-year-old female suffered from trembling legs for about six to seven years, and was diagnosed with Parkinson's disease by her Western physicians. Surgery and standard Western medicine interventions did not improve her condition. She then sought out acupuncture care. At the initial acupuncture consult, she complained of intermittent and irregular tremor of both legs two to three times a day, lasting two hours per each attack. Her facial complexion was red, and her expression dull. Her response was slow and she spoke with a weak voice. The patient's tongue was red with a thick coat, and she had a thin and slippery pulse.

According to Chinese medicine pattern diagnosis, the patient was liver- and kidney-yin deficient, with rebellious wind in the channels. Yang was not rooted, displayed by a dysfunction of the yang qiao and yin qiao meridians. The treatment principle consisted of nourishing the liver and kidneys while calming the wind and rooting the yang in order to regulate the yin and yang qiao meridians.

The patient was treated with the following protocol: Lieque (LU7), Zhaohai (KI6), Shenmai (UB62), Houxi (SI3), Fengchi (GB20), Fengfu (DU16), Baihui (DU20), Sishencong (Extra), Shenting (DU24), Benshen (GB13), Zusanli (ST36), Ganshu (UB18), Pishu (UB20) and Shenshu (UB23). The acupoints Fengchi (GB20) and Fengfu (DU16) were manipulated with reducing method, and other points were manipulated with reinforcing method; all needles were retained for thirty minutes, and the patient was treated once every other day.

On the second visit, the patient said her tremor had gradually decreased. The patient received a course of twelve treatments, then discontinuing treatment for personal reasons. However, the patient had noticed improvement, with a reduction in frequency and duration of attack to only one each day, lasting thirty minutes each time. In order to maintain the clinic effect and control the progression of disease, she was advised to continue treatment after going back to her city.

In this case, Dr. Yang holds that Parkinson's is a pathological change within the nervous system of middle-aged and elderly people. It falls under "tremor" in Chinese medicine diagnosis. Tremor, shaking and moving are dysfunctions within the tendons and vessels, caused by internal wind. As Wang Kentang mentioned in *Standards of Diagnosis and Treatment*, "Tremor is barely seen in younger people but easily seen after middle-aged, especially for the aged.

This because the aged has the deficiency of blood that is not enough to balance and resist fire. Therefore, it is hard to completely cure the disease." In this case, the patient was diagnosed with tremor in Chinese medicine and diagnosed with Parkinson's disease in Western medicine. When treating the patient, Dr. Yang believed that the disease was in brain, and thus he selected two wind points: Fengchi (GB20) and Fengfu (DU16), to calm wind for clearing the wind form the brain and three shen points: Shenting (DU24), Benshen (GB13) and Sishencong (Extra) to calm mind for stopping shaking. Dr. Yang also stated that the yin qiao meridian and yang qiao meridian govern the movement of whole body, and since the disease involves the dysfunction of movement, it is affected by the dysfunction of the yin qiao and yang qiao meridians. Therefore, he selected Lieque (LU7) and Zhaohai (KI6) to nourish kidney and liver; Shenmai (UB62) and Houxi (SI3) to clear heat and wind; and Zusanli (ST36) with back shu points to regulate qi and blood of zang-fu organs. Although it is very difficult to treat this disease, with acupuncture, it is still possible to alleviate the symptoms and to control the progression of disease.

5. Chifumi Iseki's Case [6]

Iseki and other Japanese researchers reported a case to illustrate how the nonmotor symptoms of Parkinson's disease, including pain, depression and various autonomic symptoms were alleviated by acupuncture and how the patient progress was assessed. A woman began to feel intractable pain in her lower legs when she was seventy-six. She was diagnosed as having Parkinson's disease when she was seventy-eight. The leg pain was suspected to be a symptom of Parkinson's disease after eliminating other possibilities. She also presented with nonmotor symptoms, depression, anxiety, hot flashes, and paroxysmal sweating. Though the patient had received levodopa and other medications for five years, she still suffered from the nonmotor symptoms and was referred to acupuncture, and was treated with electroacupuncture based on traditional Chinese medical principles five times per week. After two weeks, the symptoms were assessed: visual analogue scale (VAS) score of the leg pain was 16 mm (70 mm, before), Hamilton's rating scales for depression (HAM-D) score was 9 (18, before), timed 3 m Up and Go took 20 steps in 30 sec (24 steps in 38 sec, before), and the Movement Disorder Society-sponsored revision of the Unified Parkinson's Disease Rating Scale (MDS-UPDRS) Part 1 score was 13 (21, before). Autonomic symptoms, hot flashes and paroxysmal sweating, were also alleviated after the two-week course of acupuncture.

Increasing Demands

Knowledge of individual cases, common clinical presentations and traditional Chinese medicine perspectives on Parkinson's disease and related conditions reveals the need for research that both identifies conditions that create symptoms and discovers clear pathways for their resolution. This common, debilitating neuro-degenerative disorder currently knows no neuro-protective cure. Increasingly, patients with Parkinson's disease seek complementary and alternative medicine (CAM) for the abatement of symptoms and maintenance care. Researchers [7] analyzed CAM use among Parkinson's patients worldwide through a recent literature review. They found that CAM encompasses varied modalities making the generalization of data problematic. Six of the studies reviewed estimated that between 25.7% and 76% of Parkinson's patients utilize some form of CAM, and were highly responsive to treatment, (from 81%-100%). Generally employed to combat symptoms, frequently chosen modalities included acupuncture, massage and herbals, vitamins and/or nutritional supplements. Of the high rate of patients participating in CAM, only 11% to 20% had been referred by a healthcare professional. CAM use was found to be correlated with women more than men, age, age at onset of PD, longer duration of PD, level of education, affluence, rural location, comorbidity for indications, levodopa load, and more severe motor symptoms. The widespread, worldwide use of CAM among Parkinson's patients, as was observed in this study, suggest that more telling research is likely to provide useful information of direct benefit to patients seeking relief and may allow for the prevention of factors that contribute to its prevalence. Researchers remarked that increasing communication between physicians and patients about CAM participation may help coordinate care and eliminate adverse effects related to CAM or the combination of CAM and conventional medicine.

Exemplified by the various traditional Chinese medical patterns described above, Parkinson's disease may arise from distinct sets of underlying conditions. The same is true when looking at the disease through the framework of western science. Multitudes of molecular and cellular pathways potentially influence the neuro-degeneration associated with Parkinson's disease; although the exact cause and the conditions that create an opportunity for the disease to manifest are elusive. Researchers [8] at Cornell recently inquired into the mechanism by which acupuncture produces positive benefits in patients with Parkinson's. Animal experiments have shown that acupuncture protects the neuronal circuitry. By positively influencing the levels of neuroprotective agents such as brain-derived neurotrophic factor, glial-cell-line-derived neurotrophic factor and cyclophilin A. They also discovered that acupuncture inhibits cellular death processes and moderates oxidative damage on the substantia nigra dopaminergic neurons. These findings lead researchers to believe that acupuncture shows promise as a potential treatment for Parkinson's disease, suggesting that the preliminary findings, that acupuncture's mechanism of action may positively influence factors leading up to the development of Parkinson's disease, indicate that early intervention with acupuncture is the most efficacious method for its use.

In additional research on prevalence of complementary and alternative medicine (including acupuncture) use among Parkinson's patients, Pecci C. *et al.* [9], from Parkinson's Disease and Movement Disorders Unit, Hospital de Clínicas José de San Martín, Universidad de Buenos Aires, Argentina, interviewed 300 Parkinson's patients of the Movement Disorders Clinic at the Buenos Aires University Hospital. They found that 25.7% had used complementary and alternative medicine treatments to improve Parkinson's-related symptoms while 38% had received complementary and alternative medicine at least once in life for reasons other than to treat Parkinson's symptoms. With use more frequent among women and more common in the 50- to 69-year age group, referrals to complementary and alternative medicine treatments had mostly been initiated by friends and neighbors. Acupuncture, homeopathy, yoga, and therapeutic massage were among the most common modalities used, with use increasing after starting conventional interventions. Research did not show any relation to duration of the disease with complementary and alternative medicine treatments use. Researchers advised that Neurologists communicate with their Parkinson's patients about the use of complementary and alternative medicine treatments to diminish potential for harmful effects.

Observational Studies

Observational studies draw inferences about the effect of a treatment by correlating intervention with the health status among participants. Causality is not assumed; therefore, some would say that observation studies gather less compelling information than randomized controlled trials (RTCs). Observations may be made through longitudinal and/or cross-sectional assessments; cohort and case-control studies being two types of longitudinal studies commonly conducted to assess clinical interventions.

Eng *et al.* [10], conducted an observational study to evaluate the effects of sequential tui na, acupuncture, and instrument-delivered qigong on patients with Parkinson disease. Twenty-five Parkinson's patients received weekly treatments over the course of six months in an outpatient research/academic clinic for patients with Parkinson's and an acupuncture office. Researchers saw no significant improvements in clinical measures; however, there was a 2.4-point worsening in motor scores (24.0 versus 26.4, $p = 0.018$), and a 16% improvement in Parkinson's Disease Quotient-39 total score (23.2 versus 19.6, $p = 0.044$) and a 29% improvement in Beck's Depression Inventory scores (9.6 versus 6.8, $p = 0.006$). Sixteen patients self-reported moderate to marked gains and no adverse effects were seen. Researchers concluded that acupuncture is safe and well tolerated among Parkinson's patients, producing subjective benefits in most. Depression and quality of life scores reflect some benefit; however, motor scores worsened.

To compare the effect of abdominal acupuncture vs. Madopar for Parkinson's patients, Chen *et al.* [11], conducted a study in which sixty patients were randomized into either an abdominal acupuncture group or a control group. Patients in the acupuncture group were administered Madopar along with abdominal acupuncture at Zhongwan (RN12), Xiawan (RN10), Qihai (RN6) and Guanyuan (RN4) and other relevant points. Controls were administered Madopar. After three courses, effectiveness was 90.0% among patients in the acupuncture group and 83.3% among those in the control group, with a significant difference between groups ($P<0.05$). Researchers concluded that abdominal acupuncture combined with Madopar increases the beneficial effect of Madopar for Parkinson's patients while reducing its side-effects.

In a related study, Ren *et al.* [12], discovered that of fifty Parkinson's patients receiving either Madopar and acupuncture or Madopar only, a 92% effectiveness rate in motor improvement was seen in the combined treatment group; which was significantly higher than improvements among controls ($P<0.05$). This study confirmed that acupuncture can enhance therapeutic effects of medications and reduce the amount of medicine needed.

Based on years of clinical experience, Qin [13] hypothesized that needling the Du channel is primarily indicated for miscellaneous disease and diseases of the limbs. Through his knowledge of influential patterns on the scalp and Du channel effects, he created an innovative protocol combining Du channel and scalp acupuncture for Parkinson's patients. Based on the distribution of cephalic motor regions and meridians on the scalp, Qin's eight scalp needle protocol: bilateral Fengchi (GB20), Shuaigu (GB8), Toulinqi (GB15) as well as Yintang (Extra) and Baihui (DU20) has been applied to nervous system diseases, such as Parkinson's and multiple sclerosis. Researchers propose that the eight-scalp needle technique may lessen the progression of Parkinson's; improve motor function, cognitive ability and mood; ease the suffering of patients; and elevate quality of life.

Fukuda *et al.* [14], conducted a study to evaluate tongue function in terms of its clinical implications for swallowing ability in patients with Parkinson's disease from of a single acupuncture treatment. This pilot study recruited thirteen patients, aged 57-84 years. Outcome measurement included tongue pressure measured using a tongue pressure manometer, and swallowing reflex latency was measured in three of the thirteen patients. The results demonstrated that significant changes were seen after acupuncture in mean tongue pressure, which increased from 23.1 to 26.7 kPa ($p<0.01$). Reductions were observed after acupuncture in mean swallowing reflex latency (from 5.2 to 4.6 s for first saliva swallow; from 19.9 to 15.7 s for second saliva swallow; and from 10.4 to 5.7 s for third saliva swallow). This study suggested that acupuncture may be useful for improving oral cavity function.

Gait disturbance, including slower speed, shorter stride length, shorter arm swing, longer double support time, and faster cadence than in healthy individuals are some of the most common symptoms in Parkinson's disease (PD). These disturbances of gait are recognized as important motor signs affecting the quality of life of many Parkinson's patients. Fukuda *et al.* [15] from Meiji University of Integrative Medicine conducted a trial demonstrating how acupuncture can be a safe way to decrease gait disturbances. Twenty-seven outpatients participated in the study. Among them, seven participants were Hoehn-Yahr Stage I, four were Stage II, and sixteen were Stage III. The treatment principle was based on the Chinese medicine diagnosis of kidney and liver deficiency.

The acupuncture points selected for treatment were: Zusanli (ST36), Sanyinjiao (SP6), Taichong (LR3), Hegu (LI4), Quchi (LI11), Fengchi (GB20), Ganshu (BL18), and Shenshu (BL23). Gait speed, step length, floor reaction force, and cadence were assessed while walking ten meters. Gait function was measured with a portable gait rhythmogram, a small device that measures three dimensional accelerations affecting gait, associated with voluntary limb and trunk movements and those induced by step-in and kick-off. The study demonstrated that mean walking acceleration, stride length, and gait speed, indicators of gait function, increased significantly after acupuncture. No adverse effects related to the protocol were discovered.

In a prospective open-label study of combined treatment for idiopathic Parkinson's disease, Doo *et al.* [16], examined the effectiveness and safety of combined treatment using acupuncture and bee venom acupuncture (BVA) as an adjunctive treatment for idiopathic Parkinson's disease (PD). The study recruited eleven patients (seven men and four women) with idiopathic PD who had been receiving a regular dose of anti-Parkinson's medication for at least four weeks. Patients received conventional treatment for twelve weeks. They then received additional treatment with acupuncture and BVA twice a week for twelve weeks while still maintaining conventional treatment. The outcome measures included Unified Parkinson's Disease Rating Scale (UPDRS), the Parkinson's Disease Quality of Life Questionnaire (PDQL), the speed and number of steps required to walk twenty meters, and the Beck Depression Inventory (BDI). They were assessed at baseline, twelve weeks, and twenty-four weeks. Maximum excursion and directional control, measured by computerized dynamic posturography were used to assess postural stability. The study demonstrated that patients who underwent twelve weeks of twice-weekly combined treatment with acupuncture and BVA showed significant improvements in gait speed, PDQL score, activities of daily living (UPDRS part II), motor symptoms (UPDRS part III), and combined UPDRS part II+III scores compared with assessments after conventional treatment. This study warranted large-scale investigation.

Clinical Trials

Clinical trials analyze the results of specific interventions. Most researchers agree that randomly assigning study participants to groups and including controls improves the reliability of results; therefore, randomized controlled trials (RCTs) are considered the current standard in clinical research. In well-designed RCTs, differences in outcomes between groups can then be attributed to the intervention. When embarking on new or innovative research, limited patient-supply may inspire researchers to initially enroll patients into small pilot studies. Establishing safety and efficacy data may then pave the way for progressively larger-scale studies. Ideally, research is conducted according to the gold standard: randomized, double-blind, and placebo-controlled trials. Double-blind requirements can be the most difficult to meet, as both the participants and the researchers need to be unaware of whether a participant is receiving the actual intervention or a placebo. Due to belief systems and the strong psychological component within human nature, many patients will exhibit a strong placebo effect, and get better when any treatment is applied; the effect being more pronounced when a patient believes that the treatment will be effective. Including a placebo group helps researchers determine if the effects of an intervention are more dynamic than the placebo effect.

In a study to compare the effects of acupuncture to bee venom acupuncture in adjuvant care among patients with Parkinson's disease, Cho *et al.* [17], from Department of Cardiovascular and Neurologic Diseases, College of Korean Medicine, Kyung Hee University, Seoul, Republic of Korea, conducted a pilot study with forty-three patients who had been taking a consistent dose of conventional medication for a minimum of one month. Participants received acupuncture, bee venom acupuncture or no treatment for ten weeks. Patients receiving bee venom acupuncture significantly improved their ratings on the Unified Parkinson's Disease Rating Scale (overall score, part II and part III), the Berg Balance Scale, and were able to walk 30 meters at a significantly more rapid rate. They also experienced significant improvement on the Unified Parkinson's Disease Rating Scale compared with controls. Patients receiving acupuncture also showed significant improvement on the Unified Parkinson's Disease Rating Scale (part III and total scores) and the Beck Depression Inventory. Results were attributed to interventions as the control group did not show significant changes in any outcome. In this pilot study, researchers concluded that acupuncture and bee venom acupuncture both showed promise as adjuvant treatment for Parkinson's patients.

Parkinson's disease is a degenerative disorder characterized by neural defects in the substantia nigra. Previous studies have found that acupuncture point Yanglingquan (GB34), the influential point for the tendons, significantly improves Parkinson's symptoms. Functional magnetic resonance imaging (fMRI) studies have shown that Parkinson's patients exhibit diminished neuronal response in regions encompassing the putamen, thalamus, and the supplementary motor area of the brain. Yeo *et al.* [18], from the Department of Meridian & Acupoint, College of Korean Medicine, Kyung Hee University, Seoul, Korea, further researched the effects of acupuncture point GB34 on Parkinson's. They discovered that in twelve patients with Parkinson's, acupuncture at GB34, increased neural response within the substantia nigra, caudate, thalamus, and putamen; providing further confirmation that acupuncture at GB34 is an effective treatment for Parkinson's patients. The researchers suggested randomized controlled trials to substantiate these results.

Growing interest in adjuvant acupuncture care for patients with Parkinson's disease continues to spark further research. As a follow-up to earlier research, Yeo *et al.* [19], through a functional magnetic resonance imaging study, assessed Parkinson's patient response to acupuncture at right Yanglingquan (GB34). Researchers discovered that prefrontal cortex, precentral gyrus, and the putamen are activated by acupuncture at Yanglingquan (GB34). Parkinson's patients tended to show significantly higher brain activity in the prefrontal cortex and precentral gyrus, especially in the left hemisphere. Findings suggest that prefrontal cortex response as well as precentral gyrus should be assessed in future acupuncture research. This study also confirmed the effectiveness of Yanglingquan (GB34) for Parkinson's symptoms. Notably, researchers determined that acupuncture at Yanglingquan (GB34) activated the brains of Parkinson's patients differently than the brains of patients without Parkinson's.

A study [20] was conducted to explore effectiveness and mechanisms of electroacupuncture (EA) add-on treatment in Parkinson's disease (PD) patients. The study recruited fifty PD patients and they were randomly assigned to either medication plus EA (D + EA) group or medication alone (D) group. Patients in D + EA group received acupuncture stimulation on Fengfu (DU16), Fengchi (GB20), Hegu (LR3), and Dazhui (DU14). Scales for motor and nonmotor symptoms were used to evaluate the patients. Levels of neuroinflammatory factors and neurotransmitters in serum were measured. Results showed that EA add-on treatment remarkably reduced scores of Unified Parkinson's Disease Rating Scale (UPDRS) III and its subindexes of tremor, rigidity, and bradykinesia and significantly decreased UPDRS III scores in patients with bradykinesia-rigidity and mixed types and mild severity. Depression and sleep disturbances were alleviated, which were reflected by decreased scores of Hamilton Depression Rating Scale, Pittsburgh Sleep Quality Index, and elevated noradrenalin level. This study demonstrated that effects of EA add-on treatment on motor symptoms and sleep disturbances were significantly better than medication-only treatment, markedly improving life quality of PD patients. It also showed that EA add-on treatment decreased nitric oxide level in serum. The authors concluded that EA add-on treatment was effective on most motor symptoms and some nonmotor symptoms and is particularly effective in PD patients at early stage.

Acupuncture point injection is a recently-developed modality within the field of acupuncture. It has been applied to a wide range of conditions including Parkinson's diseases. Liu *et al.* [21], conducted a multicenter randomized controlled clinical trial to investigate short- and long-term benefits and safety of acupuncture point injection of kakkonein for early- or mid-stage Parkinson's disease (PD). The study recruited 135 patients with early- or mid-stage PD and 116 cases completed the study, including 40 cases in the acupuncture point injection group, 37 cases in the acupuncture group and 39 cases in the medication group. Patients in the acupuncture point injection group were treated by injection of kakkonein (2 mL) into Fengchi (GB20), once every other day for eight weeks. For acupuncture intervention, Fengchi (GB20) were needled with filiform needles, once every other day for eight weeks. Patients in the medication group were treated by oral administration of levodopa (125 mg/time, twice a day) for eight weeks. The outcome measures included Unified Parkinson's Disease Rating Scale (UPDRS) before and after treatment, and one month after the treatment.

The study showed that after the treatment, scores of psychosis, behavior and emotion, daily life activity and motor function were all significantly changed in the three groups in comparison with pre-treatment in each group ($P<0.05$), which suggested an improvement of the PD patients' conditions. Furthermore, the effects seen within the acupuncture point injection group and acupuncture group were significantly better than those of the medication group ($P<0.05$). One-month's follow-up showed that the scores of behavior-emotion and daily life activity were significantly improved in the acupuncture point injection group compared with the acupuncture and medication groups ($P<0.05$). No significant differences were found between the acupuncture group and medication group in scores of behavior-emotion, daily life activity and motor function ($P>0.05$). The study concluded that acupuncture point injection of kakkonein can improve patients' behavior, emotion, and daily life activity in early- or mid-stage PD patients and has both short- and longer-term benefits.

Comparing the effect of acupuncture and medication and obtaining data on additional benefits from acupuncture tends to attract the attention of practitioners and researchers alike. Chen *et al.* [22] conducted a study to evaluate the integrated effects of acupuncture treatment in PD patients who had received western medication. In this study, twenty patients in the acupuncture plus medication group received acupuncture treatment twice a week while twenty patients in the control group received medication only. In the short-term scenario, acupuncture treatment was performed at acupuncture points Baihui (DU20), Fengchi (GB20), Quchi (LI11), Shousanli (LI10), Hegu (LI4), Fengshi (GB31), Futu (ST32), Yanglingquan (GB34) and Yangfu (GB38) along with medication for eighteen weeks. In the long-term acupuncture treatment, thirteen patients received acupuncture treatment twice a week for 36 weeks. The outcome measures included Unified Parkinson's disease rating scale (UPDRS), Beck Anxiety Inventory

(BAI), Beck Depression Inventory-Version 2 (BDI-II), and WHO quality of life evaluation (WHOQOL). The study showed that in the short-term, a higher percentage of patients in the acupuncture group displayed an improvement in UPDRS total scores (55% vs. 15%, $p = 0.019$), sub-score of mind, behavior and mood (85% vs. 25%, $p < 0.001$), activity of daily living (65% vs. 15%, $p = 0.003$), mobility (40% vs. 15%, $p = 0.155$) and complication of treatment (75% vs. 15%, $p < 0.001$), BDI-II score (85% vs. 35%, $p = 0.003$), and WHOQOL score (65% vs. 15%, $p = 0.003$) when compared to the control group at the end of the eighteen weeks. In the long-term (36 weeks of acupuncture treatment), the mean UPDRS total scores and sub-score of mind, behavior and mood, sub-score of complications and BDI-II score decreased significantly when compared to the pretreatment baseline. The study concluded that acupuncture treatment provided additional benefits in reducing symptoms and signs related to the mind, behavior, mood, complications of therapy and depression in PD patients who were receiving medication.

Additional functional magnetic resonance imaging (fMRI) research assessed the neural mechanisms underlying the effect of acupuncture on motor function in Parkinson's patients. Significant improvement in the motor function of the affected hand occurred in patients receiving specific acupuncture. The putamen and the primary motor cortex showed increased activity with acupuncture compared with controls. Meaningful data [23] showed that the neural activation stimulated by acupuncture correlated with greater motor functionality. Expectation of acupuncture was found to activate the anterior cingulate gyrus, the superior frontal gyrus, and the superior temporal gyrus. The researchers concluded that acupuncture may increase motor functionality in patients with Parkinson's by way of the basal ganglia-thalamocortical pathway.

Systematic Reviews

Scientific compilation of clinical literature within a given domain provides an overview of the most reliable findings to date. By consolidating the results of multiple studies within a set of specific criteria, researchers can evaluate the current level of scientifically validated understandings and propose a meaningful course for further research. To complete a quality systematic review, specific steps are followed. Research generally starts with a thorough search of the literature, specifying explicitly the databases and citation indexes and criteria. Initially selected article titles and abstracts are then reviewed for alignment with criteria and relevance. Each selected study then is assessed for quality of methodological quality. Researchers also must describe an objective and transparent means for minimizing bias before employing a systematic method for coding and analyzing data. Through a systemic review, researchers can then share results of all relevant published and unpublished data in a comprehensive report. According to the *Cochrane Handbook*, eight steps are essential: *1. Defining the review question(s) and developing criteria for including studies*; *2. Searching for studies*; *3. Selecting studies and collecting data*; *4. Assessing risk of bias in included studies*; *5. Analyzing data*; *6. Addressing reporting biases*; *7. Presenting results and "summary of findings" tables*; *8. Interpreting results and drawing conclusions.* Three systematic reviews are selected on acupuncture for Parkinson's disease in this section.

Lam YC. *et al.* [24] completed a system review with the aim of comparing the efficacy and safety of acupuncture with placebo, conventional interventions, or no treatment for patients with Parkinson's disease. Relevant studies were pulled from reputable international electronic databases, journals and references. Ten randomized controlled trials (RCTs) each administering a unique acupuncture protocol (with manipulation) that compared placebo or no intervention methods were included. As is common in acupuncture research, either none of the studies were blinded or blinding was not mentioned. Only two studies mentioned the number of participants who failed to fully complete the study. Nine studies showed statistically significant benefits from acupuncture compared to controls; only one found no significant differences for all included parameters. Two studies reported accounts of adverse events. Overall researchers summarized that the review demonstrates that acupuncture is potentially effective in treating Parkinson's; however methodological flaws limit applicability of results. Lam et al., specifically suggested that "large, well-designed, placebo-controlled RCTs with rigorous methods of randomization and adequately concealed allocation, as well as intention-to-treat data analysis are needed."

Scalp acupuncture, a contemporary acupuncture method, has been found to produce positive results for a range of neurological disorders. Through systemic review, Lee *et al.* [25], from School of Korean Medicine, Pusan National University, Yangsan, South Korea, evaluated the effectiveness of scalp acupuncture in treating motor function impairments and related symptoms experienced by patients with Parkinson's disease. Randomized controlled trials that compared scalp acupuncture with conventional therapies were searched for and selected, with four meeting criteria. According to the Unified Parkinson's Disease Rating Scale, two studies showed that scalp acupuncture combined with conventional interventions provided greater benefit compared with conventional interventions alone [60 cases; weighted mean difference, -3.94; 95% confidence interval (CI), -6.05 to -1.84, P=0.01; I(2) =0%]. Three studies using the Webster scale, did not find greater improvement among patients receiving scalp acupuncture with conventional approaches compared to those receiving conventional interventions alone (154 cases; risk ratio, 1.29; 95% CI, 0.79 to 2.12, P=0.30; I(2) =84%). Unfortunately, results are difficult to assess as the quality rating of all the included trials were low. Still, Lee HS et al., concluded that the effectiveness of scalp acupuncture holds potential promise for Parkinson's patients; recommending that a sham-controlled RCT design according to CONSORT and STRICTA may improve methodology. They strongly recommended a large sample size to determine the mechanism and efficacy of scalp acupuncture in treating Parkinson's patients.

The evidence from recent clinical studies regarding the efficacy of acupuncture on Parkinson's disease was further assessed by Kim and Jeon [26]. Relevant literature was searched from thirteen databases from 2000 to 2012. Eleven studies were selected, although researchers determined that the number of trials, and total sample size were not large enough to generalize benefits. They found that five studies did not report diagnostic criteria. Two of the six RCTs neglected to describe randomization method and information on blinding. In two trials, incomplete participation or early discontinuation was not fully reported. Two of three RCTs comparing acupuncture with placebo acupuncture did not find acupuncture to be superior. One RCT reported the positive influence of “constitutional acupuncture,” but not of needle acupuncture. Three RCTs reported adjunctive benefit when combined with conventional medication; however, placebo effects were not accounted for as controls were not used in these studies. Two of four uncontrolled studies showed significant benefits within acupuncture groups. No validated acupuncture protocols were employed and lack of agreement as to correct point location was also noted by the researchers. Safety and tolerability assessment was included in only five studies; additionally, studies did not consider the enduring effects of acupuncture following cessation of the treatment. Researchers concluded that further research with well-designed studies are needed to provide more compelling information regarding acupuncture and its role in treating Parkinson's disease. There are needs for further studies with improved methodological quality.

Meta-Analysis

The ability of meta-analysis to pool data from multiple clinical trials allows for clarity to be gained in interpreting the meaning of collective research results for a given topic. The overall effectiveness as well as particular effects can be assessed across a broader scale. Meta analysis tends to provide greater precision in treatment effect; therefore, it is crucial to apply appropriate guidelines to inclusion material. Meta-analysis provides a way of looking at all participants in all included studies as if each were participants in one large, well-designed study which allows decisions based on findings to include data from all relevant quality studies. Net benefits are then revealed. The following are crucial elements of meta-analysis: *1. Systematic review methods*; *2. Calculating effect size*; *3. Coding individual studies*; *4. Aggregating effect sizes*; *5. Analyzing heterogeneity*; *6. Subgroup analysis*; *7. Conducting meta-regression*; *8. Assessing publication bias*; *9. Reporting standards*. Two studies of meta-analysis are selected on acupuncture for Parkinson's disease in this section.

To assess the clinical role of acupuncture in the treatment for Parkinson's disease, Lee *et al.* [27], reviewed the literature, (all languages) through January 2008. A meta-analysis of eleven RTCs failed to show significant effect. In six additional RCTs, a positive effect was discovered for scalp acupuncture and combined results of two further RCTs suggested beneficial effects of acupuncture vs. no treatment. Researchers qualified findings, stating that nonspecific effects were not well-controlled in studies producing positive results. Overall, researchers did not find compelling evidence to support the use of acupuncture in treating Parkinson's. They further criticized that the number of participants, quality of trials and sample size not sufficient to properly assess outcomes. Further rigorous trials were suggested. (Since this study was conducted more research has been completed; this study is currently too outdated to be of great relevance.)

Parkinson disease is a prevalent neuro-degenerative disease that may seriously restrict activities and diminish sense of quality of life for those afflicted. Zhang *et al.* [28], conducted a meta-analysis to evaluate the efficacy and safety of traditional Chinese medicine (TCM) as an adjunctive intervention for those suffering the ill effects of Parkinson's. Researchers scoured PubMed, Cochrane Controlled Trials Register, China National Knowledge Infrastructure, Chinese Scientific Journals Database and Wanfang for qualifying RCTs. Unified Parkinson's Disease Rating Scale provided means to determine effectiveness of acupuncture adjunctive care against conventional treatment as presented in twenty-seven articles with

2314 patients from 1999 to 2013. In patients who had received traditional Chinese medicine and dopamine replacement therapy compared with those who had received dopamine replacement alone, researchers found potentially remarkable improvements in overall disease rate scores.

Acupuncture adjunctive care was found to produce markedly beneficial improvements in UPDRS I-IV scores (WMD 10.96, 95%CI 5.85, 16.07). Traditional Chinese medicine alone did not improve scores; however, greater duration of adjunct intervention improved effectiveness. The intervention also was found to be safe and well-tolerated. In spite of methodological flaws, researchers found traditional Chinese medicine to be potentially superior to conventional care alone in the treatment of Parkinson's patients. Further studies with of better quality were recommended.

Acupuncture Mechanism

Acupuncture mechanism studies refer to the investigation of how acupuncture works in animals and humans. Scientific explanations for how acupuncture works could be obtained through these acupuncture mechanism studies.

To gain greater insight into the mechanism of acupuncture, specifically scalp acupuncture and its influence on dopamine regulation in Parkinson's patients, Huang *et al.* [29], conducted a pilot study in which ten patients with Parkinson's were randomly placed into one of two groups. Electro- scalp acupuncture was administered at contralateral MS6, MS4, MS8, MS9 and MS14 in patients with unilateral lesions. Those with bilateral lesions received bilateral intervention. Needles were inserted to the depth of the galea aponeurotica. Controls received oral Madopar, with dosages appropriate to severity of symptoms. Researchers found that absorption of 99mTc-TRODAT-1 increased after either intervention. Among those receiving acupuncture, the homolateral BG/OC differences before and after treatment were 1.1883 +/- 0.1471 and 1.2416 +/- 0.3146 respectively, and those in the control group were 1.1597 +/- 0.0568, 1.2053 +/- 0.1153; ratios reflecting lack of significant difference between them (P > 0.05). The contralateral BG/OC ratios before and after intervention were 0.9019 +/- 0. 1210 and 0.9496 +/- 0.2522 respectively, and 1.0436 +/- 0.1393 and 1.2972 +/- 0.2612 respectively in the controls. Contralateral BG/OC differences before and after treatment in the control groups reached significance (P<0.05). Other cerebral regions did not reflect before and after change difference according to 99mTc-TRODAT-1 SPECT.

By these measurements, researchers determined there was no difference in DAT improvement between the two groups ($P > 0.05$). Researchers concluded that electro-scalp acupuncture may diminish the loss of DAT in basal ganglia and improve DAT activity in patients with Parkinson's disease. Therefore, electro- scalp acupuncture was found to have a protective role relating to the dopamine neuron, potentially delaying or moderating the progression of Parkinson's disease while mitigating clinical symptoms.

Jiang *et al.* [30], further researched the mechanism of scalp acupuncture in Parkinson's patients. Five patients with Parkinson's were administered electro-scalp acupuncture at Dingnie Qianxiexian (MS 6), Epangxian III (MS 4), Dingpangxian I (MS 8), Dingpangxian II (MS 9) and Zhenxia Pangxian (MS 14). Contralateral needling was applied for patients with pathologic lesion on one side while bilateral needling was applied for pathologic lesion on both sides. Ratios of ST/OC on the same side as the affected extremity before and after intervention were found to be 1.19 +/- 0.15 and 1.24 +/- 0.31 respectively; while those on the opposite side were 0.90 +/- 0.12 and 0.95 +/- 0.25 respectively. Ratios increased post-intervention ($P > 0.05$). Researchers confirmed that electro-scalp acupuncture diminishes the loss of DAT while increasing the activity of striatum DAT for patients with Parkinson's disease.

Understanding the mechanism of acupuncture in Parkinson's patients gained more attention. It is believed that mechanism of action is related to moderating dopaminergic (DA) neurodegeneration in the substantia nigra (SN). To gain greater insight, Jeon *et al.* [31] conducted an animal study to determine whether acupuncture changes protein expression in the substantia nigra in a way that protects against neuronal degeneration. Mice received MPTP or a combination of MPTP and daily electro-acupuncture at Yanglingquan (GB34) for twelve consecutive days. Both interventions in MPTP mice restored behavioral impairment and protected against tyrosine hydroxylase (TH)-positive DA neurodegeneration. Researchers identified changes in twenty-two substantia nigra proteins after MPTP treatment; nine of these protein changes were restored after electro-acupuncture. Proteins affected were found to be related to cell death regulation, inflammation, or damage repair. Changes in levels of neuroprotective cyclophilin A (CypA) were not perceived in MPTP treatment; however, they were seen to increase in MPTP mice receiving electro-acupuncture. Researchers concluded that electro-acupuncture at Yanglingquan (GB34) changes protein expression within the substantia nigra, providing a protective role in DA neuronal survival for MPTP-treated mice; they suggested that electro-acupuncture may be an effective intervention for Parkinson's patients.

Adjuvant acupuncture applications in Parkinson's disease were further researched by Huang *et al.* [32] To determine cerebral effects, scalp-acupuncture with Madopar were administered to five patients, while another five received only Madopar for five weeks. PET scans among those in the electro-acupuncture group indicated increased glucose metabolisms in the parietal, temporal and occipital lobes, as well as the thalamus and the cerebellum in the light-diseased hemisphere. Glucose metabolism was also found to increase in parietal and occipital lobes of the severe-diseased hemisphere. No changes were seen among those receiving only Madopar. Researchers concluded that acupuncture in combination with Madopar seems to elevate cerebral glucose metabolism in patients with Parkinson's disease.

Parkinson's disease (PD) is closely associated with dopamine and its metabolic pathway. Loss of dopaminergic neurons in the substantia nigra (SN) and limited supply of striatal dopamine (DA) are considered primary factors in the development of the disease. To better understand the nature of acupuncture's positive action in human and animal models, Kim *et al.* [33], researched dopamine neurotransmission in a Parkinson's mouse model. Acupuncture at Yanglingquan (GB34), the influential point of the tendons, improved motor function and protected dopaminergic neurons against MPTP. Not surprisingly, acupuncture at GB34 did not restore striatal dopamine, as its function is more-closely related with influencing the liver system (which includes areas in the brain related to the function of the liver in TCM theory) and its capacity to regulate the tendons (thereby influencing tremor). Concordantly, acupuncture's mechanism was found to positively influence the initial neuronal regulators that initiate dopamine release. Downstream effects are then observed, such as greater dopamine availability in the synaptic cleft which then affects the tendons and fluidity of movement. Researchers also discovered that acupuncture served a protective role in maintaining normal function of the basal ganglia under the influence of MPTP. They suggested that acupuncture benefits may be due to an ability to increase post-synaptic dopamine neuro-transmission. Additionally, researchers concluded that acupuncture, by positively influencing synaptic dopamine levels, may combat harmful effects of MPTP.

Many nerve and neurological conditions have shown improvement with electro-acupuncture. Wang [34] performed preliminary rat studies to investigate the promise electro-acupuncture may hold for Parkinson's patients. Fifty rats were randomized into either a normal group, a control group, a model group, a pre-treatment group or a treatment group. The Parkinson's model was created by injecting rotenone. Controls received injection solution without active agent. Fengfu (DU16) and Taichong (LR3) electro-acupuncture was provided with interrupted wave, at low frequency, 1 mA in density, for 20 min. Treatment was administered once daily for 28 days. Rats in the pre-treatment group received the same electro-acupuncture as the treatment group for seven days, and then were subjected to the treatment received by the models. Abnormal manifestations such as yellow and coarse hair, the development of an arched back and slow movement, were lessened in both the treatment group and pre-treatment group. Compared with normal group and control group, the expression of Parkin, UCH-L1, UBE1, UB, TH in the model group decreased while alpha-synuclein increased (all $P<0.01$). After electro-acupuncture or pre-treatment, the expression of Parkin, UCH-L1, UBE1, UB, TH in both the treatment group and pre-treatment group was higher than in the models; expression of alpha-synuclein in the treatment group and pre-treatment group was lower than in the models (all $P<0.01$). Electro-acupuncture and pre-treatment showed both a protective function for rats with Parkinson's, and increase the effect of the ubiquitin-proteasome system. Research showed electro-acupuncture may be beneficial in both the treatment and prevention of Parkinson's via its effect on the ubiquitin-proteasome system.

Acupuncture for the treatment of Parkinson's disease has a precise clinical outcome. This study [35] investigated the effect of electroacupuncture at Fengfu (DU16) and Taichong (LR3) acupoints in rat models of Parkinson's disease induced by subcutaneous injection of rotenone into rat neck and back. Reverse transcription-PCR demonstrated that brain-derived neurotrophic factor and glial cell line-derived neurotrophic factor mRNA expression was significantly increased in the substantia nigra of rat models of Parkinson's disease, and that abnormal behavior of rats was significantly improved following electroacupuncture treatment. These results indicated that electroacupuncture treatment upregulated brain-derived neurotrophic factor and glial cell line-derived neurotrophic factor mRNA expression in the substantia nigra of rat models of Parkinson's disease. Thus, electroacupuncture may be useful in the treatment of Parkinson's disease.

Acupuncture is only one form of alternative interventions a patient with Parkinson's may use. Overall CAM use is seen approximately 40% or more of patients with Parkinson's disease. Ghaffari and Kluger [36] reviewed the frequently used alternatives, including acupuncture, tai chi, yoga, mindfulness, massage, herbal medicine, and cannabis. Researchers determined that studies on tai chi, acupuncture, cannabinoids, and music therapy lack sufficient data to substantiate the relevance or effectiveness of their use in patients with Parkinson's. They projected that most alternatives most likely treat

Parkinson's patients via generalized mechanisms, including placebo effect, reduction of stress and improving mood and sleep. Researchers also proposed that alternatives may serve to provide patients with a greater sense of control.

To gain greater insight into biochemical influences of electro-acupuncture in Parkinson's patients, Wang *et al.* [37], conducted an animal study with a rat model. Thirty-two male SD rats were randomized into control, sham-operation, model and electro-acupuncture groups. Parkinson's models were created. Electro-acupuncture was applied to Fengfu (DU16) and Taichong (LR3) daily for 20 minutes, over the course of fourteen days. Researchers found that horizontal and vertical movement scores were significantly lower in the model group than in controls; while rats receiving electro-acupuncture showed remarkably higher horizontal and vertical movement scores than those obtained by models (P<0. 05). Compared with the controls, TH protein expression in the substantia nigra in models showed significant reduction (P<0. 05); while the expression of p-ERK 1/2, TNF-α and IL-1β proteins all showed significant increases among models (P<0. 05). Electro-acupuncture was found to increase TH protein expression significantly (P<0.05), while significantly down-regulating expression of p-ERK 1/2, TNF-α and IL-1β (P<0. 05) compared to expression seen in the model group. Researchers concluded that electro-acupuncture shows signs of improvement among Parkinson's rat model ability to move. Positive effects may be due to down-regulation of the expression levels of p-ERK 1/2, TNF-α and IL-1β with concurrent up-regulation of TH expression in the substantia nigra.

Patients with Parkinson's disease often suffer from co-occurring behavioral changes that are of equal or greater disturbance than the physical symptoms. A novel study by researchers Kim *et al.* [38], revealed the underlying mechanisms of acupuncture combined with L-dopa on Parkinson's and the basal ganglia. Previously the researchers had showed that acupuncture may improve the motor function among Parkinson's disease (PD) mouse models by increasing the dopamine release and turn-over rate. In the current study, researchers predicted that the combination of L-dopa and acupuncture would have a positive effect on behavior in Parkinson's patients. Researchers discovered that half a dose of L-dopa (7.5 mg/kg) with acupuncture improved motor functioning equal to one full dose of L-dopa (15 mg/kg). Combining L-dopa and acupuncture was also found to be significantly superior in lowering AIM scores and the abnormal excess of GABA in the substantia nigra than L-dopa alone. Common side-effects of L-dopa were also reduced when administered in combination with acupuncture, reflected by blocking the abnormal expression of FosB, the gene related to L-dopa induced dyskinesia in the striatum.

In addition to obvious physical impairment, cognitive deficiencies experienced by afflicted Parkinson's patients is of great concern. Wattanathorn *et al.* [39], conducted a study to determine the effects of laser acupuncture at Shenmen (HT7) on memory, oxidative stress and the cholinergic and dopaminergic pathways in Parkinson's. A rat model was created by inducing a lesion at the right substantia nigra with 6-OHDA. Laser acupuncture was then administered continuously over the course of fourteen days. Researchers found that laser acupuncture at HT7 improved memory as well as neuronal density. A beneficial impact was also observed affecting concentrations of AChE, MAO-B, MDA, GSH-Px within the hippocampus. Researchers concluded that laser acupuncture at Shenmen (HT7) improves neuron degeneration and memory impairment in rat models of Parkinson's. Mechanism may be related to diminished oxidative stress in conjunction with optimized cholinergic and dopaminergic functioning. More research was suggested to determine the most beneficial treatment duration.

To further understand the biochemical effects of electro-acupuncture (EA) in Parkinson's patients, Li J. et al. conducted a study using a rat model. Forty-three rats were randomized into normal, model, electro-acupuncture and medication groups. The Parkinson's model was created by injecting Rotenone for twenty-eight days. The elector-acupuncture group received low-frequency, low-amp stimulation Baihui (DU20), Sanyinjiao (SP6) and Taichong (LR3) daily for ten minutes, over the course of fourteen days. Madopar suspension fluid (1.67 mg/kg) was administered daily to those in the medication group.

Researchers found that the diminished levels of SOD and GSH-Px activity, GSH contents, and excessive MDA content observed within the Substantia Nigra in the Parkinson's rats were effectively reversed by electro-acupuncture ($P < 0.05$). Medication only reversed exaggerated MDA content ($P > 0.05$). The TH immuno-activity and numbers of apoptotic cells of DA neurons were improved in both the electro-acupuncture and medication groups compared to models ($P < 0.05$), without significant differences between the electro-acupuncture and the medication groups ($P > 0.05$). Researchers also found that electro-acupuncture improved Parkinson's-induced abnormalities of the substantia nigra neurons (mild swelling of neurons with large nucleus and deranged fibers). To summarize, electro-acupuncture was found to decrease pathological changes within the substantial nigra in Parkinson's rat models. Mitigating effects were assessed to be associated with up-regulating the SOD and GSH-Px activity and GSH contents, while down-regulating MDA level, and decreasing apoptosis of DA neurons of the substantia nigra; the biochemical effects likely due to anti-oxidative action of electro-acupuncture.

In a study on the molecular mechanisms underlying acupuncture's effect on DA neuronal protection, Park *et al.* [41] demonstrated that p53 signaling mediates the protective effects of acupuncture treatment in a mouse model of PD. The study found that the acupuncture treatment in the mouse PD model results in significant recovery to the norm within the context of behavior and molecular signatures. The researchers also found that the gene network associated with p53 signaling is closely involved in the protective effects of acupuncture treatment in PD. They demonstrated that specific knockout of the p53 gene in the midbrain DA neurons abrogates the acupuncture induced protective effects in the mouse model of PD. This study suggested that p53 signaling mediates the protective effects of acupuncture treatment in PD.

In two studies, Qu *et al.* [42], explored the effects and action mechanism of electroacupuncture (EA) on Parkinson's disease (PD) with male SD rat models. Electroacupuncture (EA) was applied to "Fengfu" (DU16) and "Taichong" (LR3) at a rate of two Hz, and intensity of one mA for twenty minutes of duration in each treatment. The intervention was applied daily for twenty-eight consecutive days. In these well-designed studies with four arms (a normal group, a sham operation group, a model group and an EA group), the researchers demonstrated that electroacupuncture (EA) could improve the loss of dopaminergic neurons induced by rotenone to prevent and treat PD, (which is likely to be related to protecting the activity and expression of proteasomes in the substantia nigra).

Researchers [43] also explored the role of 26 S proteasome and nuclear factor kappa B (NFκB) within the substantia nigra and its influence on the management of Parkinson's disease (PD) by acupuncture. They further demonstrated that electroacupuncture (EA) intervention could improve PD rats' behavioral changes, which is probably related to its effects on reducing the loss of TH-positive neurons, down-regulating NFκB protein expression, and up- regulating 26 S proteasome protein expression in the substantia nigra. In another study using a similar research protocol, Wang *et al.* [44] demonstrated that the action mechanism of EA for prevention and treatment of Parkinson' s disease may be associated with inhibiting the activation of astrocytes.

In a clinical study to investigate the additional benefit of acupuncture adjunctive treatment to conventional medicine in patients with Parkinson's disease, Wang *et al.* [44] revealed that anti-neuroinflammation may be a mechanism of electroacupuncture adjunctive treatment.

Parkinson's disease (PD) is characterized by the death of dopamine-generating cells in the substantia nigra (SN). Yeo *et al.* [45] conducted a study to explore the mechanism of acupuncture stimulation in the enhanced survival of dopaminergic neurons in the substantia nigra (SN) in Parkinson's animal models. The study investigated changes in gene expression profiles. After acupuncture stimulation was applied at Yanglingquan (GB34) and Taichong (LR3), researchers discovered that acupuncture attenuated the decrease in tyrosine hydroxylase in the substantia nigra (SN) region; while stimulation at non-acupoints did not suppress this decrease. The study indicated that acupuncture may be responsible for the inhibitory effects on degeneration-related gene expression in the substantia nigra (SN) following damage induced by MPTP intoxication.

CHAPTER SIX

ACUPUNCTURE FOR STROKES

Stroke is the third leading cause of death in Western society; in China it is the second most common cause of death in cities and the third in rural areas. It is also a main cause of adult disability and dependency. Acupuncture for strokes has been used in China for thousands of years and is increasingly practiced in some Western countries. Just as Western doctors have delineated the etiology and pathology of cerebrovascular accidents in modern scientific terminology, Chinese medicine doctors developed their own theories and practice in regard to the etiology and pathology of stroke events.

This chapter on acupuncture for strokes is organized into six sections:

- Cerebrovascular Accidents from a Western medical Perspective
- Stroke Etiology, Pathology and Treatment Principles in Chinese Medicine
- Innovative Acupuncture Techniques for Stroke
- Case Reports: Treating Stroke with Acupuncture
- Modern Research: Acupuncture in Stroke Rehabilitation
- Critical Commentary on Acupuncture Therapy for Strokes, with Response

Cerebrovascular Accidents: an Introduction

A cerebrovascular accident (CVA), or stroke, occurs when the blood flow to an area of the brain is interrupted by a blood clot or ruptured artery or blood vessel. The consequent lack of oxygen and glucose supply to affected brain tissue leads to brain damage and cellular death, and often results in such attendant brain-related dysfunction as loss of motor function, speech impairment, and memory loss. In most advanced countries, stroke is the third-leading cause of death, after cardiovascular accidents and cancer.

Types of Stroke

The two principal types of stroke are ischemic stroke and hemorrhagic stroke.

Ischemic stroke occurs when a blood clot, or thrombus, blocks blood flow to part of the brain. A blood clot which has formed somewhere in the body's vascular system, and breaks off to become free-floating, is called an embolus. An embolus may be carried through the bloodstream to the brain, where it can cause an ischemic stroke. Blood clots (thrombus clots) usually occur in areas of the arteries that have been damaged by atherosclerosis and a buildup of plaques. Atherosclerosis and hypertension are the main causes of cerebral thrombosis. Causes for embolus formation include cardiac disease, cardiac surgery, atherosclerotic plaques, pulmonary venous thrombosis, and fracture of a long bone, poor circulation, and post-operative inactivity. Embolus-type blood clots are often caused by atrial fibrillation – an irregular pattern of heartbeat that leads to blood clot formation and poor blood flow. Ischemic stroke accounts for about 75% of all strokes.

A transient ischemic attack (TIA) is a temporary interruption in blood flow to part of the brain, and is often referred to as a "small stroke" or a "silent stroke." It is generally caused by micro-emboli passing into the small blood vessels leading to the brain. An acute TIA attack will cause some of the same symptoms as an ischemic stroke, depending on the part of the brain affected, but symptoms will only last from two to thirty minutes, and there is no noticeable permanent damage. A mild TIA may not produce any symptoms, but can still damage brain tissue. TIAs are most common in the middle-aged and elderly, and women are more likely to experience non-traditional stroke symptoms than men. The most significant aspect of TIAs is that they are frequently a precursor of a full-blown stroke: approximately one-third of TIA patients will experience a stroke within five years of their TIA episode.

There are two types of hemorrhagic stroke: subarachnoid hemorrhage and cerebral hemorrhage. Subarachnoid hemorrhage occurs when a blood vessel on the brain's surface ruptures and fills the space between the brain and skull with blood. Cerebral hemorrhage occurs when a defective artery inside the brain bursts and fills the surrounding tissue with blood. Both types of hemorrhage result in a lack of normal blood flow to brain cells, causing cellular death, while the extravasated blood pools into a buildup that puts too much pressure on the brain. Hemorrhagic strokes are most often caused by uncontrolled high blood pressure, a head injury, or aneurysms.

Arteriovenous malformations, infections, and tumors may also be causative factors. High blood pressure is the most common cause of cerebral hemorrhage, as it often causes small arteries inside the brain to rupture. Hemorrhagic strokes account for about 15% of all strokes.

Aneurysms are abnormal blood-filled pouches that balloon out from weak spots in the wall of an artery. Cerebral aneurysms are the most common cause of subarachnoid hemorrhage. When an aneurysm ruptures, blood spills into the space between the surfaces of the brain and skull, and blood vessels in the brain may spasm. Aneurysms are often caused or made worse by high blood pressure.

An arteriovenous malformation (AVM) is an abnormal tangle of thin-walled blood vessels that is present at birth. Hemorrhagic strokes can also result from the rupture of an AVM, but this is much less common than subarachnoid or cerebral hemorrhage.

Cerebral Arteriosclerosis is a condition of thickening or calcification of arterial walls, with loss of elasticity, which produces a decrease in cerebral blood flow, leading to tissue damage and impairment of brain function. It generally coexists with coronary and renal arteriosclerosis. Since it affects brain tissue, it produces many of the same symptoms as stroke.

Lacunar cerebral infarction is an obstruction of the blood supply of small areas of the brain resulting from the occlusion of small penetrating branches of the major cerebral arteries.

Symptoms of Stroke

Within a few minutes of having a stroke, brain cells begin to die, producing symptoms. It is important to recognize symptoms, as prompt treatment is crucial to recovery. Common symptoms include:

- Dizziness
- Trouble walking
- Loss of balance and coordination
- Hemiplegia
- Facial paralysis
- Speech problems, deviated mouth
- Hypertension
- Numbness, weakness, or paralysis on one side of the body
- Blurred, blackened, or double vision

- Sudden severe headache
- Incontinence of stools and urine

Diagnosis of Stroke

A stroke is a medical emergency. Anyone suspected of having a stroke should be taken to a hospital immediately so that tests can be run and the correct treatment can be provided as quickly as possible. Diagnostic methods employed by Western medicine include the following:

- Physical assessment: physical examination; blood pressure check; laboratory tests for cholesterol levels, blood sugar levels, and amino acid levels.
- Ultrasound imaging: high-frequency sound waves create an image of internal structures, such as arteries. An ultrasound of the carotid arteries can show any narrowing or clotting.
- Arteriography: Arteries are visualized by means of x-ray, after a dye has been introduced into the blood vessels via catheter.
- Computerized tomography (CT): An x-ray procedure which produces a three-dimensional image of internal structures. A CT scan of the brain can show aneurysms, bleeding, or abnormal vessels within the brain.
- Magnetic resonance imaging (MRI): A magnetic field generates a three-dimensional image of internal structures and tissue. An MRI of the brain assesses tissue damaged by stroke.
- CT and MRI with angiography: X-ray or magnetic-field scans are enhanced by injecting dye into the blood vessels in order to provide clearer and more detailed images.
- Echocardiography: Ultrasound waves are directed through the heart to make images of the heart. The heart can be examined for structural abnormalities and for emboli.

Treatment of Stroke

Outcomes after a stroke depend on what areas of the brain are affected and how much of the brain is affected. Smaller strokes may result in minor problems, such as weakness in an arm or leg, or difficulty speaking clearly. Larger strokes may lead to paralysis or death. Many stroke patients are left with weakness on one side of the body, difficulty speaking, incontinence, and bladder problems.

The primary goal in treating ischemic stroke is to restore blood flow to the brain. Since ischemic strokes are caused by blood clots, the first line of treatment is to administer "clot-busting" drugs such as aspirin, heparin, or tissue plasminogen activators. To be effective, these drugs must be administered within three hours of the stroke. Beyond that, surgical procedures may be performed which can open or widen arteries. These include carotid endarterectomy, which involves surgical removal of plaque from artery walls; and angioplasty, which involves introducing a balloon into an artery to widen it, then holding the artery open by implanting a metallic mesh tube called a stent.

The primary consideration in treating hemorrhagic stroke is to stop active bleeding, and then to relieve pressure on brain tissue from extravasated blood. Surgery is often used to stop bleeding. For subarachnoid hemorrhages caused by an aneurysm or an arteriovenous malformation, surgical methods include aneurysm clipping, aneurysm embolization, and arteriovenous malformation (AVM) removal. Aneurysm clipping clamps off the aneurysm to isolate it from the artery it's attached to, and keeps the aneurysm from bursting or re-bleeding. Aneurysm embolization (coiling) inserts a tiny coil into the aneurysm which fills the aneurysm and causes clotting, sealing it off from its artery. AVM removal surgically excises smaller AVMs, or AMVs that are in more accessible portions of the brain, in order to eliminate the risk of rupture. Surgery is not generally applied to cerebral hemorrhages, where the affected artery is deeper in the brain. Patients who are recovering from an acute stroke are kept immobile, in a position which avoids flexion of the head and neck, in order to promote adequate blood flow to and from the head.

Rehabilitation after a stroke event is aimed at restoring as much physiological function as possible to the patient, and helping the patient to be self-sufficient with his activities of daily living (ADLs). The ability to recover is based on the area of the brain which was affected by the stroke, and the amount of tissue that was damaged. It is common for the rehabilitation process to include speech therapy, occupational therapy, physical therapy, and family education.

Prevention of Stroke

Much of stroke prevention is based on living a healthy lifestyle. This includes:

- Being aware of and controlling hypertension
- Diagnosing atrial fibrillation
- Not smoking
- Lowering cholesterol, sodium, and fat intake
- Following a healthy diet
- Moderate alcohol consumption
- Being aware of and controlling diabetes
- Exercising regularly
- Managing stress
- Being aware of TIA symptoms
- Not using drugs

There are studies which support these additional stroke-prevention methods:

- Drinking three cups of tea per day
- Taking preventive medications such as anti-platelet and anticoagulant drugs to prevent blood clots
- Taking cholesterol-lowering drugs to prevent stroke recurrence

Risk Factors of Stroke

Anyone can suffer from stroke. Although many risk factors for stroke are out of our control, several can be kept in line through proper nutrition and medical care. Risk factors for stroke include the following:

- Over age 55
- Male
- African American, Hispanic or Asian/Pacific Islander
- A family history of stroke
- Systolic or diastolic hypertension
- High cholesterol levels, unhealthy diet
- Smoking cigarettes
- Diabetes
- Obesity and overweight
- Sedentary lifestyle
- Cardiovascular disease
- A previous stroke or transient ischemic attack (TIA)
- High levels of homocysteine (an amino acid in blood)
- Genetic defect
- Use of oral contraceptives or other hormone therapy

- Cocaine use
- Heavy alcohol consumption

Stroke Etiology, Pathology and Treatment Principles in Chinese Medicine

Innovative Ideas in Understanding Stroke

Understanding etiology and pathology of stroke has experienced three main stages in Chinese medicine. In the first stage external wind was emphasized. The analysis of Zhong Zhongjing in Han Dynasty and Chao Yuanfang in Sui Dynasty is the framework of this understanding. In Zhang Zhongjing, external wind could attack collateral, meridians, zang organs and fu organs. In Chao Yuanfang, external wind could attack heart, liver, spleen, kidneys and lung. The pathology of external wind dominates the etiological and pathological analysis of stroke for one thousand years. In the second stage starting from Song Dynasty, innovation in Chinese medicine advanced the etiology and pathology of stroke. Liu Wansu proposed the theory of heart fire explosion. Li Dongyuan suggested qi deficiency as the main mechanism of stroke. Zhu Zhenheng believed that phlegm heat is the main pathogenesis. Since China started to integrate western medicine with Chinese medicine in the 19th century, the theory of liver yang uprising, liver wind disturbance, qi and blood rebellion upward became prevalent. In contemporary Chinese medicine, obstruction of orifices became the most popular theory, especially in acupuncture. Based on this understanding, Xing Nao Kai Qiao or XNKQ, translated as Arousing the Brain and Opening the Orifices technique was developed by Dr. Shi Xuemin. The theoretical basis of XNKQ in TCM terms is based on activating and regulating the spirit, restoring qi and spirit, regulating yin/yang and qi/blood dynamics, dredging the meridians, and supplementing the marrow. The Chinese medicine etiology and pathology of stroke as follows: Fire, phlegm, blood (stasis), and deficiency are carried upward by internal wind, disturbing the sensory orifices and the spirit, and leading to blockage of the orifices and concealment of the spirit. A stroke occurs because the spirit can no longer guide qi properly. Dr. Shi combined his TCM-based theory of the origins of stroke with a thorough knowledge of the anatomy and physiology of the brain in biomedical terms.

Clinical outcomes and scientific research both show that the traditional acupuncture treatment for stroke patients has a positive effect in stabilizing the disease process and improving physical function. However, there were no clear indications as to the effects of traditional acupuncture on improving cerebral circulation and protecting brain cells from further insult.

Dr. Shi's analysis of the etiology, pathogenesis, disease location, and manifestations of stroke from a biomedical viewpoint led him to focus on the yin meridians and the Du meridian as the principal avenues of treatment in the XNKQ method. The goal of XNKQ treatment is to activate the brain, open the orifices, and nourish the Liver and Kidney. Treating the meridians and collaterals is supplementary. So far, clinical outcomes and evidence seem to indicate that the XNKQ method has a more demonstrable effect on cerebral circulation and brain cell health than traditional acupuncture for stroke.

Stroke diagnosis and treatment is based on the following theoretical constructs of TCM: yin/yang imbalance; qi and blood deficiency; circulation of qi and blood in the meridians and collaterals; zang/fu (internal organ) function; and the actions of external and internal pathogenic factors.

Symptoms or manifestations of stroke are analyzed according to the principles of TCM, and are understood as recognizable patterns, or etiologies.

Strokes are first characterized as acute or sub-acute, with three main acute patterns and five main sub-acute patterns. Whether a stroke is acute or sub-acute, it will have resulted from one of the following underlying etiological patterns:

Principal Etiology/Pathology Patterns for Stroke

1. Depletion of Qi and Blood, which is caused by complicated by emotional factors, dietary irregularities and external pathogenic factors.

- At night, yang is subordinate to yin and blood flows back to the Liver, leaving the body more susceptible to attack by internal or external pathogens.
- Deficient qi and blood allow phlegm production.
- Insufficient qi and blood in the channels and collaterals.
- Easy for pathogenic factors to invade the body.
- Blood stasis obstructs the collaterals.
- Phlegm obstructs the orifices of the heart and mists the clear orifices of the head.
- Results in hemilateral paralysis, deviation of the mouth, paralysis of the tongue and slurred speech.

2. Imbalance of Yin and Yang:

- Emotional disturbances, stress, overwork depletes Kidney and Liver yin.
- Liver yang rises and generates internal wind and/or fire.
- Mixing with fire from the Liver or Heart, wind and fire further deplete the water in the lower jiao leading to exuberant fire in the upper jiao.
- Qi and blood flow recklessly upwards.
- Phlegm turbidity is generated and obstructs the collaterals along with qi and blood.
- Results in hemiplegia.

3. Phlegm Turbidity Obstructing the Middle Jiao:

- Overindulgence in sweet and fatty foods or alcohol impairs the functions of the Spleen.
- The Spleen's transformation and transportation functions are impaired, and damp-phlegm is generated.
- Damp-phlegm causes a counter-flow of qi and stagnation.
- Damp-phlegm and stagnation can transform into heat that stirs Liver wind.
- Liver-wind, -heat or -fire combines with damp turbidity and flows upwards to harass and mist the clear orifices.
- Results in paralysis.

4. Wind-Phlegm:

- Excessive fatigue consumes qi, or a poor diet damages qi.
- Generates phlegm.
- Depletion of the yang qi.
- Pathogenic wind combines with phlegm and enters into the channels and collaterals.
- Obstruction of qi and blood.
- Results in paralysis.

5. The Brain is the House of the Spirit:

- The brain is the locus of mental functions and governs mental and intellectual activities.

- Wind-phlegm, phlegm-fire or excessive yang rising causes qi and blood to surge upwards.
- Results in syncope and loss of consciousness.

Acute-Phase Patterns of Stroke

Acute stroke episodes are related to a severe imbalance of yang or yang qi, leading to a sudden loss of consciousness. In heat patterns, internal wind drives Liver yang and turbidity upwards, blocking the sensory orifices. In cold patterns, qi movement is blocked by cold and phlegm. In the "desertion" pattern, yang qi has collapsed. Acute-phase patterns primarily affect the zang/fu organs.

1. Yang Blockage Pattern (Heat) is manifested as Sudden loss of consciousness, clenched teeth; fingers flexed into a fist; neck rigidity; constipation; enuresis; spastic limbs; red complexion; fever, restlessness; red or crimson-red tongue with a yellow coating; wiry-slippery or rapid pulse. Treatment principles include Clear Heat and Relieve Toxicity; Open Sensory Orifices; Extinguish Internal Wind; Subdue Liver Yang; Transform Turbidity; Calm Shen.

2. Yin Blockage Pattern (Cold) is manifested as Sudden loss of consciousness; clenched teeth; fingers flexed into a fist; hypertonicity; neck rigidity; constipation; enuresis; pale complexion; no spastic limbs; cold extremities; white-greasy tongue coating; deep and slippery pulse. Treatment principles include Warm Yang Qi; Open Orifices; Dispel Cold; Promote Movement of Qi; Transform Turbidity.

3. Desertion Pattern is manifested as sudden loss of consciousness; open eyes and mouth; feeble breath; relaxed fingers; cold extremities; spontaneous sweating; dizziness; incontinence of stool and urine; flaccidity of the limbs; pale tongue; faint or indistinct pulse. Treatment principles include Restore Yang; Tonify Source Qi; Rescue Qi from Collapse.

Sub-Acute Patterns of Stroke

While acute-phase patterns of stroke primarily involve the zang/fu, sub-acute patterns of stroke primarily involve an invasion of the meridians and collaterals. In the five sub-acute patterns described below, the name of the pattern describes the etiology involved.

1. Wind and Phlegm-Damp Obstruction in the Network Collaterals is manifested as sudden hemiplegia; deviation of the mouth and eye; slurred speech; deviated tongue; inability to walk; hemiplegia; numbness; weak limbs; lack of sensation in the extremities; muscle spasms; irritability; thirst; dry mouth; shortness of breath; fatigue; dizziness; headache; chest oppression; profuse phlegm; profuse urination; swollen tongue with a white-greasy coating; wiry-thin or slippery pulse. Treatment principles include Dissolve Phlegm; Extinguish Internal Wind; Clear Heat; Transform Dampness; Invigorate Blood; Nourish Qi and Blood.

2. Wind and Yang Qi Harassing Upwards is manifested as Sudden onset of heaviness and numbness or paralysis of the limbs; deviation of the mouth and eyes; stiff tongue; slurred speech; sudden headache; dizziness; loss of consciousness; red tongue with a yellow coating or no coating; wiry-rapid or slippery-rapid pulse. Treatment principles include Pacify the Liver; Subdue Liver Yang; Extinguish Internal Wind; Enrich Yin

3. Liver and Kidney Yin Deficiency is manifested as sudden hemiplegia; deviated mouth; stiff tongue with sluggish speech or drooling; aphasia; flaccidity and numbness of the limbs; dizziness; headache; tinnitus; restlessness; insomnia; red complexion and lips; red tongue with a yellow-greasy or little coating; wiry-fine and rapid pulse. Treatment principles include Enrich Liver and Kidney Yin; Extinguish Internal Wind; Nourish and Strengthen Bones and Sinews; Free Collaterals.

4. Qi Deficiency and Blood Stasis Obstruction in the Network Collaterals is manifested as Sudden onset of hemiplegia; deviation of eye and mouth; slurred speech; drooping of the mouth; flaccidity or numbness of the limbs on one side of the body; limitation of movement, or stiffness of the joints and contraction of the muscles; absentmindedness; nervousness; sallow complexion; frequent and clear urination or incontinent urination; pale-purple tongue body or with spots, white tongue coating; fine and choppy or deep and thready pulse. Treatment principles include Tonify Qi; Invigorate Blood; Remove Blood Stasis; Invigorate Circulation in the Meridians.

5. Phlegm Heat is manifested as acute onset of hemiplegia; deviation of the mouth and eye; severe headache; constipation; dizziness; stiff tongue; yellow and greasy tongue coating; wiry-rapid or slippery-rapid pulse. Treatment principles include Purge Heat; Regulate Qi; Transform Phlegm; Dredge the Channels.

Innovative Acupuncture Techniques for Stroke

In Chinese hospitals which provide traditional medical care, the stroke department is almost invariably the largest department in the hospital. Stroke therapy is one area of "traditional" Chinese medicine which has expanded significantly in the modern era, as evidenced by the enormous number of studies and research papers published in the last 50 years (mostly from China and Japan). Although there is a standard acupuncture prescription which was developed for acute-phase strokes before modern emergency medical procedures were available, acupuncture therapy is now used primarily for rehabilitative purposes.

In China and Japan, acupuncture therapy for ischemic-type strokes is started as soon as possible after a stroke, with the objective of opening blocked channels and promoting qi and blood flow. In the case of hemorrhagic strokes, it is recommended to wait several weeks until the ruptured blood vessel has clotted and stopped bleeding. This recommendation is based on studies showing that acupuncture can open blood vessels and decrease clotting and inflammation, which could aggravate a hemorrhagic condition. Post-stroke acupuncture is generally done on a daily basis in Chinese hospitals, or even several times per day. Treatment is done intensively in hospitals for several weeks, and then maintenance treatment may be continued on an outpatient basis.

This section will outline several therapeutic strategies for stroke, beginning with the traditional yangming approach, meridian connection approach, and then describing several recently-developed therapies including Xing Nao Kai Qiao, scalp acupuncture, and Jin's Three-Needling technique. A TCM acupuncture approach is presented at the end of this chapter.

1. Yangming Approach

Classical Chinese acupuncture for stroke emphasizes "using the three yang meridians to treat wind" and "using yangming meridians to treat apoplexy." Classical Chinese acupuncture texts documented a number of acupuncture prescriptions, either individual points or combined in groups. All the main points were selected from three yang meridians. For example, in *Systematic Classic of Acupuncture and Moxibustion (Zhen Jiu Jia Yi Jing)*, acupuncture points used to treat stroke include Daju (ST27), Hegu (LI4), Wangu (GB12), Zulinqi (GB41), and Jinggu (BL64). In the *Classic of Supplementing Life with Acupuncture and Moxibustion (Zhen Jiu Zi Sheng Jing*), Baihui (DU20), Xinhui (DU22), Fengchi (GB20), Jianyu (LI15), Quchi (LI11),

Hegu (LI4), Huantiao (GB30), Fengshi (GB31), Zusanli (ST36), and Juegu (GB39). In the *Classic of Magical Effective Treatment (Shen Ying Jing)*, Jianyu (LI15), Quchi (LI11), Lieque (LU7), Hegu (LI4), Shousanli (LI10), Huantiao (GB30), Fengshi (GB31), Zusanli (ST36), Weizhong (BL40), Juegu (GB39), Qiuxu (GB40), Yanglingquan (GB34), Kunlun (BL60), and Zhaohai (KI6) were prescribed for stroke. Another prescription for stroke in the *Classic of Magical Effective Treatment (Shen Ying Jing)* is Quchi (LI11), Yangxi (LI5), Hegu (LI4), Zhongdu (GB32), Zusanli (ST36), Yangfu (GB38), and Kunlun (BL60). This yangming approach was the dominant approach to stroke before XNKQ was developed.

2. Meridian Connection Method

Zhang Yuansu, who lived during the Jin Dynasty (1115-1234) was one of the four Jin/Yuan innovators in Chinese medicine history. He developed Meridian Connection Method for treating stroke which was recorded in *Treasure Mirror of Hygiene (Wei Sheng Bao Jian),* written by Luo Tianyi, who lived during the Yuan Dynasty (1206-1368). This technique is applied to the twelve Jing points. It functions to unblock the qi and blood in the twelve meridians and smoothly transition the yin and yang from meridian to meridian.

Two separate approaches were developed in the Meridian Connection Method. One is inducing yin from yang. The needling sequence is Zhiyin (BL67), Yongquan (KI1), Zhongchong (PC9), Guanchong (SJ1), Zuqiaoyin (GB41), Dadun (LR1), Shaoshang (LU11), Shangyang (LI1), Lidui (ST44), Yinbai (SP1), Shaochong (HT9), and Shaoze (SI1). The other one is inducing yang from yin. The needling sequence is Shaoshang (LU11), Shangyang (LI1), Yinbai (SP1), Shaochong (HT9), Shaoze (SI1), Zhiyin (BL67), Yongquan (LI1), Zhongchong (PC9), Guanchong (SJ1), Lidui (ST44), Zuqiaoyin (GB41), and Dadun (LR1).

3. Xing Nao Kai Qiao

Xing Nao Kai Qiao (XNKQ) was developed in 1972, opening a new and innovative approach to the treatment and rehabilitation of stroke patients. XNKQ was such a promising treatment method that it quickly developed into a standardized diagnostic and treatment system which is widely practiced today.

Acupuncture Prescription: The basic prescription of XNKQ includes Renzhong (DU26), Neiguan (PC6), Sanyinjiao (SP6), Jiquan (HT1), Chize

(LU5), and Weizhong (BL40). In this prescription, Renzhong (DU26) is the crossing point of the du, large intestine and stomach meridians. It opens the orifices, revives the spirit, and regulates viscera. Ancient doctors greatly valued Renzhong (DU26) as an important point to arouse the brain in emergency situations; it has an excitatory effect on the nervous system and it has an idiosyncratic effect of increasing blood flow in the carotid artery while improving cerebral circulation. Neiguan (PC6) is the luo-connecting point of the pericardium meridian and confluent point of the Yin Wei meridian. It nourishes the heart, calms the spirit, regulates qi and blood, and improves the cardiac output of stroke patients and improves the supply of oxygen to the brain. Sanyinjiao (PC6) is the crossing point of the spleen, liver and kidney meridians. It tonifies the kidney, generates marrow, and benefits the brain. Jiquan (HT1), Chize (LU5), and Weizhong (BL40) serve to dredge and activate meridians and collaterals, and promote circulation of qi and blood in limbs.

Supplementary acupuncture points for stroke indications include: For difficulty swallowing, add Fengchi (GB20), Wangu (GB12), Tianzhu (BL10); For slurred speech, add Shanglianquan (RN23), Jinjin (Extra), Yuye (Extra); For foot-drop, add Qiuxu (GB40) penetrating to Zhaohai (KI6); For constipation, add Fenglong (ST40), Shuidao (ST28), Guilai (ST29), Waishuidao (Extra), Waiguilai (Extra); For hypertension, add Renying (ST9), Hegu (LI4), Taichong (LR3); For retention of urine, add Shangxing (DU23) penetrating to Baihui (DU20).

Needling Techniques: The XNKQ method enforces strict attention to techniques of needle manipulation on its principal points. This insistence on uniformity and consistency of needle manipulation is a key factor in the method's effectiveness. Each point has clear specifications on needle direction and depth of insertion, and the hand techniques used in manipulation. Scientific research on the XNKQ method has studied the effectiveness of various approaches, establishing the greatest effectiveness of the techniques under study. One of the key differences between XNKQ and traditional acupuncture methods is the importance given to acupoints that arouse the spirit and open the orifices in order to achieve the effect of regulating and freeing the original spirit.

Needling Technique for Principal Points:

- Renzhong (DU26): Puncture obliquely toward nasal septum with sparrow-pecking reducing method until the eyes are full of tears.

- Neiguan (PC6): Perpendicularly puncture PC 6 on both sides, to a depth of 1-1.5 cun, with rotating and lift-thrust reducing method for 1-3 minutes.
- Sanyinjiao (SP6): Puncture obliquely to a depth of 1-1.5 cun along the border of the tibia at a 45-degree angle, then manipulate with lifting-thrusting reinforcing method, and let the leg tic three times.
- Jiquan (HT1): Puncture perpendicularly to a depth of 1-1.5 cun with lift-thrust reducing method, and let the arm tic three times.
- Weizhong (BL40): Let the patient lie on his back and raise the affected leg to about 45 degrees. Puncture Weizhong (BL40) perpendicularly, to a depth of 1-1.5 cun with lift-thrust reducing method and let the leg tic three times.

Dr. Shi refers to his needling technique as "quantitative acupuncture manipulation." The main aspects of needling which are emphasized in the XNKQ method are: Reinforcing and reducing methods of needle manipulation, with special attention to twirling and rotating of needles; Direction of applied force, which is an important factor in determining reinforcing vs. reducing; Duration of manipulation technique, which is considered best at 1 – 3 minutes for each point; Most effective interval between acupuncture sessions, which is 3 – 6 hours.

Additionally, Dr. Shi investigated commonly-applied methods of reinforcing and reducing technique in terms of frequency, range, and direction of applied force. His research on quantification of reinforcing and reducing manipulation techniques resulted in two significant definitions: 1) The Ren and Du meridians are in the center of the body, in a central position in relation to the twelve principal meridians. Using the position of the Ren and Du meridians to define the direction of needle rotation, Dr. Shi determined that directing the needle rotation towards the heart is reinforcing and directing the needle rotation away from the heart is reducing. 2) Rotating the needles within a narrow range with light force and high frequency is reinforcing; rotating needles with a wide angle, increased force and lower frequency is reducing. For reinforcing, needles are rotated within a 90-degree angle, and the frequency of rotation reaches 120 times per minute. For reducing, the angle of rotation is greater than 180 degrees, and the frequency is approximately 50-60 times per minute.

The overall recommended treatment regime is three to five consecutive courses of treatment, with one treatment course consisting of needling twice per day for ten days.

The XNKQ method has been used on more than two million stroke victims to date. Stroke patients were typically given XNKQ therapy along with other modalities such as hypertension medication, physical therapy, etc. Studies indicate marked improvement in 95 – 98 percent of those patients, which included patients in acute and sub-acute stages of stroke.

4. Scalp Acupuncture

Scalp acupuncture is a form of microacupuncture. Any system of microacupuncture, such as scalp acupuncture or auricular acupuncture, views one particular area of the body as a microcosm of the entire body. There are a number of regular acupuncture points on the head, such as Gallbladder meridian or Du meridian points, but scalp acupuncture incorporates these acupoints, as well as other points and lines, into a comprehensive system on its own terms.

Scalp acupuncture as a recognized system is a product of the twentieth century. In the 1970s, three Chinese acupuncturists independently developed scalp acupuncture systems. These systems were combined and standardized in the 1980s. However, variations on scalp acupuncture continued to be developed and practiced, including a system developed by Zhu Mingqing which is one of the most widely-practiced systems today. Dr. Zhu achieved a spectacular validation of his system in 1987 at a stroke conference in Beijing, when a seriously debilitated patient he performed acupuncture on got up and began walking around.

Two approaches to scalp acupuncture are illustrated below. The first one, "International Standardized Scalp Stimulation Areas and Indications", divides the scalp into anatomical regions, such as the frontal or parietal region, and ascribes functions and indications to the points in each region. Furthermore, different points in each scalp region can address health problems in specific areas of the body. For example, the #1 Lateral Line of the Forehead addresses lung and heart problems, while the #3 Lateral Line of the Forehead addresses genito-urinary problems. The second one, "Jiao's Style Scalp Acupuncture," locates stimulation areas on the scalp and describes them from a more functional perspective, such as motor functions or sensory functions.

Scalp acupuncture points must be needled obliquely, due to the presence of bone just beneath the skin. However, points in the scalp acupuncture system are usually needled more deeply than the regular body acupuncture points on the head. This is accomplished by inserting the needles farther into the connective tissue and manipulating the needles more intensively.

Because scalp acupuncture was developed recently (in Chinese medicine terms), it incorporates modern scientific insights into neurology and brain function. By the time scalp acupuncture was developed, for example, it was well known that one side of the brain controls the opposite side of the body. Therefore, left-sided arm paralysis is treated by needling the right side of the scalp.

International Standard of Scalp Acupuncture

In the International Standard of Scalp Acupuncture, stimulation areas for stroke include the following in the parietal region:

Middle Line of Vertex (MS5), which is located on the head, at the middle line of the head, from Baihui (DU20) to Qianding (DU21) along the Du meridian;

Anterior Oblique Line of Vertex-Temporal (MS 6) which is located from 1 cun anterior to DU20 (Baihui) to Xuanli (GB6). MS6 can be divided into 5 parts, the upper 1/5 treating the opposite leg and trunk paralysis; the middle 2/5 treating arm paralysis of the opposite side; the lower 2/5 treating the central facial palsy, motor aphasia.

Posterior Oblique Line of Vertex-Temporal (MS7), which is located 1 cun posterior to MS 6, from Baihui (DU20) to Qubin (GB7). MS7 can be divided into 5 parts, the upper 1/5 treats the opposite leg and trunk abnormal sensation; the middle 2/5 treats abnormal sensation of the opposite arm; the lower 2/5 treats abnormal sensation of the head and facial.

Lateral Line of Vertex #1 (MS 8), which is located 1.5 cun long line lateral to the middle line of vertex (MS 5), from Tongtian (BL7) draw a 1.5 cun line.

And Lateral Line of Vertex #2 (MS9), which is located 2.25 cun lateral to the middle line of the vertex (MS 5), a 1.5 cun long straight line from Zhengying (GB17) to Chengling (GB18).

And Anterior Line of Temporal (MS10) located in the temporal region, a line from Hanyan (GB4) to Xuanli (GB6).

Jiao Shunfa's Scalp Acupuncture

In Jiao Shunfa's Scalp Acupuncture, stimulation areas include:

Motor Area which is located the superior point is located 0.5 cm posterior to the midpoint of the anterior-posterior midline, the inferior point at the junction of the brow-occipital line and the anterior border of the temporal hairline, the line connecting the two points is the motor area. Indications: the upper 1/5 is for the contralateral paralysis of the lower limb; the middle 2/5 is for contralateral paralysis of the upper limb, and the lower 2/5 is for the contralateral central facial paralysis, aphemia, drooling and dysphonia.

Sensory Area which is located parallel and 1.5 cm posterior to the motor area. Indications: the upper 1/5 is for the contralateral lower back, leg pain, numbness, paresthesia, occiput pain, neck pain, vertigo, tinnitus; the middle 2/5 is for contralateral upper limb pain, numbness, paresthesia; the lower 2/5 is for the contralateral facial numbness, migraine, headache, and temporomandibular arthritis.

The Second Speech Area which is located the straight line 2.0 cm posterior to the parietal tubercle and parallel to the anterior-posterior midline, stretching 3 cm straightly and downwards.

The Third Speech Area, which is located one 4.0 cm horizontal line on each side, with the anterior end at the point 1.5 cm directly above the apex of the ear.

Application Area, which is located three lines from the parietal tubercle downward. The middle line is straight and the angle of the bilateral lines from the straight line is 40 degrees respectively. All the three lines are 3 cm in length.

Motor and Sensory Area of Foot, which is located two straight lines 3 cm stretching back 1 cm from both sides of the midpoint of the anteroposterior median line and parallel to the midline.

Balance Area, which is located a straight line 4 cm stretching downwards and 3.5 cm from both sides of the posterior point of the anteroposterior midline and parallel to the midline.

5. Jin's Three-Needle Approach

Three-Needle techniques were developed by Jin Rui, an acupuncture expert in Guangdong University of Traditional Chinese Medicine. Three-needle technique is an acupuncture technique that uniquely formulates acupuncture prescriptions and groups of acupuncture points to treat certain diseases, conditions and patterns. This technique is so-called because three acupuncture points are the core in each prescription. Therefore, the "three-needle" name refers to three acupuncture points. These points are selected from the fourteen regular meridians, extraordinary points or other points defined in specific ways.

For stroke conditions such as cerebrovascular accident sequelae, hemiplegia, deviation of eye and mouth due to brain trauma, and cerebral arteriosclerosis, the three-needle technique on the temple area (Temple Three-Needle) is recommended. The three points are Temple I, Temple II, and Temple III.

Temple I: On the temple area, 2 cun above the ear apex.
Temple II: On the temple area, 1 cun anterior to Temple I.
Temple III: On the temple area, 1 cun posterior to Temple I.
Manipulation: Oblique insertion downward along the scalp, to a depth of 1.5 cun to 2 cun, at an angle of 15-30 degrees.

6. TCM Acupuncture Approach

The traditional acupuncture treatment for acute-phase stroke patients focuses on yang imbalance, where treatment is directed to subduing Liver yang and Liver wind, and/or to restoring yang and opening the orifices. In the sub-acute and rehabilitative stages of stroke, traditional treatment is focused on clearing the meridians and collaterals of pathogens such as phlegm, wind, heat, and cold; and on restoring normal patterns of yin/yang and qi/blood.

Standard Acupuncture Treatment for Acute-Phase Stroke:

Acupuncture points selected include Shuigou (DU26), Neiguan (PC6), Xingjian (LR2), Hegu (LI4), Baihui (DU20), Shenque (RN8), and Yongquan (KI1).

Standard Acupuncture Treatment for Sub-Acute Stroke:

Acupoints along the Yangming (Large Intestine, Stomach), Taiyang (Small Intestine, Urinary Bladder), and Shaoyang (San Jiao, Gall Bladder) meridians are also selected as primary points.

1. Head acupoints include Fengfu (DU16), Fengchi (GB20), Tianzhu (BL10), Shuaigu (GB8), Taiyang (EX-HN-5) as main points, Baihui (DU20), Lianquan (RN23), Dicang (ST4), Jiache (ST6) as supplemental points. They function to treat head disorders and sensory organ disorders; Dredge channels and collaterals; invigorate qi and blood; transform stasis; Extinguish wind and prevent ascending yang qi; Transform damp-phlegm; Clear heat and relieve pain; Regulate mouth deviation and poor speech; Regulate ascending and descending yang qi.

2. Arm and Hand Acupoints include Quchi (LI11), Hegu (LI4), Waiguan (SJ5), Neiguan (PC6) as main points, Jianyu (LI15), Shousanli (LI10), Shenmen (HT7), Chize (LU5), Taiyuan (LU9), Daling (PC7) as supplemental points. They function to free the channels and collaterals in the upper limbs to regulate the movement of qi and blood; Enrich yin and subdue yang to treat limb dysfunction; Transform damp-phlegm; Strengthen qi and blood.

3. Leg and Foot Acupoints include Yanglingquan (GB34), Zusanli (ST36), Fenglong (ST40), Qiuxu (GB40), Taichong (LR3) as main points, and Xuehai (SP10), Sanyinjiao (SP6), Xuanzhong (GB39) as supplemental points. They function to Free the channels and collaterals in the lower limbs to regulate the movement of Qi and blood; Enrich yin and subdue yang to treat limb dysfunction; Transform damp-phlegm; Dredge and strengthen the sinews and invigorate blood; Strengthen qi and blood.

Case Reports from China's Leading Practitioners

The following ten cases are selected and presented as illustrative examples from China's leading contemporary practitioners. Each case represents a technique, a theory, or an innovative approach in the development of understanding stroke and treatment of stroke.

I. Case Presented by Dr. Wang Leting [1]: Treating Stoke with Penetrating Needle Technique

Male patient, age 60, complained of hemiplegia on the left side for seven months. His left arm had pain and contracture, and he could only lift it to the level of his chest. He couldn't flex and extend his fingers and had difficulty bearing weight on his left leg. Appetite, urine and feces were normal. His blood pressure was 160/90 mmHg. His tongue proper was thin white, his pulse was deep and thready.

Diagnosis: Deficiency of both qi and blood, loss of nourishment of tendons and blood vessels.

Treatment principle: Reinforce qi and blood, relax muscles and tendons, and activate the flow of qi and blood.

Acupuncture prescription: twelve penetrating points. Jianyu (LI15) to Binao (LI14), Yifeng (SJ17) to Jiafeng (Extra), Quchi (LI11) to Shaohai (HT3), Waiguan (SJ5) to Neiguan (PC6), Hegu (LI4) to Laogong (PC8), Yangchi (SJ4) to Daling (PC7), Huantiao (GB30) to Fengshi (GB31), Yangguan (DU3) to Ququan (LR8), Yanglingquan (GB34) to Yinlingquan (SP9), Jujue (GB39) to Sanyinjiao (SP6), Qiuxu (GB40) to Shenmai (BL62), Taichong (LR3) to Yongquan (KI1).

Treatment/outcome: Treat three times a week with reinforcing first, then reducing. Left arm pain diminished/stopped after five treatments, and the contracture improved. Left leg strength and mobility improved. His tongue was thin and white. The pulse was string-taut. His blood pressure was 150/90 mmHg. After more than ten treatments with the above prescription, he could walk with a cane. The flexion and extension of his fingers somewhat recovered. After a further ten treatments, he could walk several meters, lift his arm to the level of his shoulder, and manage ADLs by himself.

II. Case Presented by Dr. Shi Xuemin [1]: Treating Hemorrhage in Basal Ganglion with Xing Nao Kai Qiao

Male patient, 46, with ten-year history of hypertension. Sudden onset of difficulty in moving his right limbs, slurred speech, and left-sided migraine. Five minutes later, he experienced paraplegia of the right limbs. A lumbar puncture revealed blood in the cerebrospinal fluid, and a CT scan showed a hemorrhage of the left basal ganglion with bleeding into the cerebral chamber. The patient could respond to questions, but with slurred speech. He had complete facial paralysis on the central right side. His tongue proper was red with a thin white coating, and the pulse was irregularly intermittent. The rheoencephalogram showed that the occipitomastoid wave amplitude was low and flat. A chest x-ray showed aortic type of heart, and ECG showed chronic coronary insufficiency of blood supply and ventricular premature beat. The nervous system: Right Hoffmann's sign (+); bilateral Bard's sign (+).

Diagnosis: Excess yang qi invading upward to disturb the brain and the mind. The Treatment principle: Refresh the mind for resuscitation and dredge the meridians.

Acupuncture prescription: Neiguan (PC6), Renzhong (DU26), Sanyinjiao (SP6), Jiquan (HT1), Chize (LI5), Weizhong (BL40) and Hegu (LI4).

Treatment/Outcome: After two months' treatment with the method of refreshing the mind for resuscitation, the patient's speech and motor abilities were totally recovered. A follow-up CT scan showed the hematoma reabsorbed.

III. Case Presented by Bi Fugao [1]: Treating Yang Meridians for Sequela of Cerebral Hemorrhage

Male patient with ten-year history of hypertension. He had a cerebral hemorrhage. Two months' treatment in a hospital restored his mental clarity, but failed to treat his hemiplegia. From then on, he had deviated mouth and eyes, increased salivation, and inability to purse the mouth. An examination in November, 1976 revealed: clear mind; obese body; shortness of breath; myodynamia on the right limbs III grade; myotony weakened. The right arm could be lifted to the chest, hand grasping force was 0. The lower limbs were weak: he could lift his leg, but could not walk without help. Shallow nasolabial groove; inability to purse the mouth; salivation; string-taut, rolling pulse; flabby tongue with tooth marks, yellow sticky coating. BP 118/80 mmHg.

Diagnosis: Sequela of stroke with the involvement of zang-fu organs.

Differentiation: Phlegm-damp resulted from obese constitution. Too much stress caused yang to be hyperactive in the upper portion of the body, and yin to be deficient in the lower portion. Liver wind in combination with phlegm attacked the mind. Resulting symptoms: loss of consciousness; obstruction of the meridians; qi and blood blockage leading to deviation of mouth and eyes; and paralysis of the limbs.

Acupuncture prescription: Jiaji point on lumbar region, Jianyu (LI15), Quchi (LI11), Hegu (LI4), Liangqiu (ST21), Yanglingquan (GB34), Xuanzhong (GB39), Bafeng (Extra), Shangmiantanxue (Extra), Xiamiantanxue (Extra).

Treatment /outcome: Treated once a day, for a course of thirty treatments. After the first ten treatments improvement could be seen on the right leg, and the patient could walk three to five steps with a cane. After 60 treatments, the patient could purse his mouth and lift his right arm over his shoulder. He could walk five meters without any help. Ten days later, his facial paralysis was relieved and he could stretch or flex the right arm and walk stably on the right leg. The blood pressure remained 150/80 mmHg.

Commentary: Jiaji points can activate the qi of zang-fu organs and the Du meridian, resolving phlegm and dampness. The combined use of two Miantan points (Extra) can dredge the meridians and collaterals on the face. For facial paralysis, the points are mainly selected from Foot Yangming, Foot Shaoyin and three Hand Yang Meridians. Jiangyu (LI15), a crossing point of the Yangming and Yangqiao Meridians, can treat contracture, obstruction and flaccidity of the upper limbs. Hegu (LI4), a Yuan-source point of Hand Yangming, is able to regulate the general functions and to activate the qi flow of the meridians. Quchi (LI11), the He-Sea point of Hand Yangming Meridians, where the meridian qi infuses, can connect qi of the fu organs, promote qi flow, and dredge the meridians. The combined use of Hegu (LI4) and Quchi (LI11) can treat facial paralysis, as well as paralysis of the upper limbs. Yanglingquan (GB34), the he-sea point of foot shaoyang, is able to reduce the liver and subdue wind, activate tendons and collaterals. Xuanzhong (GB39), the major connecting point of the three-foot yang meridians and the influential point of marrow, in combination with Bafeng (Extra), can treat difficulty in walking.

IV. Case Presented by Xu Bin [1]: Treating Yang Meridians for Cerebral Thrombosis

Male, 49, complained of sudden onset of slurred speech, deviated mouth and eyes, numbness of left limbs and loss of consciousness. Hospital examination showed: blood pressure, 140/100 mmHg; mild slurred speech; wry tongue; salivation; 10 cm raise of the left arm; hemiplegia of the left leg; hyperactive deep reflex and dull shallow reflex of the left limbs.

Diagnosis: Windstroke or cerebral thrombosis due to long deficiency of the pectoral qi, disturbance of qi flow and malnutrition of limbs.

Treatment principle: Promote qi flow in the meridians and eliminate wind.

Acupuncture prescription: The upper and lower lightning points, Quchi (LI11), Hegu (LI4), penetrating towards Houxi (SI3), Yanglingquan (GB34), Yinlingquan (SP9), Zusanli (ST36), Sanyinjiao (SP6) and Jiexi (ST41).

Treatment/outcome: Deep perpendicular or oblique puncture was applied with the lift-thrust and sparrow-pecking techniques. Strong manipulations were given to the upper and lower lightning points to transmit the needing sensation to the toes and fingers tips. Generally, the needle was retained fifteen to twenty-five minutes. Treatment was given once a day, with ten treatments being a course. After the first course of treatment the patient was able to raise his hand over his head and walk normally. The second course of treatment resolved all the symptoms and restored the function of the left limbs. A follow-up survey showed that he was entirely recovered.

Commentary: The upper and lower lightning points were selected to treat hemiplegia with strong stimulation and reducing method to get rid of the pathogenic factors in the three yin and yang meridians. Physical build varies: for weak, hypertensive, or nervous patients, moderate stimulation is suggested.

V. Case Presented by Dr. Jiao Shunfa [1]: Treating Cerebral Hemorrhage with Scalp Acupuncture

Female, 34, complained of frequent headache and nausea. Upon awakening one morning, she felt dizziness for twenty minutes, then lost consciousness. She woke an hour later with complete hemiplegia on the left side. She came to the clinic on the sixth day. Lumbar puncture revealed CSF pressure of 320 mm H2O, with yellowish spinal fluid containing 785/MM RBC. There was no improvement following a course of IV fluids, and she was transferred to the acupuncture department. Examination eighteen days after the stroke event revealed: Blood pressure 100/70 mmHg; clear consciousness; normal speech; normal cranial nerves; normal extension and flexion of right hand; grasping force 4 kg (34kg for left hand); Hoffmann's sign (-); right arm could elevate to the xyphoid process; complete paralysis of the right leg; increase of muscle tonicity; hyperactivity of the knee reflex; Babinski's sign (-); the temperature, pain and cortical sensation of the right side normal; the cardiac rhythm normal; heart rate 70/min. Examination of fundi: bilateral congestion of the optic disc, their margins not clear, more severe on the left side, 3 to 4 D. higher than the retina, dilatation and curvature of the vein, the artery normal, A:V=1:2, no crossing pressure of the vein by the artery, no bleeding or exudation, clear central reflex of the macula.

Acupuncture prescription: Upper 3/5 of the left Motor Area and Foot Motor Sensory Area were needled once daily.

Treatment/outcome: Improved noted after six treatments. Her right arm could elevate normally, the grasping force of the right hand was 26 kg, the movement of her right leg was within normal range. She could walk four to five steps. After fifteen treatments, the muscle power of her right hand recovered to normal range, her grasping force was 32 kg, and all joints of her right leg could move except ankle and toes.

VI. Case Presented by Dr. Yang Jiasan: Combining Reinforcing and Reducing for Treating Stroke

Male, 58, complained of weakness on the right side of the body for six days, with stiffness of tongue, right arm numbness, and right-side body weakness. His condition was controlled with herbal medicine, without pathological development. However, he continued to complain of: distended feeling in the head; dizziness; weakness of the right side of his body, especially the right arm; slurring of speech; stiffness of tongue; distention and dryness of eyes; dry mouth but without desire to drink; and difficulty in falling asleep. Blood pressure was unstable, 130-150/80-110 mmHg. The patient had a dark red tongue with moist white coating; wiry pulse slightly rolling.

Diagnosis: Windstroke (attack on channels and collaterals), Liver yang transformed into wind.

Treatment Principle: Replenish yin, subdue yang, calm the mind. It is to clear the upper part. reinforce/tonify the lower part, and calm the mind.

Acupuncture prescription: Qianding (DU21), Houding (DU19), Baihui (DU20), Tongtian (BL7), Fengchi (GB20), Hegu (LI 4), Lieque (LU7), Zhigou (SJ6), Juegu (GB 39), Taichong (LR3).

Discussion: The points on head, Qianding (DU21), Houding (DU19), Baihui (DU20), Tongtian (BL7) function to replenish marrow, strengthen the brain and calm the mind. Fengchi (GB20) dispels wind of Upper Burner. Hegu (LI4) and Zusanli (ST36) remove obstruction of the intestines, permitting the clean to ascend and the turbid to descend. Quchi (LI11) and Zusanli (ST 36) bring down the rebellious Qi. Hegu (LI4) and Taichong (LR3), Yuan-Source points, soften the Liver to stop wind, replenish yin, and clear heat. Lieque (LU7) induces Kidney water to nourish genuine yin, and combines with Juegu (GB39) to increase Kidney Essence. Juegu (GB39) and Taichong (LR3) increase Liver and Kidney Essence. This prescription reinforces the lower and clears the upper.

Treatment/outcome: Qianding (DU21), Houlding (DU19), Baihui (DU20), Tongtian (BL7) were reinforced with mild stimulation. Lieque (LU7), Zhigou (SJ6), Juegu (GB39), and Taichong (LR3) were reinforced with medium stimulation. Other points were reduced with medium stimulation. Three month's treatment made the numbness of the right side of his body disappear, and his speech basically returned to normal.

This is a syndrome of yin deficiency and yang hyperactivity transformed into wind blocking in the brain, manifested as weakness of right side of his body, especially the right arm, slurring of speech, stiffness of tongue, and wiry rolling pulse. Distention and dryness of eyes, and dry mouth but without desire to drink are the signs of yin deficiency. It is the syndrome of upper-body excess and lower-body deficiency.

VII. Case Presented by Dr. Cheng Xinnong [2]: Treating Stroke by Reducing Yang Meridians and Reinforcing Yin Meridians

Female, 73, complained of weakness of the right limbs for two days. After getting angry with her family, she suddenly had weakness of her right limbs and sluggish movement. She presented with weakness of the right limbs; sluggish movement; irritability; dry mouth; poor appetite; sleep almost normal; no dizziness; tinnitus; shortness of breath on exertion; occasional incontinence of urine. Tongue tip red, with dry yellow coating; deep thready pulse.

Diagnosis: Liver and Kidney deficiency, with qi and blood deficiency and Liver qi stagnation.

Treatment principle: Reinforce Liver and Kidney, regulate qi and blood.

Acupuncture prescription: Baihui (DU20), Fengchi (GB20), Guanyuan (RN4), Hegu (LI4), Taichong (LR3). Zusanli (ST36), Sanyinjiao (SP6), Taixi (KI3), Yongquan (KI1). Right side: Jianyu (LI15), Quchi (LI11), Waiguan (SJ 5), Yanglingquan (GB34), Xuanzhong (GB39).

Discussion: Baihui (DU20) regulates yin and yang to circulate qi and blood. Fengchi (GB20) dispels wind. Taichong (LR3) pacifies Liver to subdue yang. Guanyuan (RN4) reinforces Yuan-Source qi. Zusanli (ST36) strengthens the Middle Burner. Sanyinjiao (SP6) replenishes yin to subdue yang. Taixi (KI 3) replenishes water to irrigate wood. Yongquan (KI1) conducts fire downward. Jianyu (LI15), Quchi (LI11), Waiguan (SJ5), Hegu (LI4), Yanglingquan (GB34), and Xuanzhong (GB39) remove obstruction of channels and balance yin and yang.

Treatment/outcome: Fengchi (GB20) and Taichong (LR3) were reduced; Guanyuan (RN4), Zusanli (ST36), Sanyinjiao (SP6) and Taixi (KI3) were reinforced; even method was employed for the other points. After three treatments, there was great relief of the numbness and weakness of the right limbs, and movement was no longer sluggish. Her condition was maintained with ten treatments. The follow-up found no recurrence.

This patient is elderly, with Liver and Kidney deficiency, qi and blood insufficiency, and Liver qi stagnation due to anger, so the limbs lack nourishment and are sluggish in movement. With Kidney yin deficiency, body fluids fail to distribute upward, so the mouth is dry. Yin deficiency leads to internal heat, so the patient displays red tongue with yellow coating, and thread, rapid pulse. Kidneys are deficient and not receiving qi, so there is shortness of breath on exertion. The bladder is out of control owing to Kidney qi not being consolidated enough, so there is incontinence of urine.

VIII. Case Presented by Dr. Yang Jiebin [2]: Treating Stroke with Bleeding on Jing-Well Points

Female, 55, suddenly fell down and lost consciousness for half a day. She had suffered from blurred vision and dizziness for many years, along with occasional numbness of the fingers, and had been diagnosed with hypertension. On examination, the patient was unconscious, with phlegm gurgling in her throat, abrupt respirations, left limbs paralyzed, staring eyes, flushed face, and closed mouth. BP 160/130 mmHg. Slightly red tongue with yellow sticky coating; rolling rapid pulse.

Diagnosis: Windstroke (attack on Zang Fu Organs, tense syndrome). This is a case of Liver yang transformed into fire with wind produced. Wind brought phlegm-damp upward, disturbing the brain and flowing to the channels and collaterals. Yellow sticky tongue coating and rolling rapid pulse imply that phlegm-heat is misting the Heart, which is the cause of unconsciousness, staring eyes, and closed mouth.

Treatment principle: Promote resuscitation, pacify the liver to stop wind, resolve phlegm, and clear fire.

Acupuncture Prescription: Five Center Points [Renzhong (DU26), Yongquan (KI1), Laogong (PC8)], Jing-Well points, Fenglong (ST40), Hegu (LI 4), Taichong (LR3).

Treatment/outcome: Five Centers and Jing-Well points were pricked for bleeding. Renzhong (DU26) was punctured with a thick filiform needle and manipulated with sparrow-picking method for 10 minutes. Fenglong (ST40), Hegu (LI4) and Taichong (LR3) were reduced heavily. The needles were retained for five minutes and manipulated once every five minutes. After the first treatment, her respirations became more normal and the restlessness was relieved. On the following day, the same treatment was applied and her consciousness was restored. With another three treatments given in succession, her left limbs could move. Acupuncture was continued for three months, and her movement became normal again.

Commentary: For windstroke, first-aid treatment should be given as quickly as possible. In differentiation of acute-phase strokes, flaccid or tense syndrome should be clearly diagnosed. In cases where the patient has staring eyes, mouth agape, clenched jaws, stiff limbs, coarse breathing, flushed face, and big floating pulse, it will be a case of qi and fire floating upward. If phlegm is rattling in the throat, it will be excess tense syndromes. Promoting resuscitation and clearing heat are the principles of treatment in these cases. Pricking to cause bleeding from the 'Five Centers [Renzhong (DU26), Yongquan (KI1), Laogong (PC8)]' is important to save the patient from unconsciousness. Renzhong (DU26), Hegu (LI4) and Shixuan (EX-UE11) are stimulated to restore consciousness. Fenglong (ST40) sends down and dissolves phlegm; and Taichong (LR 3) pacifies to stop wind.

IX. Case Presented by Dr. Jin Rui [3]: Treating Cerebral Thrombosis with Three-Needle Technique

Male, 60, with a six-month history of cerebral thrombosis. His symptoms included salivation, feeble voice, slurred speech, hemiplegia on the right side of the body, swollen fingers and wrist, and numbness of the right leg with swollen ankle. When he was brought in for treatment, the CT scan indicated cerebral thrombosis. BP was 19/14kPa. His tongue and the nasolabial groove deviated toward the left. Right arm and right leg grade II. Slow response to shallow stimulation; lack of response to deep stimulation. Hoffmann's sign (+), bilateral Bard's sign (+).

Treatment/outcome: Treatment with Temple Three-Needle was performed. Two sides were alternated, with Yinlingquan (SP9) and Sanyinjiao (SP6) added to reduce water retention. After thirty treatments, salivation and edema were alleviated. Muscle strength was improved to grade V. Responses to stimulation were symmetric. Pathological reflexes were negative.

Modern Research: Acupuncture in Stroke Rehabilitation

We collected a selection of acupuncture researches on stroke conducted recently. This is a growing field of research. More rigorous studies are always expected.

I. A Clinical Study on Acupuncture with "Xing Nao Kai Qiao" Method for Treatment of Apoplexy [4]

Apoplexy is a common encountered disease with high mobility and sequelae. It is necessary to establish effective therapies for the disease.

The authors have established an acupuncture method called Xing Nao Kai Qiao (XNKQ) to treat the pathogenic factors of apoplexy. In the XNKQ method, points on the Yin meridians and the Governor Vessel are the primary ones selected, and emphasis has been made on the quantity of acupuncture maneuvers. According to traditional Chinese medicine theory, blood stagnation, liver wind, and phlegm-turbidity causing blockage of the aperture of the heart resulting in Qi stagnation are the pathogenic factors of apoplexy.

This study reported the following results: Since 1972, 9005 cases of hospitalized apoplexy patients have been treated with XNKQ method. Among them, 5337 cases (59.27%) were cured; 2085 cases (23.15%) markedly improved, 1453 cases (16.14%) improved, 40 cases (0.44%) were unimproved, and 9 cases (1.0%) died. This is an effective rate of 98.56%.

In addition, 270 apoplexy patients at the acute stage were divided into a XNKQ group (Group 1), a conventional acupuncture group (Group 2), and a conventional drug group (Group 3), with 90 cases in each group. A comparison made among the 3 groups showed that the therapeutic effect in Group1 was considerably better than that in either Group 2 or Group 3. At the same time, 30 cases of acute encephalorrhagia and cerebral infarction were chosen for observing changes of certain neurochemical indices. It was found that the XNKQ method acupuncture maneuver reduced the contents of lipid peroxide (LPO) and thromboxane (TXA2) in study group patients, and increased the activity of superoxide dismutase (SOD) and the level of prostacyclin (PGI2). These studies indicated that XNKQ acupuncture method influences various pathological processes in apoplexy.

XNKQ acupuncture method is an effective therapy for treating apoplexy. It functions to involve various pathological links. It has beneficial regulative function on unnormalized hemodynamics. It can provide inhibition on free radical damage, as well as protection of the structures and functions of the brain by way of elevating SOD activity and alleviating neural injury induced by lipid peroxidation. PGI2 and TXA2 are important factors for maintaining normal blood circulation and preventing thrombosis formation. The results indicate that XNKQ acupuncture method can obviously enhance the depressed PGI2, and reduce the increased TXA2 to balance the value of PGI2/ TXA2.

II. Acupuncture Improves Recovery, Physical Functioning in Stroke Patients [5]

This pilot study was to address inconsistencies in the published literature with regard to whether acupuncture improves physical and mental abilities of stroke patients when combined with traditional Western rehabilitation procedures. While some trials have suggested that acupuncture provides no additional benefit in the rehabilitation of stroke patients, other studies have reported that stroke patients receiving acupuncture have demonstrated significant improvements in certain aspects, such as recovery of motor skills and overall physical functioning.

The study was conducted at the Daniel Freeman Rehabilitation Center's inpatient stroke rehabilitation unit in Los Angeles by practitioners from Emperor's College of Traditional Oriental Medicine. In the trial, 29 patients who had suffered a stroke within the previous 60 days that resulted in hemiparesis (weakness on one side of the body) were randomized to either a control group or an acupuncture group. The control group received conventional stroke rehabilitation care (consisting of three hours of physical, occupational, and/or speech therapy, six days per week) for the duration of the inpatient stay. The acupuncture group received the same care as the control group, along with an additional 30 minutes of acupuncture therapy, seven days per week, for two weeks during the inpatient stay. Acupuncture was provided by eight licensed acupuncturists who had trained at Emperor's College and had a minimum of one year of clinical experience.

To ensure consistency, a standardized treatment protocol was used among all patients in the acupuncture group. Needles were inserted into specific points on the affected limb. Acupuncture points included Renzhong (DU20), Houding (DU19), Qianding (DU21), Tongtian (UB7), Baihui (GB20), Dazhui (DU14), Qihai (RN6), Zhongwan (RN12) and Tianshu (ST25). Supplementary points for the upper limbs Jianyu (LI15), Quchi (LI11), Waiguan (SJ5), Hegu (LI4), and Lieque (LU7) and lower limbs Fengshi (GB31), Zusanli (ST36), Yanglingquan (GB34), Sanyinjiao (SP6), Weizhong

(ST40), Jiexi (ST41), and Taichong (LR3) were selected depending on the patient's condition. Within two weeks of the stroke episode, the acupuncturists added Bafeng (Extra), Lianquan (RN23) and Tongli (HT5) for aphasia; Dicang (ST4), Quanliao (SI18) and Jiache (ST6) for facial paralysis; and UB 6 (Chengguang) and GB 37 (Guangming) for vision problems.

To measure the effects acupuncture might have, the researchers used a tool that assessed aspects of physical performance in a person's upper and lower extremities, along with a functional independence scale that evaluated a person's ability to complete certain activities of daily living without assistance. Patients were evaluated at baseline (within three days of being admitted to the stroke rehabilitation unit) and after being discharged. At baseline and after the completion of the study, evaluations were performed by therapists who were blinded as to the randomization of each patient.

This study produced the following results: While a general analysis of the data appeared to show no real difference in physical performance scores between patients in the control and acupuncture groups, closer inspection revealed that acupuncture patients experienced "significantly greater" lower extremity motor function compared to the control group. Acupuncture patients also fared slightly better than control patients in terms of lower extremity joint pain.

Other improvements were seen when the researchers compared functional independence scores. While the average score of patients in the control group increased 8.5 points between baseline and discharge, the average score of acupuncture patients increased 11.2 points. In all seven activities of daily living measured on the scale, the average score of patients receiving acupuncture was between .1 and .8 points higher than control patients. The authors noted that "patients who received acupuncture as an adjunct to standard rehabilitation demonstrated significantly greater improvement in tub/shower transfer mobility and a trend for greater improvement in toilet transfer mobility."

III. Acupuncture Effective in Treatment of Post-Stroke Hand Movement [6]

This research demonstrates that acupuncture is effective for the treatment of post-stroke hand movement and walking dysfunction. Researchers from the China Rehabilitation Research Center of Rehabilitation (College of Capital Medicine University, Beijing) investigated the use of acupuncture points

Zhongzhu (SJ3) and Waiguan (SJ5) in relation to restoring hand function following a stroke. A randomized trial of 60 patients was divided into a treatment group and a control group. Both groups received physical therapy, occupational therapy, and other standard rehabilitative procedures. Both groups were evaluated with the National Institutes of Health Stroke Scale (NIHSS) to measure changes in walking, hand function, and activities of daily living (ADL). The group receiving acupuncture at Zhongzhu (SJ3) and Waiguan (SJ5) showed significant improvement over the control group in all areas of measurement. The acupuncture group demonstrated superior hand function, greater walking ability, and enhanced ADL. The researchers conclude that the combination of acupuncture with routine post-stroke recovery procedures produces significantly improved patient outcomes.

IV. Acupuncture Improves Swallowing Difficulties after a Stroke [7]

Stroke is an event marked by either loss of blood flow to or bleeding into an area of the brain. The affected area of the brain is damaged, resulting in some degree of loss of body functions controlled by nerves associated with the damaged area. The swallowing reflex is frequently affected and dysphagia occurs in 30 to 50% of people who have experienced stroke. In most cases, recovery occurs without treatment, but in some it is slow or does not occur. Those who do not recover will require long-term nursing care. People with dysphagia are at high risk of dehydration, malnutrition, choking, and pneumonia.

Several therapies have been used to treat dysphagia. Applications of cold to the inside of the throat (thermal treatments) and electrical stimulation to specific points on the neck have both been used to give some immediate but temporary relief from dysphagia. One study comparing these treatments found that thermal treatments applied for one hour every day were not as effective as electrical stimulation. In another preliminary study, electrical stimulation was applied across a specific muscle in the neck that was found to be weak in all of the participants. Electrical stimulation was applied for four hours every day until improvement in swallowing was achieved. Treatment was effective for 20 of 23 people in this study, and the number of days of treatment ranged from 2 to 30 days. Dysphagia returned within nine months in 30% of those who responded to the treatment, but they all improved again after a second course of electrical stimulation.

In the current study, 41 people with dysphagia following a stroke were treated with acupuncture. A single 15-minute treatment with acupuncture was applied to both legs at two points that were chosen following traditional

Chinese medicine practices. The swallowing reflex was triggered by placing 1 ml of water into the throat and the time between introduction of the water and the onset of swallowing was measured. This measurement was taken before and 30 minutes after treatment with acupuncture. The average time to onset of swallowing was 10.2 seconds before treatment and 4.5 seconds after treatment, an improvement of more than 55%. In a subset of participants who were retested after seven days, the improvement in swallowing was found to persist.

The current study shows that a single, short application of acupuncture has beneficial effects for people with dysphagia due to a stroke. The effect of longer or more frequent treatment and the length of time its benefits are sustained are unknown and should be addressed in future studies.

V. Effect of Electro-Acupuncture on Impaired Cognitive Function of Stroke Patients [8]

This study was to investigate the effect of electroacupuncture on cognitive function and health-related quality of life in patients who have had a stroke.

This clinical trial employed a prospective, randomized, single-blind design. The study was conducted at the department of rehabilitation medicine, Tri-Service General Hospital, Taipei, Taiwan.

Thirty-eight (38) participants were recruited, but only 33 completed the study. Seventeen (17) stroke participants with cognitive impairment were assigned to the treatment group and 16 were assigned to the control group. Electroacupuncture was applied to acupuncture points Neiguan (PC6) and Shenmen (HT7) for 20 minutes twice a week for eight weeks in the treatment group, while participants in each group continued rehabilitation. Cognitive assessment (LOTCA-G) and quality-of-life assessment (SF-36 and SS-QOL) were carried out in each group at baseline, and at eight weeks after treatment.

This study produced the following results: Significant improvement was detected in four subtests of LOTCA-G: orientation, perception, praxis, and attention ($p<0.05$) between treatment and control groups. Significant improvement was also indicated in subscales of SF-36 (RP, VT, SF, RE, MH, MCS) and SS-QOL (language) ($p<0.05$). No correlation was noted between the variables of LOTCA-G and SF-36/SS-QOL except four matches: Memory (LOTCA-G) and Mental Component Summary (SF-36): $r=0.492$; Memory (LOTCA-G) and Personality (SS-QOL): $r=0.485$; Praxis

(LOTCA-G) and Language (SS-QOL): r=0.616; Orientation (LOTCA-G), and Language (SS-QOL): r=0.534.

The results of this study confirm a positive effect of electroacupuncture on cognition and quality of life in patients who had a stroke. Future research will be required to evaluate potential mechanisms and potential long-term benefits.

VI. Clinical Trial of Electrical Acupuncture on Hemiplegic Stroke Patients [9]

This clinical trial was to assess the efficacy of electrical acupuncture in the rehabilitation of patients with hemiplegia in stroke, we randomized 128 patients within 2 wk of stroke onset to receive either comprehensive rehabilitation plus electrical acupuncture (*n*= 59) or comprehensive rehabilitation only (*n* = 59). Electrical acupuncture was administered by electrical stimulation of acupuncture points through adhesive surface electrodes five times per week. Neurological status (Brunnstrom's stage) and the Chinese version of the Functional Independence Measure were assessed before treatment and at discharge. Patients treated with electrical acupuncture had a shorter duration of hospital stay for rehabilitation and better neurological and functional outcomes than the control group had, with a significant difference in scores for self-care and locomotion (P = 0.02). This result did not postulate the previous study that acupuncture therapy for stroke patients should depend on needle manual and "de qi" response. We suggest that electrical acupuncture through adhesive surface electrodes in conjunction with current optimal rehabilitation programs is a convenient and effective therapy for stroke patients.

VII. A Randomized Controlled Trial on the Treatment for Acute Partial Ischemic Stroke with Acupuncture [10]

The effectiveness of acupuncture in acute stroke remains largely untested and unproved. A randomized, controlled trial was carried out to study the feasibility of acupuncture in combination with conventional supportive treatment for acute stroke patients. A total of 30 patients, aged 46-74, with the onset of symptoms within 36 h were enrolled into the study after appropriate screening. All patients gave informed consent. Basing on the same supportive treatment, patients were randomly assigned to a treatment with or without acupuncture. The procedure and acupoint selection were discussed and decided through several meetings of a group of senior acupuncture doctors in Taiwan. Acupuncture was applied 3 times/ week for

4 weeks. During the study period, there were no problems in conducting this trial in terms of patient availability and acceptance, and physician cooperation. A significantly better neurologic outcome was observed in the acupuncture group on day 28 and day 90. The improvement in neurologic status was greatest in patients with a poor neurologic score at baseline. There were no important side effects except for one episode of dizziness related to acupuncture treatment. The data and results of this study will be used as a guideline for planning a full-scale clinical trial, e.g. sample size calculation, method of randomization with stratification of prognostic factors, choosing acupuncture points and technique of acupuncture.

VIII. Treating Spastic Paralysis after Stroke with Different Methods of Acupuncture Therapy [11]

Acupuncture is an important method for the treatment of stroke, and its clinical efficacy is precise. But different doctors use different approaches based on their different experiences. The objective of this study was to observe the effects of three different acupuncture therapy methods to see how effective they were in treating spastic paralysis after stroke, and to see if any of the methods were clearly superior to the others. The three treatment methods selected for study were: needling tendon method, harmonizing yin and yang method, and Jin's 3-needling method. The study was conducted from January 2009 to March 2010 in the Acupuncture and Moxibustion Department of the First Affiliated Hospital of Guangzhou University of Traditional Chinese Medicine. Sixty patients were randomly assigned to a needling tendon method group, harmonizing yin and yang group, or Jin's 3-needling group in a 1:1:1 ratio. Acupuncture was performed over a 28-day period, with treatments given daily for five days, a 2-day rest, and then resumed. At the same time, patients continued their basic treatments for controlling blood pressure and blood sugar, and other therapy. Patients were assessed before and after treatment with ADL scales and the Fugl-Meyer scale to test their activities of daily living and motor function. All the data were analyzed with SPSS16.0 package.

This study produced the following results: 1.) According to statistical results of ADL, all three experimental groups had significant statistical difference after treatment ($P<0.01$), but differences in the efficacy of treatment between groups was not statistically significant ($P>0.05$). 2.) According to statistical results of the Fugl-Meyer Scale, the three experimental groups had significant statistical difference after treatment ($P<0.01$). Between groups, the needling tendon method group and the Jin's 3 needle group showed a significant difference ($P<0.01$), but there was no statistically significant difference between the needling tendon method group and the harmonizing yin and yang method group ($P > 0.05$). The data show that: Jin's 3 needle method is more effective than harmonizing yin and yang method, and harmonizing yin and yang method is more effective than the needling tendon method.

After a course of treatment, all three acupuncture methods were effective to treat spastic paralysis after stroke. 1) To improve patient ADLs, all three types of acupuncture methods had a significant effect. The effective rate of improvement of the Jin's 3 needle group was 95%, and the improvement rate of the needling tendon method group and the harmonizing yin and yang method group was 90%. 2) To improve motor function, all three acupuncture methods again had significant positive effects. Comparing the three methods, Jin-3 needle group members had the best results, and results for the harmonizing yin and yang method group were better than the needling tendon method group.

IX. An fMRI Study Showing the Effect of Acupuncture in Chronic Stage Stroke Patients with Aphasia [12]

Acupuncture is used as a treatment in stroke patients with aphasia, yet the underlying neural mechanisms are unknown. This study aims to examine the relationship between changes in language function and brain activation using functional magnetic resonance imaging in chronic stroke patients with aphasia who underwent an 8-week acupuncture protocol.

Seven chronic stroke patients were identified from a stroke database of a regional acute hospital in Hong Kong between January and July 2007. Patients were treated three times a week over a period of 8 weeks. Four acupoints were stimulated on the weak side of the patient's body. No other rehabilitation was given during the study period. Changes in language function were measured by aphasia quotient (AQ) of Cantonese Aphasia Battery (CAB). Functional magnetic resonance imaging blood oxygen level dependent signals were used to demonstrate the correlation between changes in AQ and brain activation after treatment. The patients were divided into well-recovered and poorly- recovered groups based on their CAB scores at entry.

This study produced the following results: The well-recovered group showed significant improvement in CAB scores after receiving acupuncture treatment. A significant correlation between changes in AQ and blood oxygen level dependent activation in the lesioned Wernicke's speech area was found. These preliminary results suggest that acupuncture may be beneficial to language recovery in chronic stroke patients.

X. Acupuncture Stimulation Causes Bilaterally Different Microcirculatory Effects in Stroke Patients [13]

The aim of this study was to determine the effects of acupuncture stimulation (AS) in stroke patients by analyzing the pulsatile waveform and frequency content of skin blood-flow signals recorded simultaneously on the bilateral skin surface of the head.

Laser Doppler flowmetry (LDF) signals were obtained in 18 stroke patients. Each assessment involved a 20-minute baseline recording, a 20-minute AS, and a further 20-minute recording. Significant bilateral differences in LDF parameters were noted following AS, with an increased pulsatile component of the microcirculatory blood flow (MBF), decreased blood-flow resistance, and decreased MBF variability in the vascular beds on the stroke-affected side. Spectral analysis revealed that the vasodilation on the stroke-affected side could be partly attributed to decreased sympathetic neural activity.

This study made the following conclusion: This is the first study to demonstrate the feasibility of evaluating the cerebral MBF conditions induced by AS in stroke patients by noninvasive LDF measurement. The present skull-intact measurement setup could aid the development of noninvasive detection techniques for determining bilateral differences in the cerebral MBF, and could thus become useful for the efficacy evaluation of treatment techniques for stroke. It might also promote understanding of the mechanisms underlying the responses and possible treatment efficacy of AS as applied to stroke patients.

XI. An fMRI Study of Acupuncture-Induced Brain Activation of Aphasia Stroke Patients [14]

This investigation aims to test the effect of acupuncture on word generation activation (WGA) in post-stroke aphasia patients. Seven vascular aphasia patients and 14 control subjects were studied using functional magnetic resonance imaging (fMRI). Each performed: (1) a word generation (WG) task alone, followed by (2) repeating WG after insertion of acupuncture needles (WGN) into Sanyangluo (SJ8), a language-implicated acupoint, followed by (3) repeating WGN reinforced by electrical stimulation (WGA) of Sanyangluo (SJ8), and finally (4) electrical stimulation (ES) of Sanyangluo (SJ8) alone. Significant activation was found in the opercular, triangular, or insula during the ES stimulation in patients when comparing each patient to 14 normal controls. For the WG task, significant activation was found in the inferior frontal gyrus when comparing each patient to 14 normal controls. The signal induced by acupuncture was larger than that of the WG task in the left middle frontal gyrus with the comparison of WGA vs. WGN in seven patients. Further, main significant effects in the right insula in patients were observed when comparing seven patients to 14 normal controls. The activation induced by ES stimulation was only found on the left side in controls. This activation was observed on the lesion side of superior and middle frontal gyrus (SMFG) in patients. This study demonstrates for the first time that language-deficit-implicated acupoint stimulation can selectively activate the brain on the lesion side in post-stroke aphasia patients. These results suggest that acupuncture may have therapeutic benefits in post-stroke aphasia patients.

Critical Commentary on Acupuncture Therapy for Stroke, with Response

I. Acupuncture in Post-Stroke Rehabilitation: A Systematic Review and Meta-analysis of Randomized Trials [15]

Acupuncture is a low-risk treatment with purported claims of effectiveness for poststroke rehabilitation. To comprehensively assess the efficacy of acupuncture in poststroke rehabilitation, a systematic review and meta-analysis of all randomized clinical trials of acupuncture for poststroke rehabilitation was conducted.

This study searched 7 English and 2 Chinese databases from inception to September 2009. Eligible studies included randomized clinical trials that evaluated the clinical efficacy of acupuncture in adult patients with disability after stroke. A meta-regression was conducted to determine if specific covariates explained heterogeneity.

The following results are produced: Thirty-five articles written in Chinese and 21 articles written in English were included. The overall quality of the studies was "fair" and most studies were small (median n=86; range, 16 to 241). The majority (80%) of the studies reported a significant benefit from acupuncture; however, there was some evidence of publication bias. In 38 trials, data were available for meta-analysis and meta-regression, yielding an OR in favor of acupuncture compared with controls (OR=4.33, 95% CI: 3.09 to 6.08; I2=72.4%). Randomization, modes of delivery, method of control, study source country, and reporting of randomization may explain some of the heterogeneity observed between the studies.

Randomized clinical trials demonstrate that acupuncture may be effective in the treatment of poststroke rehabilitation. Poor study quality and the possibility of publication bias hinder the strength of this recommendation and argue for a large, transparent, well-conducted randomized clinical trial to support this claim and implement changes to clinical practice.

II. Assessing the Effectiveness of Acupuncture for Acute Stroke [16]

Acupuncture-like sensory stimulation activates multiple efferent (nerve) pathways leading to altered activity in numerous neural systems. Acupuncture is widely accepted by Chinese people and it is increasingly requested by patients and their relatives in Western countries. This study is to assess the effectiveness and safety of acupuncture in patients with acute stroke.

The authors searched the Cochrane Stroke Group trials register (last searched August 2003), the Chinese Stroke Trials Register (August 2003) and the Chinese Acupuncture Trials Register (August 2003). Electronic searches were performed in the Cochrane Controlled Trials Register (The Cochrane Library, Issue 3, 2003), MEDLINE (1966 to 2003), EMBASE (1980 to 2003), Alternative Medicine Database (1985 to 2003), CINAHL (1982 to 2003) and the Chinese Biological Medicine Database (1981 to 2003). Reference lists of systematic reviews and identified trials were hand searched. Randomized and quasi-randomized trials of acupuncture started within 30 days of stroke onset, compared with placebo/sham acupuncture or open control in patients with acute ischemic and/or hemorrhagic stroke. Needling into skin was required for acupuncture.

Two reviewers selected trials for inclusion, assessed trial quality, and extracted the data independently. Authors of trials were contacted for missing data. The following results are produced: Fourteen trials involving 1208 patients were included. Ten trials included patients with only ischemic stroke. When acupuncture was compared with sham acupuncture or open control, there was a borderline significant trend towards fewer patients being dead or dependent (Odds ratio (OR) 0.66, 95% confidence interval (CI) 0.43 to 0.99), and significantly fewer being dead or needing institutional care (OR 0.58, 95% CI 0.35 to 0.96) in the acupuncture group after three months or more. There was also a significant difference favoring acupuncture in the mean change of global neurological deficit score during the treatment period (standardized mean difference (SMD) 1.17, 95% CI 0.30 to 2.04). Comparison of acupuncture with sham acupuncture only showed a statistically significant difference on death or requiring institutional care (OR 0.49, 95% CI 0.25 to 0.96), but not on death or dependency (OR 0.67, 95% CI 0.40 to 1.12), or change of global neurological deficit score (SMD 0.01, 95% CI -0.55 to 0.57). Severe adverse events with acupuncture (dizziness, intolerable pain and infection of acupoints) were rare (6/386, 1.55%).

The authors concluded that acupuncture appeared to be safe but without clear evidence of benefit. The number of patients is too small to be certain whether acupuncture is effective for treatment of acute ischemic or hemorrhagic stroke. Larger, methodologically-sound trials are required.

III. Assessing the Effectiveness of Acupuncture for Stroke Rehabilitation [17]

This study is to assess the efficacy and safety of acupuncture for patients with stroke in the subacute or chronic stage.

The authors searched the Cochrane Stroke Group Trials Register (November 2005), the Cochrane Complementary Medicine Field Trials Register (November 2005), the Cochrane Central Register of Controlled Trials (The Cochrane Library Issue 3, 2005), MEDLINE (1966 to November 2005), EMBASE (1980 to November 2005), CINAHL (1982 to November 2005), AMED (1985 to November 2005), the Chinese Stroke Trials Register (November 2005), the Chinese Acupuncture Trials Register (November 2005), the Chinese Biological Medicine Database (1977 to November 2005), the National Center for Complementary and Alternative Medicine Register (November 2005), and the National Institute of Health Clinical Trials Database (November 2005). The authors hand-searched four Chinese journals and checked reference lists of all papers identified for further trials.

The authors selected truly randomized unconfounded clinical trials among patients with ischemic or hemorrhagic stroke, in the subacute or chronic stage, which compared acupuncture involving needling with either placebo acupuncture, sham acupuncture or no acupuncture.

Two review authors independently selected trials for inclusion, assessed quality, and extracted and cross-checked the data. The authors produced the following results: Five trials (368 patients) met the inclusion criteria. Methodological quality was considered inadequate in all trials. Although the overall estimate from four trials suggested the odds of improvement in global neurological deficit was higher in the acupuncture group compared with the control group (odds ratio (OR) 6.55, 95% confidence interval (CI) 1.89 to 22.76), this estimate may not be reliable since there was substantial heterogeneity (I(2)= 68%). One trial showed no significant improvement of motor function between the real acupuncture group and the sham acupuncture group (OR 9.00, 95% CI 0.40 to 203.30), but the confidence interval was wide and included clinically significant effects in both directions. No data on death, dependency, and institutional care, change of neurological deficit score, quality of life or adverse events were available.

The authors concluded that currently there is no clear evidence on the effects of acupuncture on subacute or chronic stroke. Large, methodologically-sound trials are required.

Response to Critical Commentary

In a commentary, "Does Acupuncture Work for Stroke Rehabilitation: What Do Recent Clinical Trials Really Show?" Shiflett [18] stated: A number of randomized controlled trials of acupuncture for stroke recovery were critically reviewed, beginning with an existing systematic review and meta-analysis. A number of these clinical studies suffered from methodological flaws that tended to obscure and reduce the reported effect size. These flaws included inadequate statistical analysis, failure to adequately account for differences in baseline stroke severity, and the use of an inadequate post-treatment assessment period. These three flaws, taken individually or in combination, resulted in the underreporting of acupuncture effects in five of the randomized controlled trials reviewed.

By informally adjusting study results for these limitations, it was possible to demonstrate that acupuncture is probably much more effective in assisting stroke recovery than has generally been reported, especially when the stroke is in the moderately severe range. The negative impact of well-intended but inappropriate exclusion criteria in the meta-analysis was also illustrated. The importance of giving more attention to ancillary results, such as walking speed and mortality, was illustrated as a way to gain a deeper understanding of the true impact of a still poorly-understood therapy such as acupuncture. The general conclusion of the re-analysis presented here is that there is in fact substantial evidence that acupuncture is effective as an adjunctive treatment for facilitating stroke recovery.

In a statement to *Acupuncture Today* (April 2005), a group of acupuncture researchers on stroke elaborated on the results of their research, and outlined ways that future studies that examine the effectiveness of acupuncture in the rehabilitation of stroke patients should be conducted.

"This study provides important insight into the design of future post-stroke acupuncture clinical trials, particularly the selection of appropriate outcome measures," they wrote. "We believe that one of the problems in past investigations of acupuncture effectiveness after stroke is that outcome measures are used that look at gross changes in motor or functional ability that may be too far removed from the underlying mechanisms that may account for acupuncture effectiveness. Recent studies that are trying to understand the mechanisms that could explain how acupuncture works after stroke suggest that acupuncture induces changes in blood flow to the brain or may stimulate the production of growth factors that can help neurons survive. If that is the case, then studies need to use outcome measures that are more sensitive and can detect relevant changes in motor control that may lead to improved function. Our study demonstrated that when more sensitive measures are used, these types of motor and functional changes can be detected."

Does acupuncture really work to help stroke victims improve? Many studies involving thousands of patients have been published in China and Japan, and two of three studies from Scandinavia demonstrated significant help. These studies indicate that patients get well faster, perform better in self-care, require less nursing and rehabilitation therapy, and use fewer healthcare dollars. However, since most studies come from China, they get little credence from the Western medical community because researchers in China do not appear to be published unless their results are highly positive, so publication bias is possible. And, no money has been made available in the United States for studies needed to confirm the claims of experts in China and Japan of indeed helping stroke patients. Such studies, if done well, demand significant funding; sources of such money are difficult to find. Most physicians, including rehabilitation experts, have appeared unwilling to consider acupuncture therapy, not due to bias but because the published studies do not necessarily meet research study criteria for the United States.

Acupuncture is a safe therapy, and my experience has taught that this is especially true when helping stroke victims. Even discomfort is generally minimal. If one compares the possible positive help to be obtained with the risks associated with acupuncture, my contention is that acupuncture is worthy to attempt for stroke therapy. Studies are needed in the United States to prove this to medical skeptics. It will be important for such studies to involve skilled acupuncturists with experience in stroke therapy.

Chapter Seven

Acupuncture for Hypertension

Hypertension is a systemic disease marked by persistent elevation of the arterial blood pressure, which may be attributed to disorders of the heart, brain and or blood vessels. Hypertension can exist as a primary condition independent of any other pathology or manifest as a secondary symptom of another disease or disorder. The manifestation of primary hypertension is often influenced by a combination of factors including genetics, occupation and environment, diet, sodium concentration, cholesterol levels, electrolyte and mineral balance, age, sex, obesity and stress. Secondary hypertension is high blood pressure that's caused by another medical condition that affects the kidneys, arteries, heart or endocrine system. It can also occur during pregnancy.

Chinese Medicine on Hypertension

In traditional Chinese medicine theory, hypertension often falls under the symptom of "dizziness," or "headache," two of its most common outward expressions. Although hypertension may arise from many diverse patterns, it frequently coincides with stagnant liver qi, improper diet, internal injury of zang fu organs, pathogenic phlegm or fire with impairment of the liver, kidney and spleen, etc. A body with a yang constitution, or long-standing anxiety or anger, tends to accumulate stagnant liver qi. Prolonged stagnation produces heat, the excess heat and pressure then creates fire. Over time, fire consumes liver yin; when yin is depleted, fire easily generates wind, which stirs, carrying liver yang upwards; the clinical manifestation is elevated blood pressure or hypertension. Improper diet, especially excessive intake of fatty and greasy food, raises blood pressure through a different mechanism. Fatty and greasy foods create damp-phlegm or damp-heat that impairs the spleen and stomach. Phlegm-dampness or damp-heat accumulates causing blockages and increased pressure within the vessels; liver-wind can then easily carry the pathology upwards causing dizziness and confusion. In the elderly, weak, thin and frail, dehydrated, or those recovering from prolonged illness, kidney-yin deficiency may exacerbate liver-yin deficiency, in turn giving rise to hypertension due to hyperactivity of liver yang.

In Chinese medical theory, co-occurring symptoms are grouped into patterns. The grouping then becomes the basis for syndrome differential diagnosis as well as the therapeutic target. Although Chinese medicine originated before blood pressure could be measured objectively, hypertension was effectively treated by resolving the pattern of signs and symptoms expressed in various types of hypertensions. When the signs and symptoms of hypertension no longer express themselves, the condition is considered to be controlled or resolved. To illustrate, it may be detected that a patient is likely to have objectively measurable hypertension by observing the most common clinical manifestations such as dizziness, headache (especially vertex or migraine with pressure behind the eyes, or a feeling that the head is in a vice-lock), emotional outbursts, short-temper, ringing in the ears, fatigue, shortness of breath, lassitude, pain in the loins and knees, memory loss, dry or red eyes, palpitation, tendency toward tendonitis or muscle strains and floating or excessive pulse. When these manifestations are eliminated, it is likely that the underlying conditions causing the hypertension has been controlled or resolved.

Some cases of hypertension fall under "vertigo" in Chinese medicine. The main pathologies underlying cases of vertigo due to hypertension include wind, stagnation of phlegm, excess of liver yang, deficiency of qi and blood, liver- and kidney-yin deficiency and blood stagnation. According to the Shang Han Lun, hypertensive vertigo may also present with excessive fluid and pathogenic factor in the shaoyang meridians. Dizziness arising from excessive fluid syndrome is nearly always accompanied by a sense of distress in the chest, palpitation, nausea, and vomiting. Shaoyang syndromes typically exhibit paroxysmal dizziness; when accompanied by heat and excessive fluid, shaoyang pathologies are also are marked by persistent dizziness, headache, nausea, and vomiting.

Syndrome differentiation of headache is similar to that of vertigo. The main conditions leading up to hypertensive headache are liver-yang excess, deficiency of qi and blood, kidney deficiency and stagnation of phlegm and blood. Flaring-up of liver fire is also common in patients with hypertension. Flaring-up of stomach, intestinal and meridian fire may also coincide with hypertension. Severe, boring, unrelenting headache suggests blood stasis; therefore, blood-activating and stasis-dissolving Chinese herbal medicinals are first-line agents that may offer the quickest route to pain relief.

Contrarily, cold accumulation in the liver and stomach may also provoke a severe headache in hypertensive patients.

Weakness and fatigue are extremely common in hypertensive patients as the deficiency of qi, blood, yin or yang is what allows for a relative excess to go unchecked. Deficiencies generally seen in hypertensive patients are not the characteristic symptoms of deficiency syndrome. Some result from an inner accumulation of dampness and water. Pathogenic damp, being weighty and sticky, leads to stagnation of the functional qi, while excess fluid stagnation consumes yang qi; this combined pathogenic excess pattern leads to weakness, fatigue, heaviness in head and body, and lassitude in the loins and limbs.

Identification of the specific hypertension etiologies and pathogeneses from a TCM perspective directly determines which differential pattern the particular syndrome falls under and which therapeutic approach to take. According to one traditional viewpoint, the pathogenesis of hypertension originates from yin deficiency, then progresses to include yang hyperactivity which manifests superficially, while phlegm-dampness and blood stasis infiltrate all through the meridians; in this case, the treatment principle consists of supplementing qi and nourishing yin. However, due to the ubiquitous use of antihypertensive agents, the progression of the disease is most often blocked, which greatly changes the natural course and pathogenesis of the disease. Given the wide-spread use of anti-hypertensive medication, contemporary patient-specific delineation of pathogenesis and differentiation of syndromes factors-in the presenting signs and symptoms derived from the original syndrome, along with the medication effects and side-effects. The overall treatment principle then relies on current layers of symptoms.

Although hypertension due to yin deficiency with yang hyperactivity is a classic presentation, there is variance among hypertensive patterns. Clinical experience and contemporary texts verify the prevalence of other contributing pathogenic factors along stages of disease etiology and progression such as heat, excessive fluid, and deficiency, occurring either independently or in concert with one- another. Pernicious heat can be detected at various stages of hypertension progression, especially when the target organ is healthy, showing no sign yet of damage. Extreme heat may lead to fire, commonly afflicting the liver, heart, stomach and/or intestines. Liver fire blazing is demarcated by vertigo, headache, facial flush with perspiration, conjunctival congestion yellowish in color, bitter taste in the mouth, severe irritability or agitation, wiry, rapid, overflowing, strong, excessive pulse, or powerful superficial liver pulse, or wiry and long pulse even well beyond the liver position. Patients with heart- fire syndrome often present with sensations of or intolerance to heat, extreme restlessness, fidgeting, and distraction, distress and fullness in the chest, sense of vexation or panic around the heart and within the mind, strong palpitations or pounding of the heart, excessive nervous energy, insomnia with tossing and turning and vivid dream-disturbed sleep or nightmares, difficulty falling asleep, inability to stay asleep and waking easily.

Zhi Zi Chi Tang (Decoction of Gardenia and Lobster Sauce) and Huang Lian Jie Du Tang (Detoxicant Decoction of Coptis) both can be used for clearing away heart fire and lowering blood pressure. Patients with exuberant stomach fire may have a dry mouth, irritated or sore throat, painful gums, heartburn, palpitations, hiccup, loud belching, burning stomach pains, ulcers, spitting blood, burning projectile vomit, intense thirst with desire for large amounts of cold drinks, extreme hunger, fast metabolism, loud voice, talkativeness, rapid speech, sweaty or warm forehead, frontal headache, foul breath, strong-smelling stool that may burn with defecation, burning muscular pain and inflammation, mania, aggressiveness, hatefulness, cravings, insomnia and excessive flooding or full stomach- pulse, which may flood into the heart pulse, and long, red tongue with a dry, yellow coat. Chinese herbal formula, Bai Hu Tang (*White Tiger Decoction*), can be used to cool heat, drain stomach fire and lower blood pressure in this case.

Often co-existing with stomach fire, signs and symptoms of blazing intestinal fire include foul breath; dry stool with strong odor; constipation; hot, explosive, foul diarrhea; hemorrhoids, fresh blood in the stool; abdominal distension, cramping and pain; strong and deep, hidden, flooding, forceful, warm pulse. Da Chai Hu Tang (*Major Bupleurum Decoction*) may drain intestinal fire, dredge the intestines, and descend and expel turbid waste. When liver fire and heart fire appear simultaneously, exacerbation of hyperactive fire occurs. Hyperactivity of liver, stomach, and intestinal fire occurs when the liver restricts the spleen and stomach.

Hypertension due to fluid retention, is divided into specific categories, all may include aversion to or dislike of water or fluids (taken internally, exposed to, or being submerged in). The main categories include: morbid fluid retained in the shang jiao (upper burner), zhong jiao (middle burner) and/or xia jiao (lower burner); retention of cold fluids; fluid retention transforming into heat syndrome; and downward draining damp-heat syndrome. Morbid fluid retained in the shang jiao affects the upper body including the heart and lungs and is more closely associated with the external as opposed to the internal layer. This type of hypertension coincides with heavy-headedness and dizziness aggravated by body position change; morbid thoughts; excess watery saliva or spit; difficulty speaking due to a sense of pressure or blockage in the throat, words may be easily drowned out; shallow breathing compounded by distressed, overwhelmed and drowning sensation in the chest; submerged palpitations or heavy pounding sensations; watery or congested cough or coughing up fluids, post-nasal drip or watery, runny nose; ears may be clogged or congested. The pulse may be flooding and overflowing especially at the heart and lung positions; tongue may be overly wet, flaccid, dusky with large amplitude and the anterior third may be swollen.

Morbid fluid retained in the zhong jiao manifests with gastric pressure, fullness, and distension; borborygmus with swishing, gurgling sounds; abdominal distension and pain worse with pressure; belching or a desire to belch or vomit; vomiting copious fluids; nausea, poor appetite or craving for small amounts of dry spicy food; thirst without desire to or ability to drink, lack of thirst, aversion to liquids or refusing to drink; difficulty swallowing due to epigastric pressure and fullness; daytime sleepiness and heavy eyelids; heavy and slow body; bloated appearance; limbs swollen with water-weight and lack of productivity or concentration. The tongue may be overly wet, dusky, bloated, enlarged with teeth marks and covered with greasy fur-like coating. The pulse may be overflowing or flooding and full in the liver and spleen positions at mid-depth.

Morbid fluid retained in the xia jiao can be identified by sore and painful low back and knees with lumbar heaviness; weakness and heaviness in the lower extremities; asthma worse with humidity or dampness; edema with or without pitting, especially in the legs and ankles; excessive watery leucorrhea; dysuria, turbid or copious urine or difficult urination; watery stool; low motivation and slow movements. The tongue may be enlarged, swollen in the rear, and wet with thick-greasy fur at the root. The pulse may be submerged, soggy, or full at the kidney position.

Hypertension due to retention of cold fluids can be differentiated by perceived coldness with aversion and dislike of cold and damp conditions; lack of thirst or preferring to sip warm fluids; nausea, retching, or vomiting liquids, possibly aggravated by ingesting even small amounts of fluid; cold and excruciatingly painful sensations in the kidneys, low back and whole spine; agonizing headache; constricted body, muscles and organs; and fainting or dysphoria with cold, damp hands and feet and skin. The tongue may be short/retracted, purple and enlarged with watery or excess coat. The pulse may by tight, full, sinking and/or submerged.

In cases where hypertension is related to fluid retention transforming into damp-heat that flows downward, many signs and symptoms may involve the spleen, kidneys, urination and bowels. Pattern differentiation includes: down-bearing sensation or burning pains and heavy sensations of the lower extremities; thirst for small amounts of cold drinks; yellow and thick leukorrhea; excess sweating with sweet or strong odor; beriberi; distended abdomen; foul stool that may vary between sticky, watery and constipated; turbid, dark excessive, difficult or burning urination and feeling sluggish, overly warm, bothered, resentful, depressed, betrayed, drained or tired. The tongue may be enlarged with toothmarks and a thick-greasy yellow fur in the center or at the root. The pulse may be obstructed, rapid, soggy, submerged and/or full from the spleen to the kidney position.

Ze Xie Tang (Decoction of American water Plantain), Fu Ling Xing Ren Gan Cao Tang (Decoction of Poria cocos, Apricot Kernal and Licorice), Wu Ling San (Wuling Powder), Ling Gui Zhu Gan Tang (Decoction of Poria cocos, Cinnamon Twig, Atractylodes macrocephala and Licorice), Ban Xia Bai Zhu Tian Ma Tang (Decoction of Pinellia ternata, Atractylodes Macrocephala and Gastrodia elata), Wu Zhu Yu Tang (Decoction of Evodia rutaecarpa), Er Miao Wan (Ermiao Pill), and Si Miao Wan (Simiao Pill) all can be selectively used for dissipating excessive fluid.

Hypertension due to deficiency often falls under spleen and kidney deficiency syndromes. As the spleen promotes transportation and transformation of dampness, spleen deficiency often leads to excessive fluid retention. Cang Zhu (Rhizoma Atractylodes), Bai Zhu (Atractylodes macrocephala), Fu Ling (Poria cocos), Ze Xie (American water Plantain), and Gan Cao (Glycyrrhiza) can all be used to remove dampness by strengthening the spleen and replenishing the qi. Hypertension arising from kidney deficiency syndrome includes both kidney-yin deficiency syndrome and kidney-yang deficiency syndrome, especially in prolonged disease. The longer the illness endures, the higher the incidence rate of kidney deficiency syndrome. Furthermore, antihypertensive medications can further contribute to kidney deficiency. Diuretics and β-blockers have greater impact on sexual function than other antihypertensive medications, with effects being more pronounced with sustained use lasting more than ten years. Chinese herbal formulas that may be applied to reinforce the kidneys include: Liu Wei Di Huang Wan (Rehmannia Pill), Shen Qi Wan (Kidney Qi Pill), Qi Ju Di Huang Wan (Pill of Chinese Wolfberry, Chrysanthemum, and Rehmannia) and Ji Sheng Shen Qi Wan (Pill for Reinforcing Kidney Qi).

Acupuncture on Hypertension

Acupuncture treatments for hypertension are presented for the following four common Chinese medicine patterns:

Hyperactivity of liver yang: marked by dizziness, tinnitus, distending headache and irritability.

Obstruction of phlegm dampness in the middle jiao: marked by dizziness, headache, heaviness of head, chest stuffiness.

Deficiency of liver yin and kidney yin: marked by dizziness tinnitus, soreness and weakness of lower back and legs.

Deficiency of qi and blood: marked by dizziness, exacerbated by movement, with pale complexion and lassitude.

Three special acupuncture points are essential for treating hypertension: Taichong (LV3), Fenglong (ST40), and Yanglingquan (GB34). With clinical manifestations from different patterns, acupuncture prescriptions are modified.

Hyperactivity of Liver Yang: Manifestations include dizziness, tinnitus with high-pitched ringing, distended headache, irritability, impatience or anger, heat sensation in the upper body and head, restless sleep, red face and eyes, inflammation of the tendons and bitter taste in the mouth. Tongue: Red sides with yellow coating. Pulse: Wiry. Acupuncture prescription includes points: Fengchi (GB20), Xingjian (LR2), Taichong (LR3), Jiaxi (ST40), Ganshu (BL18), and Shenshu BL23).

Obstruction of Phlegm Dampness in the Middle Jiao: Manifestations include dizziness, headache, cloudy thinking, heaviness of head, vertigo, distended abdomen, slow metabolism, bloating, nausea, vomiting with thick fluid, tastelessness in the mouth, poor appetite, tired, does not feel rested upon waking and grogginess. Tongue: White greasy tongue coating. Pulse: Wiry slippery. Acupuncture prescription includes points: Neiguan (PC6), Fenglong (ST40), Zhongwan (RN12), Touwei (ST8), Jiexi (ST41), Yanglingquan (GB34), and Yinlingquan (SP9).

Deficiency of Liver Yin and Kidney Yin: Manifestations include dizziness, tinnitus, soreness and weakness in the lower back and knees, blurred vision, dry eyes, dry skin, dry hair, slight thirst, hotness in the palms, soles and chest, listlessness, lassitude, insomnia with intermittent waking, hot flashes, night sweats and long-term forgetfulness. Tongue: Red, peeled tongue with cracks. Pulse: Wiry fine. Acupuncture prescription includes points: Ganshu (BL18), Shenshu (BL23), Sanyinjiao (SP6), Fengchi (GB20), Taichong (LR3), Taixi (KI3), Guanyuan (RN4), and Neiguan (PC6).

Deficiency of Both Qi and Blood: Manifestations include dizziness, more severe with movement or exertion, pale complexion, listless, lassitude, weakness, palpitation, insomnia, pale lips and nails, poor appetite, quiet, forgetfulness, and lack of concentration. Tongue: Pale listless tongue with thin whitish coating. Pulse: Fine, empty and weak. Acupuncture prescription includes points: Pishu (BL20), Zhongwan (RN12), Guanyuan (RN4), Zusanli (ST36), Ququan (LR8), Geshu (BL17), Sanyinjiao (SP6), Hegu (LI4), Taichong (LR3), Tanzhong (RN17).

Clinical Studies

The following clinical studies are collected to demonstrate the effectiveness of acupuncture on treating high blood pressure. They show the diversity of acupuncture treatment protocols, research designs and assessment tools.

Globally, blindness, or poor vision, frequently stems from glaucoma, with high individual intraocular pressure a strong contributing factor. Glaucoma often co-occurs with hypertension as overall blood pressure can be a source of ocular pressure. To address these concerns, researchers designed an observational study to determine the effects of acupuncture on patients with glaucoma or ocular hypertension. Eighteen patients, three with glaucoma and fifteen with ocular hypertension were observed [1]. Patients received one session of a standardized acupuncture protocol: Taichong (LR3), Hegu (LI4) and Guangming (GB37). Compatibility and change in intraocular pressure were assessed. Intraocular pressure was measured fifteen minutes before, fifteen minutes after, and twenty-four hours after acupuncture. Compared with average intraocular pressure in both eyes before the treatment (21.94 +/- 2.4 mm Hg), patients showed a significant decrease fifteen minutes after treatment (-2.67 +/- 1.34 mm Hg) as well as twenty-four hours after treatment (-2.5 +/- 2.13 mm Hg). No significant difference was found between the mean intraocular pressure at fifteen minutes after treatment and at twenty-four hours after treatment. Adverse events were not seen. Researchers concluded that acupuncture shows potential as an effective treatment option for glaucoma and ocular hypertension patients. Further randomized studies were recommended.

Wu *et al.* [2], examined the mechanism of acupuncture in hypertension patients and its influence on Angiotensin Converting Enzyme (ACE) and Endothelin (ET). Two acupuncture protocols were included for study, Taichong (LR3) and Quchi (LI11). Sixty hypertension patients were randomized into the Taichong group, Quchi group or the medication control group (Captopril). Research revealed that at fifteen minutes after acupuncture, those in the Quchi group showed greater lowering of systolic pressure than those in the Taichong group ($P < 0.01$). However, 120 minutes following acupuncture, the Taichong group showed greater lowering of the systolic than the Quchi group ($P < 0.05$). Following one course of treatment, both those who had received needling at Quchi (LI11) and those in the medication group showed greater improvement than those in the Taichong group ($P < 0.05$ and $P < 0.01$). Furthermore, serum ACE showed a significant increase in the Quchi group while plasma ET significantly decreased among those in the Taichong group, with values showing significant difference between the two groups, (all $P < 0.01$). Overall researchers reported that needling both Quchi point and Taichong point produce antihypertensive effects, Quchi-point needling having a greater antihypertensive effect than needling Taichong points. Both acupuncture groups effectively regulated blood levels of ACE and ET and positively influenced protection and repair of vascular endothelial cells. Researchers affirmed the positive actions of both acupuncture groups, although they proposed the underlying mechanisms of each may be different.

Gao *et al.* [3], sought to discover the blood-pressure-lowering action of auricular point Jiangyagou in patients with hypertension. One hundred and twenty-nine hypertension patients received electro-stimulation at auricular point Jiangyagou, for 20-30 minutes daily for three weeks. Of the 129 patients, forty-four showed markedly improvement, seventy-three patients showed some improvement and twelve showed no improvement; the total effective rate being 90.70%. Average systolic pressure decreased by (18.64 +/- 1.48) mmHg and the diastolic pressure was lowered by (8.01 +/- 0.68) mmHg, showing high significant differences between before and after auricular electro-stimulation at Jiangyagou in both systolic and diastolic readings. Researchers concluded that electric pulse stimulation of Jiangyagou effectively decreases both the systolic pressure and diastolic pressure in the hypertensive patient.

Hypertension is a primary risk factor leading up to both heart attack and stroke; with an estimated 25% of those afflicted not able to effectively manage the condition. Demographic disparities in the prevalence, treatment and control of hypertension have been addressed by the Joint National Committee on Prevention, Detection, Evaluation and Treatment of high BP (JNC 7 report), which offers lifestyle modification recommendations including yoga, meditation, acupressure and acupuncture with or without medicinal intervention. Historically, traditional Chinese medicine practitioners have been successfully treating hypertension as well other cardiovascular concerns for roughly 3000 years. Previous animal and human studies affirm the efficacy of acupuncture's long history of lowering both acute and chronic hypertension. Escalating interest from the United States as well as other western nations continues to spur research growth that may further reveal the specific effects of acupuncture applications as well as diverse accompanying mechanisms of action. Researchers Zhou and Longhurst [4] compiled existing research on acupuncture's capacity to regulate cardiovascular function, especially hypertension, finding widespread confirmation that acupuncture possesses potential as a non-pharmaceutical intervention in hypertension care.

When phlegm (in traditional Chinese medicine terminology) blocks the collaterals, the occlusion leads to elevated arterial pressure, thus hypertension ensues, (as in cases of high cholesterol). Researchers Huang *et al.* [5], observed the effects and assessed potential mechanisms of acupuncture in cases of phlegm-stasis-induced hypertension. Acupuncture protocol Fengchi (GB20), Quchi (LI11), Neiguan (PC6), Zusanli (ST36), Fenglong (ST40), Taichong (LR3) was administered to the intervention group along with oral administration of Captori; controls received medication without acupuncture. After four courses of treatment, significantly lower blood pressure values were seen in those who had received acupuncture; CRP, TC, TG and LDHD values were lowered as well. Benefits were also observed in hemorheological components and HDL values. Measurements relating to total symptomology as well as each individual symptom reflected significant improvement; with substantial significant differences seen as compared with pre-treatment status. Markedly significant differences were also seen compared with those taking medication alone ($P<0.01$). Researchers concluded that adjunctive acupuncture profoundly impacts blood pressure and cholesterol levels. It shows great promise in even reversing or delaying the progression of atherosclerosis. Mechanism of action may be associated with providing protection to the integrity of the vascular endothelium.

Acupuncture is endlessly diverse in its applications and effects. In addition to generalized hypertension, by varying point selection, traditional Chinese medicine can also treat cervical hypertension. In a randomized controlled trial, Cao *et al.* [6], treated thirty patients with bilateral cervical Jiaji points (EX-B 2), while thirty patients in the control group received acupuncture at Fengchi (GB20), Taichong (LR3), Quchi (LI11), Zusanli (ST36) and Yinlingquan (SP9). Among those who received acupuncture, 60.0% achieved a substantial reduction in blood pressure, compared with 43.3% in controls. Points 10 (33.3%) and 9 (30.0%) had a hypotensive effect, 2 (6.7%) and 8 (26.7%) had no apparent changes in blood pressure; 12 (40.0%) and 5 (16.7%) experienced marked improvement in clinical symptoms, 15 (50.0%) and 16 (53.3%) were effective, 3 (10.0%) and 9 (30.0%) failed in the treatment, with the effective rates being 90.0% and 70.0% respectively.

The therapeutic effect of the treatment group was apparently superior to that of the control group in lowering blood pressure and the cumulative scores of clinical symptoms and in improving clinical symptoms ($P < 0.05, 0.01$). This study concludes that acupuncture of Jiaji (EX-B 2) is an effective therapy in the treatment of cervical hypertension.

Whether acupuncture is best applied as an alternative or adjunct to standard pharmaceutical or lifestyle interventions is debatable. To gather more information on integrative approaches among pre-hypertensive or hypertensive patients, a randomized, double-blind, placebo-controlled trial was performed through Kyung Hee University Hospital [7]. Patients with systolic blood pressure greater than or equal to 120 mmHg, or diastolic BP greater than or equal to 80 mmHg received either actual or sham acupuncture. Of the thirty who completed the study, all were already taking medication and continued as directed. Acupuncture points were chosen according to Saam acupuncture protocols while the control group received Park's sham protocols.

Average blood pressure values showed no significant changes among controls; however, eight weeks post-intervention, patients who had received Saam acupuncture protocols exhibited a significant decrease ($p<0.01$) in average blood pressure values, averages falling from 136.8/83.7 to 122.1/76.8 mmHg.

Hypertension is linked with many detrimental and debilitating effects, often posing life-threatening risks. Though many cases are successfully managed with pharmaceuticals and other existing interventions, many are not. In searching for a wider array of options, and options with improved outcomes,

Flachskampf *et al.* [8], designed a study to gauge the ability of traditional Chinese medical acupuncture in lowering blood pressure. They conducted a single-blind randomized study in which approximately three-quarters of the one-hundred-forty participants who completed the study were taking stable prescriptions throughout. Results revealed that in patients receiving acupuncture, there was a significant post-treatment reduction in blood pressure by 5.4 mmHg (95% CI, 3.2 to 7.6); patients receiving sham acupuncture showed a drop of 3.0 mmHg (95% CI, 1.5 to 4.6). At three- and six-months post-intervention, systolic and diastolic values reverted to baseline levels in those who had received genuine acupuncture. Average 24-hour ambulatory blood pressures showed improvements after a six-week course of TCM acupuncture, whereas sham acupuncture did not. Improvements did not persist over time once acupuncture was discontinued.

Renal hypertension is a common concern in chronic kidney disease. Song YH [9], sought out to gather more information on potential acupuncture benefits for this population. In a randomized trial, acupuncture with medication was tested against medication alone. Balance points "Jiangya" and "Shenbing" were among the primary points administered to the combined method test-group. Small doses of hypotensor, Irbesartan were administered to this group as well; while oral administration of Irbesartan and Fosinopril were given to the medication group. Approximately fifty-six percent of the seventy-six participants in the combined method group hit the target-value, diastolic blood pressure less than or equal to 84.96 mm Hg, compared to approximately 54% of those taking medication alone; significant difference was not observed between groups ($P > 0.05$).

At both eight and twenty-four weeks the improvement in the combined method group was superior to the medication group ($P < 0.01$). Less protein was detected in the urine of those receiving combination treatment; concurrently blood creatine levels decreased. Elevation of the clearance rate of endogenous creatinine increased in both groups, showing significant differences ($P < 0.01$). Researchers concluded that acupuncture using primarily the Jianya (Extra) and Shenbing (Extra) points, combined with small doses of hypotensor and Irbestan produced similar clinical benefits as Irbesartan and Fosinopril on renal hypertension in patients with chronic kidney disease. After eight weeks, the combined method surpassed benefits seen in patients taking only medication.

Another study [10] was conducted to determine the effects and mechanism of electroacupuncture at specific points on hypertension and blood plasma catecholamines. In a randomized controlled trial, thirty patients with essential hypertension received electroacupuncture at Quchi (LI11), while thirty patients received medication (Nicardipine). After the intervention, researchers measured a significant decrease in systolic and diastolic blood pressure in those receiving electroacupuncture and the controls ($P < 0.01$). Adrenaline and noradrenaline levels significantly decreased as well ($P < 0.01$). Neither group showed significant differences in dopamine ($P > 0.05$). Effective rates were similar among groups, reaching 66.7% for electroacupuncture patients and 70.0% in controls ($P > 0.05$). Overall, the study demonstrated that electroacupuncture at Quchi (LI11) and Nicardipine produce positive effects on blood plasma catecholamines and HTN.

Hans electroacupuncture and its effects on hypertension were further studied by Zhang *et al* [11]. Over the course of five weeks, twenty-seven male participants averaging 25 +/- 5 years of age received thirty-minute bi-weekly Hans electroacupuncture at two points. A decrease in systolic pressure was observed; dropping form an average of 117.8 +/- 4.2 mmHg to 110.8 +/- 5.5 mm Hg ($P < 0.05$) during week three, then reaching 110.1 +/- 5.8 mmHg during week five ($P <0.05$). Diastolic measurements descended somewhat; from 78.1 +/- 5.0 mmHg to 77.4 +/- 4.3 mmHg ($P >0.05$) during week three, then reaching 74.8 +/- 4.3 mmHg ($P >0.05$) during week five. For controls, average systolic pressure dropped from 115.6 +/- 13.3 mmHg to 113.0 +/- 12.6 mmHg ($P > 0.05$) during week three, then reached 112.2 +/- 10.3 mmHg during week five ($P >0.05$). Average diastolic pressure dropped from 76.4 +/- 7.9 mmHg to 76.5 +/- 6.9 mmHg ($P >0.05$) during week three, before reaching 73.9 +/- 5.4 mmHg ($P > 0.05$) during week five.

Patients often notice beneficial effects of acupuncture as soon as needles are inserted or shortly thereafter. Some notice the sensation of de qi more than others, or some patients may feel de qi at some points and not at others. In 2006, researchers [12] surveyed patients as to their acupuncture experience, with specific focus placed on these two elements and their relationship to adverse reactions. Outpatients, 1095 in all, averaging fifty-eight years in age, from the East-West NEO Medical Center, and the Kyung Hee Medical Center were treated by acupuncturists who were also Korean medicine doctors with more than ten years of experience. Immediate benefits were experienced by 80.2% of the patients while 6.8% reported negative reactions. Of those reporting positive responses to acupuncture, 43.1% felt relaxed, 8.2% noticed a reduction in pain, 1.5% felt like they had more energy, 2.4% felt sensations such as tingling, heat or cold. Pain, tiredness and dizziness were among the negative reactions reported.

Traditionally, the sensation of de qi is sensed as a distended, pulling, sore, heavy, achy or numb feeling at the acupuncture point, that may travel up the channel, or create distal sensations. De qi was perceived by 39.7% of patients, under forty years old; while the greatest percentage of those with no reaction were among the those over seventy years old. Conditions being treated by acupuncture included stroke, headache, hypertension and dizziness. Bleeding, (which is not unusual when piercing the skin) was the only adverse event. Researchers assessed acupuncture to be very safe when, as in this study, acupuncturists are well educated, and experienced; with immediate benefits far out-weighing negative responses. Patients also reported high levels of satisfaction.

Chen, *et al* [13]. researched the potential mechanisms involved when combining acupuncture with orally administered Felodipine medication for patients with essential hypertension. They found that blood pressure was reduced in all sixty patients, who had been equally divided between the combined treatment and mediation only groups. The combined group exhibited a higher level of effectiveness, 86.7%, as compared to 73.3% in those who received only Filodipine. Plasma Es and iNOS was significantly lowered in all patients as well (both $P < 0.01$), with plasma Es values showing greater improvement among those in the combined group ($P < 0.01$). Patients receiving combined treatment also produced elevated concentrations of eNOS ($P < 0.01$). The mechanism of blood-pressure lowering effects seemed to correlate with improving cellular function within the vascular endothelium. Researchers concluded that acupuncture in conjunction with Filodipine improves Es, iNOS and eNOS expression. Optimal values of these markers tend to correlate with normal blood pressure.

Auricular acupuncture points are known to produce strong regulatory effects that may offer relief of acute symptoms as well as constitutional support. Researchers [14] tested the response of sixty-seven patients with arterial hypertension to trans-auricular low-frequency electroacupuncture. After one course, in addition to achieving lowered arterial blood pressure, a noticeable reduction in stress ensued, witnesses as less anxiousness, improved neurohumoral regulation of arterial pressure and central hemodynamics, greater ability to handle controlled psycho-emotional loading, enhanced cerebral blood circulation, and better lipid and electrolyte metabolism. Results bode well for auricular electroacupuncture's role in treating patients with arterial hypertension.

Electroacupuncture is known to be effective in certain conditions, to determine its effects in comparison to anti-hypertension medications, Yang [15] conducted a study with sixty young patients who had high blood pressure. After fourteen days, the response to electroacupuncture at Quchi (LI11) and Taichong (LR3) was compared with the response to taking oral Captoril. It was found that both diastolic and systolic pressures were lowered at various times (all $P < 0.01$). Compared with those who had taken Captoril, results were not statistically different (all $P > 0.05$). Standard deviations of systolic pressure and diastolic pressure at various times after electroacupuncture at Quchi (LI11) and Taichong (LR3) also diminished significantly ($P < 0.01$, $P < 0.05$). The blood-pressure lowering response in those who had received electroacupuncture at Quchi (LI 11) and Taichong (LR3) persisted over time and was seen to moderate fluctuations in day-night rhythm variation in the study population of young patients with hypertension.

Chen *et al.* [16], conducted a randomized controlled trial to determining the efficacy of a specific acupuncture protocol in regulating high blood pressure. The protocol consisted of typical acupuncture points for hypertension such as Fengchi (GB20), Quchi (LI11), Taichong (LR3); combined with Xingjian (LR2), Xiaxi (GB43) to settle liver-yang; and in cases of excessive phlegm-damp Ganshu (BL18) and Fuliu (KI7). Guanyuan (RN4) and Shenshu (BL23) was also added for patients with both yin and yang deficiency. Treatments were provided daily, Monday-Friday over the course of thirty consecutive days; while those in the control group were given 80 mg of Diovan medication per day. Significant reduction in blood pressure was seen in both groups, 45.0% in the acupuncture group and 67.5% in the Diovan group. Effective rates reached 80.0% in those who had received a course of acupuncture, and 95.0% in those receiving medication. Overall, researchers reported that those who had received hypertension-specific acupuncture excelled in lowering acupuncture compared with those who had received Diovan ($P < 0.05$).

Park *et al.* [17], designed a study to more accurately identify which acupuncture points possess the greatest positive potential in influencing dysfunctional endothelium in patients with hypertension. To ensure quality design and applicability of results, researchers conducted a randomized, placebo-controlled, double-blind, crossover trial. Fifteen patients assigned to the acupuncture group received four fifteen-minute acupuncture treatment phases, spaced seven days apart at bilateral Zusanli (ST36), Neiguan (PC6), Zusanli (ST36) plus Neiguan (PC6) and placebo points. At Zusanli (ST36), researchers observed a significant increase in flow-mediated dilation (0.266 +/- 0.078 mm to 0.306 +/- 0.077 mm, $p = 0.003$) which showed a significant change as compared to placebo ($p<0.05$). Acupuncture at Zusanli (ST36) plus Neiguan (PC6) also produced a significant increase (0.284 +/- 0.098 mm to 0.332 +/- 0.103 mm, $p < 0.001$); however, researchers found that flow-mediated dilation was unchanged after treating acupuncture point Neiguan (PC6) or the placebo points. Researchers concluded that endothelial dysfunction is immediately improved by acupuncture, and therefore, may limit cardiovascular disease-progression. Long-term effects of acupuncture in these cases require more long-term analysis.

Xing *et al.* [18], researched the efficacy of syndrome-specific acupuncture and its mechanism in cases of primary hypertension. All patients received daily acupuncture for fifteen days at Fengchi (GB20), Quchi (LI11), Zusanli (ST36) and Sanyinjiao (SP6). In addition to the previous points, the observation group also received acupuncture points consistent with individualized traditional Chinese medicine pattern diagnosis. After fifteen days, researchers discovered that the nail fold microcirculation increased in both groups. Blood-flow state integrals, peripheral capillary and total integral showed improvements as well, and were more significant among those who received syndrome-specific acupuncture than controls (all $P<0.05$). Overall, researchers found acupuncture to be an effective treatment modality in cases of primary hypertension. Syndrome-specific acupuncture was shown to increase the efficacy, and increased microcirculation was witnessed as the mechanism producing an important lessening in peripheral vascular resistance.

In the field of acupuncture, empirical points exist that alone seem to resolve a very specific condition or symptom. The mechanism by which an empirical point effects a condition is not always known and there may be no mention of the empirical function in any of the classic texts on point indications. Its use in a certain case may also fall outside of the point's seeming domain of influence. Clinically an empirical point is recognized over time; by direct verification. Research [19] was recently conducted to verify the immediate and long-term effects of empirical point Renying (ST9) on hypertension patients. Seventy patients with primary hypertension received acupuncture protocol: Renying (ST9), Hegu (LI4), Taichong (LR3), Quchi (LI11) and Zusanli (ST36) between 2pm-4pm. Patients received acupuncture over the course of three months. Researchers found that diastolic pressures at each time-point on the 1st, 15th, 30th and 60th days of acupuncture were significantly decreased compared with pressure before beginning the course of acupuncture (all $P < 0.05$). During the three-month treatment interval, the systolic and diastolic pressure before treatment every fifteen days was lower than before the start of acupuncture on day one (all $P < 0.05$). Researchers determined that acupuncture decreases blood pressure in hypertensive patients immediately following treatment; the anti-hypertensive effect remained stable over time. Acupuncture may be an effective modality for producing long-term benefit in hypertension patients.

Acupuncture needle-retention time can be varied for different purposes. Points on the scalp and ears are unusual in that they can be retained while individuals are engaged in mobile activities. This can be useful as points on the head and ears often have profound impact on the brain, nervous system and the organs themselves. Duration of needle-retention at Baihui (DU20) and Sishencong (EX-HN 1) were assessed according to impact on blood pressure in hypertension patients. Researchers [20] randomly assigned twenty-four HTN patients to either an acupuncture group, receiving needle stimulation for ten seconds (to achieve de qi) at Baihui (DU20) and Sishencong (EX-HN 1). Needles were then retained for eight hours. Nifedipine tablets (20 mg) were given to those in the control group. Systolic and diastolic pressure in the acupuncture patients and pressures were taken at the same point in time among controls, showed reductions in both groups ($P<0.05$, $P<0.01$). When monitored at thirty minutes and at eight hours post-intervention, the blood-pressure lowering effect was greater in the medication group ($P<0.01$); at two, four- and six-hours post-intervention significant differences leveled out. At thirty minutes, two, four, six- and eight-hours post-intervention, differences between diastolic lowering effects leveled out ($P>0.05$). Researchers summarized that retaining needles at Baihui (DU20) and Sishencong (EX-HN 1) reduces blood pressure in patients with hypertension, although medication acts more quickly and has a longer acting capability than the retained-needle method.

Blood pressure measurements tend to fluctuate according to activity level and the body's own natural rhythm. To gain greater understanding of how acupuncture affects blood pressure changes due to circadian rhythms, researchers [21] conducted a double-blind RCT. Thirty-three hypertension patients were administered a bi-weekly, eight-week course of either acupuncture at Zusanli (ST36) and Neiguan (PC6), or sham (placebo) acupuncture. The sham acupuncture group lacked a night-time drop in diastolic blood pressure, whereas night-time diastolic blood pressure did drop in patients who received real acupuncture (10.20 ± 7.56 mm Hg versus 5.21 ± 10.19 mm Hg, $p=0.038$). The number of patients who displayed a drop in nocturnal diastolic pressure also showed an increase from four to eight among those who received acupuncture. Researchers concluded that acupuncture may help regulate the circadian rhythm effects on blood pressure in patients with hypertension.

Acupuncture's role in mediating nitric oxide (NO) in patients with hypertension was recently studied [22]. Thirty-two patients from 32-65 years of age taking anti-hypertensive medication were provided ten acupuncture treatments over a course of ten weeks. Acupuncture was administered at points commonly used in hypertensive patients: Yintang (EX-HN), Taixi (KI3), Taichong (LR3), Yinlingquan (SP9), Hegu (LI4), Shenmen (HT7), Zusanli (ST36) and Sanyinjiao (SP6). Researchers found that after ten weeks of consistent treatment, systolic and diastolic pressures dropped following the first and tenth treatment ($p<0.05$). A rise in blood concentrations of NO was seen also at the first (71.5%) and tenth treatment (184.6%) ($p<0.05$).

The resting brain network and its relationship to cardiac function in hypertension was explored by assessing the role of acupuncture in affecting the hypothalamus [23]. Thirty right-handed patients, (approximately half male and half female) either received a five-consecutive-day course of acupuncture or became part of the control group. All received fMRI scans and twenty-four-hour blood pressure monitoring. Among patients who had received verum acupuncture, both blood pressure and heart rate averages fell immediately following the intervention, however the values did not reflect a significant change from baseline levels or between groups. According to scores on the SF-36, body pain ($P = 0.005$) was relieved while vitality ($P = 0.036$) improved compared to starting values. With respect to the hypothalamus-related brain network, those who had received acupuncture demonstrated greater functionality in the form of enhanced communication with the medulla, brainstem, cerebellum, limbic system, thalamus, and frontal lobes. Overall, researchers found that short-term acupuncture did not reach statistically significant reductions in blood pressure or heart rate. Patients reported relief from body pain and greater vitality. It was proposed by the researchers that the mechanism of action may be associated with effects on the cortex of the brain, hypothalamus, and brainstem.

Blood pressure control helps protect the heart and vascular system from further damage and disease. Although many cases of hypertension can be effectively managed, improved treatments and more options are needed. Sometimes, even creatively-combined medication prescriptions do not provide adequate aid, and prolonged use may produce harmful side effects. Some common side effects experienced by those on anti-hypertensives include fatigue, dizziness, weakness, headache and migraines, joint aches and pain, insomnia, cold extremities, edema and weight gain and low energy and feelings of depression. Researchers Cevik et al. [24], studied the effects of acupuncture on those who had been taking HTN medication such as ACE inhibitors, diuretics and beta blockers for a minimum of two years. Patients in the study received acupuncture protocol: Taixi (KI3), Taichong (LR3), Yinlingquan (SP9), Hegu (LI4), Shenmen (HT7), Zusanli (ST36), Sanyinjiao (SP6), Fuliu (KI7) and Taiyuan (LU9) every other day for one month. The protocol was found to have a lowering effect on both systolic (from 163.14 +/- 19.33 to 129.49 +/- 18.52) and diastolic (from 94.37 +/- 19.70 to 79.31 +/- 7.87) values. Researchers concluded that acupuncture in conjunction with current anti-hypertensive medications lessened complaints of side effects and that acupuncture be adopted into current standard treatment guidelines as its widespread use appears to be beneficial.

Concerns regarding hypertension-related heart disease span the globe. With widespread use of anti-hypertensive medication, the demand for non-pharmacological options have increased. Acupuncture point Quchi (LI11) is often included when treating hypertensive patients. To assess whether there are lateral effects of acupuncture when treating this population, either right or left Quchi (LI11) acupoints were needled in sixty hypertensive patients of average age approximately fifty-six years of age [25]. Researchers detected a significant lowering ($P<0.05$) in fHR immediately following needle stimulation. A rise in total HRV was seen immediately following insertion with significance seen at the end of stimulation and post-removal. Insignificant differences were noticed between the left and the right Quchi (LI11) acupuncture point. Researchers concluded that acupuncture at Quchi (LI11) improved heart rate variability in patients with high blood pressure and there may be some lateral effects.

An observational study was conducted to assess the clinical efficacy of acupuncture at Hegu (LI4), Taichong (LR3), Quchi (LI11) and Xingjian (LR2). In a randomized trial [26], sixty patients with essential hypertension received either acupuncture at Hegu (LI4) and Taichong (LR3), acupuncture at Quchi (LI11) and Xingjian (LR2) or medication for twenty-one consecutive days. Those in the medication group received twenty-five mg of Captopril. Researchers found that blood pressure was significantly lowered ($P<0.01$) in both acupuncture groups. Significant decreases in diastolic pressures were seen in the Captoril group after days, while it took twenty-one days to significantly reduce diastolic pressures in those who had received acupuncture (both $P < 0.01$). Those who received acupuncture also experienced significantly greater improvements in ratings of dizziness, soreness and weakness of waist and knees, and palpitations compared with those who took Captoril (all P < 0.05). Adverse events were also less frequently observed in the acupuncture group as compared with controls (P < 0.05). Overall, the study demonstrated that acupuncture at Hegu (LI4) and Taichong (LV3), Quchi (LI11) and Xingjian (LR2) lowers blood pressure and shows superior ability to lower diastolic pressure than oral Captopril. Acupuncture showed additional benefits of a reduction in symptoms commonly occurring with hypertension, such as dizziness, soreness and weakness of waist and knees, and palpitations.

Blood stagnation is often seen in patients with hypertension. Exercise helps circulate the blood and is often considered to protect against heart disease; it is often incorporated into a maintenance regimen for those who have high blood pressure. Certain Chinese herbals have blood-moving, cholesterol-lowering and other properties associated with blood-pressure lowering effects. A recent study [27] by Li sought to differentiate the benefits of acupuncture without herbal support and acupuncture with antihypertensive herbal patches in borderline cases of hypertension. A randomized trial was conducted in which thirty patients received acupuncture once per day for five consecutive days per week for four weeks at Fengchi (GB20), Taichong (LR3) and other points commonly used in hypertension protocols. The combined method group received the same acupuncture protocol and an herbal plaster, consisting of Chuanxiong (ligusticum wallichii) and Wuzhuyu (fructus evodiae) combined at a one-to-one ratio, ground into a fine powder and mixed with vinegar. Every other day, the Chinese herbal plaster was applied at the umbilicus, acupoint Ren 8.

It was discovered that both interventions reduced systolic and diastolic pressure (all P<0.001); with those in the combined method group showing significant difference compared with those who received acupuncture without the herbal plaster (P<0.01, P<0.05). Syndrome symptoms also improved in both groups; however, a significant difference was not observed between groups (both P<0.001 and P>0.05, respectively). Total effectiveness at a three-month follow-up (of effective and markedly effective cases), was 89.3% among those who had received acupuncture and herbal plaster; while it was 60.0% in those who received acupuncture without the Chinese medical plaster, with significant difference between groups measured at (P<0.05). Results positively indicated the use of acupuncture at specified points along with the Chinese herbal plaster, chuanxiong and wuzhuyu with vinegar, to protect against and treat patients with borderline hypertension. Benefits persisted over time for both acupuncture alone and the combined treatment method as described above;

with superior improvement in syndrome-related symptoms among those receiving the combined method.

The effects of acupuncture compared to Captopril medication was assessed in ninety patients with primary hypertension [28]. Patients were randomized into either an orally administered Captopril group or combined method group, receiving acupuncture and 12.5 mg Captopril twice per day. Daily acupuncture at Renying (ST9), Fengchi (GB20) and Baihui (DU20), with auricular Shenmen (TF4), Xin (CO15), Jiangyagou and Jiaogan (AH6a), was provided over the course of four weeks. At the study's conclusion, ambulatory blood pressure (24-hour) had improved for both groups ($P<0.01$, $P<0.05$); with relatively greater improvement in the combined method group ($P<0.05$). Variation coefficients were lowered in the two groups; in the combination group, variation within twenty-four-hour ambulatory blood pressure as well as systolic pressure was lowered to a greater degree in the combined method group as compared with the medication group (both $P<0.05$). Although both groups experienced a reduction in serum angiotensin II, plasma creatinine levels and TCM syndrome scores ($P<0.05$), greater improvements were seen in patients who received acupuncture in conjunction with Captoplil ($P<0.05$). Researchers also found that the combined method to be 95.6%, while Captopril alone was found to be 71.1% effective ($P<0.05$).

Overall, the acupuncture protocol, including auricular points Shenmen, Jiangyagou and Jiaogan was highly effective for patients with primary hypertension; eliciting greater improvements in twenty-four-hour ambulatory blood pressure, angiotensin II and creatinine levels than Captopril alone. Those in the acupuncture plus medication group also saw a reduction in TCM pattern symptoms, such as dizziness, palpitations and other related symptoms.

To gauge the ability of acupuncture to lower blood pressure in patients with borderline hypertension, Liu *et al.* [29], conducted a randomized, controlled pilot study. Thirty patients with systolic and diastolic blood pressures measuring between 120-159mmHg and 80-99mmHg received either acupuncture or no treatment. The acupuncture groups received bi-weekly sessions for eight weeks. After the intervention, researchers found that there was a significant difference between diastolic blood pressure (-5.7mmHg; $P=0.025$), but not systolic blood pressure (-6.0mmHg; $P=0.123$), between those who had received acupuncture and those who had not. However, four weeks after intervention conclusion, significant difference between groups was seen in both diastolic blood pressure (-7.8mmHg; $P=0.004$) and systolic blood pressure (-8.6mmHg; P=0.031). Significant differences were also seen in high frequency power between the those who had received acupuncture and those who had not after four and eight weeks (P=0.047 and P=0.030, respectively). Groups achieved similar Euro Quality of Life scores, body mass index scores and lipid profiles. Researchers concluded that the pilot indicates that acupuncture may have the potential to lower blood pressure in borderline hypertension cases, however a larger randomized controlled trial is needed with one hundred and ninety-four participants to confirm.

Researchers Li *et al.* [30], conducted a study to determine the effects of point-specific electroacupuncture on hypertension. Over the course of eight weeks, sixty-five hypertensive patients received weekly electroacupuncture at either PC 5-6+ST 36-37 or LI 6-7+GB 37-39. The interventions were administered by a single-blinded team of four acupuncturists. At termination of the intervention, assessment of scores was completed by a double-blinded evaluation. Scores showed a significant difference in lowering effect on peak and average systolic and diastolic pressures in those who had received electroacupuncture at PC 5-6+ST 36-37, compared with those in the control group who had received electroacupuncture at LI 6-7+GB 37-39. Fourteen patients demonstrated a long-term reduction in blood pressure with four more weeks of electroacupuncture at PC 5-6+ST 36-37; plasma norepinephrine levels, which had been elevated, also fell 41%; renin levels were reduced by 67% and aldosterone concentration dropped by 22%. Researchers concluded that electroacupuncture at select acupoints did reduce both systolic and diastolic blood pressure. Longer acting effects were attributed to sympathetic and renin-aldosterone influences.

Systematic Reviews and Meta-Analysis

The literature was reviewed to consolidate the collective findings regarding the effects of acupuncture on blood pressure in hypertensive patients. We selected the following six systematic reviews and meta-analysis.

Lee *et al.* [31] searched six electronic databases for randomized controlled trials through June 2007, with no language exclusions. Eleven trials of uneven quality met criteria; with lack of good reporting a commonality. Combined results from three trials, which were sham-controlled, did not find significant difference in systolic blood pressures with an average difference of 5 mm Hg, 95% CI (-12, 1), P = 0.12); while the pooled data also showed that acupuncture lowered diastolic blood pressure 3 mm Hg (95% CI (-6, 0), P = 0.05). Greater improvements were seen when acupuncture was provided with blood-pressure lowering pharmaceuticals, with significant systolic lowering of 8 mm Hg, 95% CI (-10, -5), ($P < 0.00001$); and diastolic lowering of 4 mm Hg, 95% CI (-6, -2), ($P < 0.0001$), with no heterogeneity between studies.

Four studies found acupuncture to be similar to pharmaceutical interventions in ability to lower blood pressure, although sample sizes did not meet standards to justify equivalence and researchers judged the studies to be of inferior quality. Studies evaluating groups who had received acupuncture or different types of controls had varied results and were difficult to validate as the majority were not of high quality. Researchers determined that lack of compelling data and poor study quality rendered them unable to make any strong statement regarding the efficacy of acupuncture in lowering blood pressure. They suggested that quality studies with greater rigor would be needed to make a scientific assessment.

The efficacy of acupuncture depends on applying protocols that address the individual's specific set of symptoms. In traditional Chinese medicine theory, hypertension may take on many different forms, each with varying co-symptoms. In a recent literature review [32], researchers compiled data on the treatment of hypertension with acupuncture according to "syndrome differentiation." Databases searched included: Medline, Embase, Cochrane Central Register, and China National Knowledge Infrastructure through September 2008. Randomized, controlled trials comparing acupuncture with controls such as sham acupuncture were selected. Those comparing acupuncture to other eastern and western interventions such as antihypertensive medications, Chinese herbal formulas, or exercise were also selected. After independent review for quality and high confidence intervals, twenty trials were selected. Out of the twenty, researchers assessed three of the trials to be more rigorous while the remaining seventeen did not adhere to strict methodology guidelines. With these factors in consideration, the compiled data of nineteen trials showed that acupuncture significantly regulated blood pressure compared to controls. Systolic blood pressure was reduced by a mean difference of 4.23 mmHg, diastolic blood pressure was reduced by 2.53 mmHg; groups were found to be significantly heterogeneous. Greater positive effects were seen as quality of trials increased. In two trials, acupuncture plus antihypertensive medications were found to significantly lower blood systolic and diastolic pressure averages compared with sham-acupuncture plus antihypertensive medications by 5.72 and 2.80, respectively; with no significant heterogeneity detected. Benefits increased further with the application of acupuncture according to syndrome differentiation. In data collected from eleven trials, average systolic (-6.46 mmHg) and diastolic (-3.07 mmHg) blood pressures were significantly reduced as compared with controls; no significant heterogeneity was found between groups. A significant reduction in blood pressure was not seen in compiled data of eight trials that did not apply syndrome differentiation protocols compared with controls. In these trials, acupuncture reduced the average systolic pressure by 1.55 mmHg and diastolic pressure by 2.12 mmHg; significant heterogenicity was observed between groups. Researchers concluded that greater number of rigorous studies are needed to more effectively evaluate the effects of acupuncture on hypertensive patients.

A literature review [33] on acupuncture and hypertension including data through January of 2013, was conducted by Wang J et al. Randomized, controlled trials on the effects of acupuncture compared with western modalities, sham acupuncture or lifestyle modification in hypertensive cases were gathered from PubMed, EMBASE, the Chinese Biomedical Literature Database (CBM), the Chinese National Knowledge Infrastructure (CNKI), the Chinese Scientific Journal Database (VIP), and the Wan-fang Data in the Cochrane Library. Language restrictions were not applied in the search. Cochrane standards were upheld throughout the process, which produced thirty-five trials totaling 2539 patients. Trials overall, were assessed to be of low methodological quality. Two trials comparing the effects of acupuncture and sham acupuncture with western medicine showed significant lowering of both systolic (-7.47 mmHg, $P<0.00001$) and diastolic pressure (-4.22 mmHg, $P<0.0001$); heterogeneity between studies was not detected. Many of the studies were difficult to assess relevance of results due to poor quality and small sample size. Five of the trials reported and described adverse effects. Researchers concluded that acupuncture may have potential benefits for patients with hypertension, however higher quality larger trials are needed to confirm positive findings.

The tonifying application of moxibustion has been studied for its use in cases of essential hypertension. To gather the collective data on this traditional Chinese medical intervention, researchers searched relevant databases for randomized, controlled trials on moxibustion and antihypertensive medications through March of 2013. Cochrane standards were adhered to throughout the inclusion process. In the five selected studies, data showed that moxibustion was no more effective than antihypertensive medications in lowering blood pressure. Moxibustion combined with antihypertensive medications did produce a lowering effect on systolic and diastolic pressures, which dropped an average of 9.57 mmHg and 4.08 mmHg, respectively, (both $P<0.00001$). The majority of trials did not report adverse events, leaving the safety of moxibustion as yet to be determined. Study methodology was deemed to be poor, limiting applicability of results. Researchers [34] concluded that more rigorous trials are needed to assess the use and safety of moxibustion as an adjunctive treatment for patients with essential hypertension.

Acupuncture is frequently used to treat cases of hypertension; however, the effectiveness of acupuncture is these cases had not been fully evaluated. Although sham acupuncture tends to be a controversial method of attaining meaningful data, researchers gathered the current information comparing acupuncture and sham acupuncture in cases of hypertension. Researchers Li *et al.* [35], searched relevant randomized, controlled trials via PubMed, the Cochrane Library, EMBASE, and the Chinese databases Sino-Med, CNKI, WanFang, and VIP through November of 2012. Of the four trials meeting the criteria, researchers found that acupuncture did not show greater reductions in systolic pressure than sham acupuncture, which dropped an average of 3.80 mmHg; however, a significant drop compared to sham acupuncture in average diastolic pressure of 2.82 mmHg was observed. The combined effect of acupuncture plus antihypertensive medication produced a significant reduction in both systolic and diastolic numbers. Of the adverse events reported, only minor events were associated with acupuncture. The results confirmed acupuncture's ability to significantly reduce blood pressure when combined with antihypertensive medications. Significant reductions were not found when acupuncture alone was administered to hypertensive patients.

The efficacy of acupuncture for hypertension was further reviewed by Xiao *et al.* [36]. Relevant databases were searched for randomized, controlled trials through mid-April of 2014. Twenty-three trials totaling 1788 patients met study criteria; researchers noted that among chosen studies, there may have been some bias concerning allocation, blinding, incomplete outcome data and selective reporting. Results of two trials comparing acupuncture to sham acupuncture plus medication, showed that adjunctive acupuncture with medication produced greater reductions in both systolic and diastolic blood pressure averages, which dropped 7.47 mmHg and 4.22 mm Hg respectively. Results from four of the trials confirmed that acupuncture combined with medication was more efficacious. The results from seven trials showed that acupuncture without medication was not more effective than medication alone in lowering systolic or diastolic values. Safety assessment remains inconclusive as specific and accurate information on adverse events was lacking among most of the RCTs. Researchers concluded that acupuncture is potentially beneficial as an adjunctive intervention with antihypertensive medication. Larger scale high quality studies are needed to determine the effectiveness of acupuncture alone in lowering blood pressure in patients with hypertension.

Mechanism

Empirical acupuncture points for lowering blood pressure have been identified, however the mechanism of most remains a mystery. To understand the mechanisms behind the blood pressure lowering effects of acupuncture at Zusanli (ST36), researchers [37] conducted a study. Current knowledge suggests that needling at Zusanli (ST36) activates nitric oxide synthase signaling mechanisms, thus affecting blood pressure. In an animal study, researchers used the two-kidney, one-clip renal hypertension (2K1C) hamster model to test the effects of electroacupuncture treatment on arterial pressure, nitric oxide concentration and nitric oxide synthase. Electroacupuncture was administered at Zusanli (ST36) over the course of five days. Researchers found that arterial pressures were more effectively reduced in hamsters receiving electroacupuncture at Zusanli (ST36) in than those receiving sham acupuncture. Electroacupuncture at Zusanli (ST36) was also found to increase periarteriolar nitric oxide from 309.0 +/- 21.7 nM to 417.9 +/- 20.9 nM in the hamster models. Compared to sham controls, a reduction in endothelial nitric oxide synthase (eNOS) as well as neuronal nitric oxide synthase (nNOS) was seen in tissues along the stomach meridian among those in the treatment group. Researchers found that electroacupuncture lowered eNOS and hypertension-related nNOS; with results more elevated in tissues along the stomach channel, than in the sham controls. Liver tissue did not show the same changes in eNOS and nNOS; indicating that effects do not necessarily extend beyond the stomach meridian. Researchers concluded that the antihypertensive effects of electroacupuncture at Zusanli (ST36) appears to be associated with reductions in eNOS and nNOS along the stomach meridian.

Although there have been many advancements in pharmacological regimens, many have unwanted side effects, and there are always those cases that do not respond. To improve results, or mitigate side effects of medication, acupuncture is often used in conjunction with pharmaceuticals. Stress is a strong indicator and risk factor for elevated blood pressure; via negative effects on the sympathetic nervous system and the adrenals. In some cases, AT1 receptors in the rostral ventrolateral medulla (rVLM) has been found to suppress the sympathetic system and lower blood pressure. Whereas hyperactivity of the angiotensin system in this nucleus may serve to moderate blood pressure. Past experimental studies have shown that electroacupuncture has an activating effect on arcuate nucleus, ventrolateral gray, and nucleus raphe neurons, which then decreases neural activation in the rVLM among hypertensive models. Researchers [38] suggested that greater understanding of the effects of acupuncture on structures in the brain, central nervous system and the endocrine system will positively impact the way acupuncture may be used in treatment of hypertension.

The effect of electroacupuncture on hypertension via neuronal regulation was researched by Li *et al* [39]. Experimental studies have shown that electroacupuncture inhibits sympathetic neurons within the cardiovascular system in stimulated models. This mechanism was found to act through arcuate nucleus neuronal activation within the hypothalamus, through vlPAG in the midbrain and through NRP in the medulla. This activation then has an inhibitory effect on premotor sympathetic neurons in the rVLM. Endorphins, glutamate, acetylcholine, opioids, GABA, nociceptin, serotonin and endocannabinoids may all contribute to the blood-pressure lowering effect of electroacupuncture. Through this complex response, researchers found that low-current/frequency electroacupuncture at Jianshi (PC5)-Neiguan (PC6) and Zusanli (ST36)-Shangjuxu (ST37) may reduce hypertension in approximately 70% of patients with borderline hypertension. They found the onset of effect to be slow but persistent. Although many potential mechanisms of electroacupuncture's effect on hypertension and cardiovascular function have been identified, further avenues of research into this area may provide more specific and meaningful information.

Acupuncture and moxibustion's mechanisms of actions on hypertension have been studied to some degree. Studies on mechanisms affecting the regulation of the nervous system, humoral artery and peripheral vessel resistance in relation to hypertension were recently reviewed. Researchers [40] found that more information needs to be gathered through studies on blood pressure-lowering point combinations, understanding optimal time-effect and dose-effects and illuminating mechanisms related to the nervous, endocrine and immune systems.

Given the individualized nature of treatment protocols and multitude of potential acupuncture applications and approaches, the field lends itself to great variance in study design. To determine benefits of various designs, acupuncture and moxibustion studies were compared with regards to their use in hypertension. Through the process of document retrieval, clinical research on the treatment of hypertension with acupuncture and moxibustion have already been published. Although these studies were high in quality, applications were limited due to design variability. Researchers [41] suggested that high quality design proposals which follow standard acupuncture-moxibustion procedures, and are accepted by western medicine are needed to gauge the advantages of acupuncture-moxibustion on TCM pattern symptoms as well as clinical outcomes. They suggested improved standards on measuring the blood pressure, they also suggested standardizing sample size calculation, selection of the control measurements, stochastic method and implementation of the blind methods.

Analgesic and cardiovascular effects of acupuncture have increasingly become a topic of interest in the growing field of acupuncture research. Studies and clinical experience have shown that manual and low-frequency, low-intensity electroacupuncture produce favorable effects on blood pressure and cardiovascular effects in patients with hypertension. Effects seem to be the result of a compilation of mechanisms. Stimulation at acupoints is thought to activate underlying sensory neural pathways that interconnect with the central nervous system (CNS). Activation of structures and pathways within the hypothalamus, midbrain, and medulla then moderates cardiovascular function and blood pressure. Somatic effects on neurotransmitters impact autonomic systems, such as those that regulate blood pressure. Lowering of elevated blood pressure has also been attributed to acupuncture's effects on the thoracic spinal cord. Sympathetic and parasympathetic nuclei effects in the medulla are also produced through electroacupuncture. Researchers [42] assessed that the autonomic effects, such as moderation of blood pressure, to be slow in onset but long-lasting. Researchers propose that findings suggest that acupuncture has potential to treat a range of cardiac diseases related to sympathetic system hyperactivity, such as myocardial ischemia and elevated blood pressure.

Essential hypertension may affect many areas of health, and the state of the immune system may strongly influence the emergence and progression of hypertension. Yu *et al.* [43], proposed taking a closer look at cellular immune factors as well as body fluid immune factors that influence hypertension. They also suggested researching the effects of acupuncture on natural killer cell activity, exercise-induced immunosuppression, concentration of circulating inflammatory markers and cytokine concentration. Research has shown that TNF-alpha, IL-6, matrix reduction, metalloproteinases-9, angiotensin convertase and endothelin concentration tend to show reductions in response to acupuncture while serum opioid peptide content and other factors that relieve inflammation within the cardiovascular system tend to increase. Further research in these areas may bring about a greater level of understanding of acupuncture's positive effects on essential hypertension and provide insight into its connection with the immune system.

Chapter Eight

Acupuncture for Schizophrenia

Understanding Schizophrenia

A person suffering from schizophrenia may feel both cursed and blessed, as the mind may be plagued with dark thoughts, hallucinations, delusions or confusion one moment, and then display some form of unspeakable genius the next. On one end of the spectrum, altered, distorted and twisted messages; the essence of which may be so dark, maniacal, menacing, torturous, condescending, hateful; that mental capacities may be overwhelmed to the brink of either constant agony, or the acting out of some horribly regretful compulsion. Contrarily, many individuals with Schizophrenic tendencies also experience supremely inspired states of heightened awareness that may yield glorious masterpieces in the fields of art, science or mathematics that deeply reach into the heart and minds of humanity, profoundly uplifting whole populations. Schizophrenia is not as rare as one might think, although outward signs and symptoms can be suppressed or go unnoticed for lengths of time. An estimated 1.0-1.5 percent of people in the U.S. are said to suffer from schizophrenia at some point in life.

A cascade of symptoms leads up to the expression of schizophrenia; generally proceeding from subtle shifts in thought patterns to physical expressions of grossly abnormal behavior. Rational, organized and meaningful thought may deteriorate progressively during the disease, escalating to a point where the separation from reality and non-reality becomes indistinguishable. Disconnected or loose associations give way to meaningless speech and impaired ability to process what is heard; making fluid conversation impossible. Delusional states may take the form of conspiracy plots that infiltrate every aspect of life. Feelings of being watched, followed, surveilled, undermined, sabotaged, mocked or ostracized may invoke a constant sense of unbearable paranoia. A person with schizophrenia may feel a lack of privacy even of thought, sensing that what is held in mind is being "broadcast" and can be heard by other people. Visual, audible or tactile hallucinations may haunt an afflicted person, making it difficult to distinguish between what is actually happening and that which is delusional. Most often, auditory hallucinations take the form of voices heard only by the afflicted person. An auditory hallucination may take the form of a constant running commentary on the person's every thought, feeling or movement; may threaten the person or command the person to do harm to self or others; may encourage paranoia by engendering a sense of imminent danger; or may harass or torment the individual. Some may hear multiple voices. Schizophrenia is also characterized by the absence of certain normal traits, such as the lack of expressed emotion, or blunted affect, lack of motivation or apathy and social isolation. In traditional Chinese medicine, schizophrenia is considered Dian Xian.

Schizophrenia is a disorder that originates in the brain. With billions of neurons firing chemical signals via the neurotransmitters, the relay of messages is orchestrated without conscious effort. In schizophrenia, these messages are disordered or altered in some way. Multiple genes have been identified as pre-indicators for schizophrenia. Developmental factors such as prenatal trauma due to malnutrition, viral infections, complications, various forms of stress throughout life, brain chemistry and constitution each may influence the expression of schizophrenia.

Human genome studies indicate that chromosomes 13 and 6 may play a role in schizophrenia, although further study is needed. Current research in brain chemistry has also revealed that the neurotransmitters dopamine and glutamate may be involved in the illness. Neuroimaging technology has provided a gateway by which brain activity can be observed in living individuals. Although many studies detect slight abnormalities in brain physiology or activity in some people with schizophrenia, the changes are not universal among all those with schizophrenia and therefore must not be determining factors; some of these variances are witnessed in people without schizophrenia as well. Histology research shows slight abnormalities in the amount and distribution of neurons; the appearance of which may arise before or after onset of the condition. During the fetal stages of development, neurons may have formed abnormal connections, producing effects in early adolescence as the brain chemistry naturally shifts. Brain-imaging has also revealed that early alterations in biochemistry may be detected before the onset of symptoms.

Although there is no known cure for schizophrenia, many afflicted are able to manage the symptoms with medication. Anti-psychotics, anti-depressants and anxiolytics are often given in combination as well as anti-hypertensives in many cases to address the dynamic thought and mood fluctuations and complexities related to Schizophrenia. Risperidone, (Risperdal), Olanzapine

(Zyprexa), Quetiapine (Seroquel), Ziprasidone (Geodon), and Clozapine (Clozaril) are examples of some medications commonly used in the treatment of those with Schizophrenia.

Risperidone (Risperdal) has been prescribed in the United States since 1994. Although less tranquilizing than other atypical anti-psychotic medications, a greater likelihood of extra-pyramidal effects suggest it may not be well-tolerated by those who struggle with coordination. As its mechanism of action tends to have a dampening effect, watery weight gain, excessive mucous production, edema and diabetes are potential side effects. Two years later, in 1996, American physicians began prescribing Olanzapine (Zyprexa) for schizophrenia. Compared with Risperidone, pyrimidal side-effects were found to be less of a problem. Although Zyprexa may enliven the affect in some people with schizophrenia; excessive weight gain and increased risk of diabetes are deterrents to its use. Quetiapine (Seroquel) arrived in the United States in 1997. Extrapyramidal effects were found to be less common than with Risperidone; and, weight gain and diabetes may potentiate at a lower rate than with Clozapine or Olanzapine. Ziprasidone (Geodon) was introduced to Americans in 2001. Not likely to induce extrapyramidal effects, or be as likely to induce weight gain and diabetes as are atypical antipsychotics, cardiac arrhythmia may be exacerbated. Therefore, the use of Geodon is not advised with other medications that may alter the rhythm of the heart. Clozapine (Clozaril) has been prescribed for schizophrenia in America since the 1990s. It is often used when other treatments have failed; often employed to reduce the risk of suicide. White blood cells may be affected by the use of Clozaril and need to be monitored throughout treatment. Weight gain and diabetes are common side effects.

Although they may be effective in moderating some symptoms, taking large amounts of anti-psychotic medications has been linked to brain tissue deterioration. The *American Journal of Psychiatry* has published studies that reveal the effects of anti-psychotics on the brains of schizophrenic patients [1]. A longitudinal study, was conducted to monitor brain changes associated with extended use of anti-psychotic medications. Initial evaluation was taken after the first Schizophrenic episode, which continued periodically over the subsequent fifteen years. Researchers tracked neuro-deterioration via scans taken every six months. With higher doses, researchers found a concordantly higher loss of functional tissue.

Schizophrenia can be devastating and frequent episodes may be associated with a greater incidence of brain loss; however, studies have not fully confirmed this supposition. Researchers assessed MRIs from 202 patients taken periodically over an average of seven years. By analyzing data over the course of treatment, researchers noticed an increase in brain loss among those who had received more intensified medical interventions. The researchers confirmed that prolonged schizophrenic episodes may be destructive to neuronal tissues, and suggested increasing focus on protective measures and encouraging compliance with maintenance therapies. As with many conditions, there seems to be a delicate balance between protecting the integrity of the physicality from the negative impact of episodes while limiting negative impact of pharmaceutical interventions. Treating with the lowest necessary dose may be one method of maximizing benefits while minimizing side effects of treatment.

Incorporating acupuncture and Chinese medical modalities may provide a means by which to reduce the amount of medication needed and; therefore, limit brain loss in those suffering from schizophrenia. To gather scientific data on the effects of adjunct acupuncture treatment, patients with schizophrenia, depression and sleep disorders were assessed. Researchers expressed the importance of differential diagnosis in determining a treatment principle; as, in traditional Chinese medicine, one western psychiatric diagnosis may encompass many individual patterns of expression requiring different treatment approaches. Insomnia and sleep disturbance is common in conditions such as schizophrenia and depression. Determining the underlying pattern and applying the correct treatment principle in each case is one way to increase effectiveness of treatment for the main condition and the co-existing type of sleep disorder. Researchers also underlined the potential benefit of resolving the sleep issue as a means to alleviate mood symptoms.

Western Diagnosis

Schizophrenia in western medicine is defined by episodes in which unusual states manifest as psychosis. Auditory, visual or tactile hallucinations may be experienced as if real. Delusional thoughts or speech that take on a grandiose nature and abnormal or disconnected thinking in which the patient often draws loose associations between unrelated events, people, places or things may also predominate. In addition to fluctuating periods of withdrawn or isolated preference to overly social or invasive relations; the afflicted may express a blunt affect, little motivation or a disturbed, confused or disorganized demeanor. Work and social situations may be difficult to manage and navigate; productivity and cooperation may be limited. Western Psychiatric Symptom Subtypes:

Western medicine also recognizes the distinct categories within the schizophrenic spectrum. The paranoid subtype is dominated by delusions or hallucinations, without disorganized thought patterns or catatonia. In fact, this person may display an obsessively high degree of organization; however, the attention may be focused on delusional phenomena.

The disorganized subtype may not be overtly paranoid, rather the speech may be incoherent, broken or non-intelligible. Actions may also display a lack of organization. Catatonia is absent in this group. The catatonic subtype is so withdrawn that immobility may be accompanied by mutism; or the person may move as if in a driven trance, oblivious to the external world. A person in a catatonic state may exude negativity, may parrot words of others or repeat certain words or phrases hypnotically; a patient displaying the catatonic subtype may also copy or mimic the actions of others or perform a certain action repeatedly. The undifferentiated subtype simply expresses the general aspects included in the Schizophrenic spectrum; while the residual subtype exhibits only some undifferentiated symptoms.

A person may display characteristics similar to those seen in schizophrenia; however, symptoms are not compelling enough to meet the full criteria of schizophrenia. Schizophreniform disorder is one such manifestation. In a schizophreniform condition, the same symptom pattern is displayed; however, the duration of symptoms has spanned at least one month, but not yet six months. In a brief psychotic disorder, the pattern mimics the psychosis seen in schizophrenia; however, symptoms are limited in duration, lasting more than one day, yet less than one month. Delusional disorders may be expressed in which mild delusions predominate for at least one month, yet never meet the criteria required for schizophrenia. A closer approximation to schizophrenia, a patient with a schizoaffective disorder will display a pattern of mania and depression while experiencing a psychotic episode. When experiencing a substance-induced psychotic disorder, psychotic symptoms associated with a mind-altering substance are expressed only while intoxicated.

Secondary Psychosis

In certain circumstances, psychotic symptoms may be related to, or coincide with, another medical condition. Diseases of the brain such as CNS lesions and brain tumors may physically or chemically alter specific brain features, inducing states and symptoms similar to those seen in schizophrenia. Disorders that either accelerate or decelerate metabolic processes such as hyper- or hypo-thyroidism may generate manic or catatonic states. Systemic Lupus Erythematosus (SLE) and Multiple Sclerosis (MS) are two illnesses that may affect the ability to think rationally and stay connected to reality. States of generalized delirium or dementia of any etiology may occur along with many medical conditions. Mind-altering substances such as alcohol or street drugs may induce a temporary psychotic state; while persistent use may alter the brain chemistry such that a psychotic condition becomes ingrained. Psychoactive medications, including steroids, L-DOPA and opiates may also bring on a psychotic episode or condition.

Etiology and Pathogenesis from a TCM Perspective

When the emotions are out of balance, and the mind is conflicted, physical signs and symptoms may progress to a diseased state if left unresolved. In TCM theory, Schizophrenia is said to arise from over-activity of the five minds and excesses of the seven affects. Overly expressed anger, fear, and terror or obsessive thoughts disrupt the normal flow of qi in the channels and eventually damage specific organ systems. Yin and Yang become imbalanced, leading to a host of potential ills. Lack of ability to resolve emotional states as they arise may then lead to maladaptive patterns such as qi depression, phlegm stagnation, pathogenic fire or blood stasis. Any emotion can distress the heart, cloud the orifices and disturb the spirit. Normal brilliance fades and psychological integrity may diminish; further deterioration may ensue progressively. Of course, individual constitutional strength from birth, as well as that developed during the lifetime, will determine how deeply any stress affects the mind and spirit. If the upright qi is intact and the Yin is abiding while Yang is replete, stressful events or challenges may upset the overall balance peripherally; however, disease will not take root in a resilient person. If a person's constitution is chronically weak, or if Yin or Yang are in a constant state of relative imbalance, reactivity to perceived stress may easily disrupt the spirit, withdrawal or mania may then be resorted to as coping mechanisms.

Individuals with schizophrenia frequently display neurologic deficiencies, including loss of dexterity or coordination and increased blinking of the eyelids. Inability in following a sequence of steps may be due to disturbance affecting the right parietal lobe. Neuro-psychological exam and functional brain-imaging suggest that the temporal and frontal lobes are especially affected in patients with schizophrenia; thus, language and executive functioning, as well as abstract reasoning may be limited.

TCM Differentiation: Divergent manifestations of schizophrenia fall under specific categories in traditional Chinese medicine. When a withdrawn personality alternates with manic episodes, the disease is called "Dian Kuang;" when the condition is purely manic, it is termed "Kuang Zheng" and when the condition is more sedate, marked by lack of mental responsiveness, it is considered, "Chi Dai."

TCM Pattern Differentiation

In many cases a patient exhibits a combined pattern or multiple patterns simultaneously. Paranoid schizophrenia is often the result of both qi stagnation and blood stasis. The classic symptoms defining schizophrenia are visual hallucinations, auditory hallucinations, forming loose associations, intense emotional fluctuations or bizarre behavior. In order to meet standard diagnostic criteria, a patient needs to expresses at least three of five hallmark symptoms; or, two of the symptoms must be severe. Also, manifestation of symptoms must last the duration of at least one month. The tongue may be purple, dark or dusky; and the veins on the underside of the tongue will be gorged and purple or dark. The pulse will be uneven or wiry and full. The most crucial acupuncture points to include in this case are Xuehai (SP10) and Geshu (BL17).

Disorganized schizophrenic states generally arise when phlegm and fire combine. Harassment of the spirit or heart is inevitable. Diagnosis of disorganized-type schizophrenia also requires that three of five hallmark characteristics be displayed; or, two are severe. For disorganized psychosis, the five most important symptoms to observe are: chaotic thoughts, vivid hallucinations that make distinctions between the real and unreal difficult to discern, extreme sensitivity, immature or strange behavior and manic states with compulsive behavior. Here also, symptoms must manifest continuously for at least one month to meet diagnostic criteria. Dissolving phlegm to unblock the orifices and clearing heat are the primary treatment principles for this type of schizophrenia. The tongue may be bright or deep red with a thick, slimy or sticky yellow coat; while the pulse may be slippery and rapid with force at the skin surface.

Acupuncture protocols may center on fire points and stomach source points, including such points as: Tongli (HT5), Xiangu (ST43), Weishu (BL21), Zhongwan (RN12), Xingjian (LR2), Lidui (ST45), Shaochong (HT9),

Waiguan (TB5), Zulinqi (GB41), Houxi (SI3), Shenmai (BL62) and Neiting (ST44).

Catatonic schizophrenia often coincides with Yin deficiency that has given rise to fire blazing.

As in other types of schizophrenia, diagnosis depends on the presence of three of the hallmark signs; or extreme manifestations of two of the characteristics. The five definitive characteristics for catatonic schizophrenia are: delusions and hallucinations, suspicious and hostile behavior; blunted affect interspersed with bouts of excitability, loneliness with tendency to withdraw and isolate, states of non-responsiveness which may be interrupted by spontaneous excitation. To meet diagnostic criteria, symptoms must persist for at least thirty consecutive days. The tongue will be bright or dark red, with little or no coat; while the pulse will be slippery, thin at the deep level and forceful at the surface.

One way to resolve this type of catatonic schizophrenia is to nourish the Yin and extinguish the fire. Front-mu points may be combined with points that drain the fire and nourish Yin, including such points as: Chengjiang (RN24), Shangxing (DU23), Fuliu (KI7), Zusanli (ST36), Guanyuan (RN4), Lieque (LU7), Zhaohai (KI6), Quchi (LI11) and Yanglingquan (GB34).

Uncomplicated schizophrenia is generally due to obstruction of phlegm-dampness. As with other types of schizophrenia, three of the five hallmark symptoms need to be present in order to attain a diagnosis; or two characteristics must be pronounced. To meet criteria, symptoms need to endure for a continuous two-year span. The hallmark symptoms for simple Schizophrenia are: blankness of mind, lack of emotions, apathy or a passive attitude, lack of motivation or will and lack of social engagement. The tongue will be puffy, enlarged and flabby with toothmarks and a thick white slimy coat; while the pulse will be slippery, soft, submerged or moderate.

To resolve schizophrenic patterns that emerge from prolonged phlegm-damp, acupuncture points may be selected that target the affected organs and channels along with points that tonify the spleen's ability to metabolize damp. An acupuncture protocol may contain: Yinlingquan (SP9), Zusanli (ST36), Fenglong (ST40), Taichong (LR3), Zhongwan (RN12) and Fengchi (GB20).

Chronic schizophrenia is often due to Yang deficiency. Three out of five of the following characteristic need to be met to meet diagnosis criteria: blankness of mind or floating thoughts, blunted affect or catatonia, low motivation or will, isolation or withdrawal, and reluctance to speak or mutism. In order to meet criteria, symptoms must also persist continuously for a minimum duration of two years. The tongue will be pale, dark or greyish with a thin white coat; while the pulse will be deep and deficient. Acupuncture points that include the front-mu or back-shu of the kidney, heart and spleen, mingmen, and those that tonify qi may be selected; an appropriate prescription may include: Ligou (LR5), Taixi (KI3), Guanyuan (RN4), Baihui (DU20), Hegu (LI4), Zusanli (ST36), Tanzhong (RN17), Jujue (RN14), Zhongwan (RN12), Taichong (LR3), Neiguan (PC6) and Gongsun (SP4).

Some of the most effective points for treating many forms of Schizophrenia: Fenglong (ST40), Sanyinjiao (SP6), Jianshi (PC5) toward Zhigou (SJ6), Daying (RN5) with Qihu (RN13), Baihui (DU20) with Si Shen Cong, Yongquan (KI1), Xinshu (BL15), Ganshu (BL18), Pishu (BL20), Dingshen, Shenmen (HT7), Fengchi (GB20).

The following points may also provide substantial benefit: Renzhong (DU26), Neiguan (PC6), Yintang, Shentang (BL44), Shenting (DU24), Yanglingquan (GB34), Dazhong (KI4), Daling (PC7), Tianchuang (SI16), Ligou (LR5), Zusanli (ST36), Zhongwan (RN12), Bizhong, Jianli (RN11) and Tongli (HT5).

Additional points may be added according to individual manifestation.

For manic episodes, points may be selected from: Dadun (LR1), Qiangjian (DU18), Jiuwei (RN15), Laogong (PC8), Shaoshang (LU11), Taichong (LR3), Renzhong (DU26), Ligou (LR5), Neiguan (PC6), Quchi (LI11), Ququan (LR8), Yinxi (HT6), Chengjiang (RN24), Yinbai (SP1), Shangxing (DU23) toward Baihui (DU20), Hegu (LI4) toward Houxi (SI3) and Taixi (KI3) toward Yongquan (KI1).

For depression, points may include: Xinshu (BL15), Ganshu (BL18), Pishu (BL20), Shenshu (BL23), Jujue (RN14), Daling (PC7), Laogong (PC8), Yongquan (KI1), Tanzhong (RN17), Taichong (LR3), Xingjian (LR2), Yin Tang, Neiguan (PC6) toward Waiguan (SJ5), Hegu (LI4) toward Laogong (PC8).

To revive conscious awareness in unresponsive patients with Schizophrenia: Baihui (DU20), Shenting (DU24) toward Shangxing (DU23).

To eliminate verbal auditory hallucinations: Tinggong (SI19), Tinghui (GB2), Zhongzhu (SJ3), Yifeng (SJ17) and Gongsun (SP4).

To eliminate visual hallucinations: Yifeng (SJ17), Jingming (BL1) and Yuyao.

Excessive anxiety or worry may be treated with: Neiguan (PC6), Taichong (LR3), Laogong (PC8) and Jujue (RN14).

Obsessive thoughts, or over-thinking may be diminished with: Baihui (DU20), Tai Yang, and Yin Tang.

To treat loss of short-term memory or forgetfulness: Shendao (DU11) and Neiguan (PC6).

Emotional reactions to stress, such as aggravation, irritability and excitability may be harmonized by treating Taichong (LR3).

For fear, timidity and fright; a sense of security may be instilled with: Danshu (BL19), Ximen (PC4) and Jujue (RN14).

To restore the appetite, add Zusanli (ST36). When antipsychotics produce side-effects of headache with dizziness, add: Baihui (DU20), Taiyang, Yintang, Hegu (LI4) and Ashi points on the head.

When antipsychotic medications produce side-effects such as dizziness with ringing in the ears, accompanied by flaccidity, sore low back and knees, add: Shenshu (BL23) and Taixi (KI3).

When antipsychotic medications produce side-effects such as amenorrhea and lactation, add: Guanyuan (RN4), Pishu (BL20), Shenshu (BL23), Zusanli (ST36), Hegu (LI4), Taichong (LR3) and Zhongji (RN3).

Auricular points may empower any treatment through their direct connection to the brain's regulatory systems. Additionally, they are convenient points of access in patients who are not able to be still for the duration of an acupuncture treatment. They also provide a means by which to treat patients whose mood may fluctuate drastically or suddenly. Ear seeds can then be placed to extend the therapeutic effect. The most essential points may include: Kidney, Occiput, Heart, Stomach, Ear Shen Men, Central Rim, Subcortex, Sympathetic, Endocrine, and Heart of Posterior Surface. Additional support may be gained by needling points: Brain Stem, Adrenal Gland, External Ear, Internal Ear, Lesser Occipital Nerve and the Neurasthenia Region.

Pathogenesis of Schizophrenia

Schizophrenia may be differentiated into various patterns depending on presentation, and is often the manifestation of a combination of patterns according to traditional Chinese medicine. Some common patterns are described below.

Heart-Phlegm: Schizophrenia often begins with some manifestation related to phlegm-fire. Phlegm will follow the movement of qi. When the heart's capacity to house and anchor the spirit is diminished, a disorganized state may occur; when severe, a dissociative condition, such as schizophrenia may predominate. Phlegm may exist on its own, confusing the heart, mind and spirit; or be combined with blood stasis, often manifesting as depression; it may also exhibit fire, which often leads to manic states.

When the regular, smooth flow of qi and blood is disrupted by phlegm, stasis, fire or a combination of any of these, clear and lucid thought becomes clouded; aggravated or emotional states may ensue and the spirit will not be able to rest.

Differential Diagnosis

Obstruction by phlegm and dampness: Phlegm may combine with damp, compounding the problem. The additional heaviness and turbidity may present with inability to focus or concentrate, confusion, lack of coordination, low motivation, slow digestion, slowed-down movements, indifference, lack of animated facial expression, hallucinations and delusions.

Phlegm-fire: When phlegm combines with fire, turbulent wind is also often involved that stirs the phlegm and fire upwards. The heart or head may then be harassed, manifesting as excessive activity, unnecessary movements, irrational speech and agitated outbursts.

Yin deficiency with fire blazing: When an underlying yin deficiency leads to fire; or fire burns up fluids and yin, the patient will show signs of deficiency and excess such as lack of energy and motivation with an emaciated appearance and flushed, dry cheeks. The patient may also be thirsty for cold fluids, yet drink in sips or not be able to get water down. The throat may also be dry and lips may be dry and cracked. The tongue may be red and cracked without coating.

Qi and blood stagnation: When stagnation or stasis leads to schizophrenia, the pathogenic accumulation often affects the brain, heart or pericardium and their associated channels and collaterals. An individual may present with severe agitation, depression, a sense of oppression, a sense of mental or spiritual disconnect, feelings of suffocation, morbid thoughts or demeanor, impulsive or strange behavior as well as auditory, visual or tactile hallucinations. A dark complexion may accompany a choppy or wiry pulse and dusky tongue.

Yang deficiency: When a patient is relatively low on yang, an internalized, withdrawn or introverted character may develop. The patient may seem confused, unresponsive and slow. Loathing of cold and dislike of speaking may also predominate. Clinically, the schizophrenic patient with yang deficiency may tend toward catatonia, or extreme somnolence.

Treatment According to Patterns

Once a schizophrenic condition has been differentiated according to traditional Chinese medical pattern, a well-suited treatment plan can be established. Some potential patterns and plans are included here.

Phlegm-Damp Obstruction: Signs and Symptoms include inability to concentrate, slowness, lack of facial expression, or response to another's facial expression, hallucinations, heavy-headedness, lack of desire for physical activity, reduced appetite, a puffy, enlarged tongue with teeth marks and a white, thick greasy coating, and a slippery, or deep, soft pulse.

Acupuncture Protocol: Points may be selected that tonify the spleen, dissolve phlegm and damp, calm spirit, clarify the mind and regulate and move qi, such as: Sanyinjiao (SP6), Yinlingquan (SP9), Zusanli (ST36), Fenglong (ST40), Zhongwan (RN12), Hegu (LI4), Neiguan (PC6), Baihui (DU20).

Phlegm-Fire: Signs and symptoms include overly excited, illogical and incessant speech, red cheeks or a red complexion, red eyes (especially the inner corners), erratic mood, inability to be still or sleep, desire for cold food and drink, a red or purple tongue with a thick or sticky yellow coating and a slippery, rapid, forceful or overflowing surface pulse which is soft at the deeper levels.

Acupuncture Protocol: Fenglong (ST40), Xingjian (LR2), Jiaxi (GB44), Hegu (LI4), Qichi (LI11), Zhongwan (RN12), Baihui (DU20).

Yin Deficiency with Hyperactive Fire: Signs and symptoms include prolonged Yin deficiency may lead to accumulation of heat which then creates fire. Deficiency signs of lassitude, low motivation, emaciation or a dry withered appearance, flushed cheeks or face, dry mouth and parched throat absent of desire for drinking, a red, dry, cracked tongue without coating, and a thready, rapid pulse. Manic bouts may be interspersed with fatigue or exhaustion.

Acupuncture Protocol: Yongquan (KI1), Taixi (KI3), Taichong (LR3), Sanyinjiao (SP6), Baiui (DU20), Shenting (DU24).

Qi Stagnation and Blood Stasis: Signs and symptoms include restlessness, agitation, irritability, moodiness, a desire to move, impulsiveness, strange behavior, dark complexion, hallucinations, amenorrhea or dark menses with clots in women, a purple or dusky tongue, gorged veins on the underside of the tongue and a wiry or unsmooth pulse.

Acupuncture Protocol: Hegu (LI4), Qichi (LI11), Sanyinjiao (SP6), Taichong (LR3), Baihui (DU20), Shenting (DU24).

Yang Deficiency: Signs and symptoms include confusion, slowness, lassitude, reluctance to speak, low appetite, or desire for warm food and drink, fatigue, a pale or white complexion, loathing of cold, cool limbs, clod back and bones, a pale or greyish tongue with white coating, and a deep, thready, slow pulse.

Acupuncture Protocol: Taixi (KI3), Taichong (LR3), Guanyuan (RN4), Shenshu (BL23), Mingmen (DU4), Baihui (DU20).

The above prescriptions are some of the most common and effective in treating the various patterns within the schizophrenia spectrum. To further illustrate the clinical relevance of Chinese medicine in schizophrenia, case reports are included below.

During Active Psychotic Episodes

In psychosis that erupts from a Yang pattern, giddiness may be combined with excitement, agitation, hallucinations, delusions, lack of mental clarity, mental disturbance, disorganized thought or behavior, eccentricity, a red face and eyes and dry stool. In this case, the tongue will be red with a yellow coat; and the pulse may be bowstring, rapid and with force. To resolve the condition, drain fire, dissolve phlegm, invigorate the blood and break up stasis, anchor the yang and calm the spirit. The relative excess may be drained via acupuncture on the front and back; alternatively, Huantiao (GB30) may be added for additional calming of the spirit and anchoring of the Yang. On the front side, Zhongwan (RN12), Shenmen (HT7) and Sanyinjiao (SP6) will ground the center, calm the spirit and nourish the Yin. On the back, back-shu points of the heart, liver and spleen will ground and harmonize the organs; these may be combined with ST40, in order to resolve phlegm. A variety of herbal formulas may be chosen from, depending on specific pattern. When the liver and gallbladder fire is blazing, showing signs of excessive over-stimulated energy, emotions or movement; *Long Dan Xie Gan Tang* will drain the excess. When a patient is overwhelmed with pathogenic phlegm obstructing heart orifices, and turbid qi mists the mind, *Di Dan Tang* will dissolve the excess phlegm; thereby, clarifying the mind. When heat has congealed the blood; causing stasis, agitation and delusions, *Dian Kuang Meng Xing Tang* may be prescribed to invigorate and move the blood. If phlegm-fire is harassing the heart. The patient may toggle between a preference for isolation and withdrawal, interrupted by agitated, manic episodes. *Sheng Tie Luo Yin* will dissolve the phlegm and drain the fire.

Yin Disease Pattern

When psychosis arises from a relative Yin excess; the affect may be blunted, slowness, weak will, difficulty or inability to think, lassitude, empty demeanor, weakness, timidity, laconic speech, a melancholy expression and white or pale complexion are common. The tongue may be pale or greyish; the pulse, deep and thready. The condition may improve when the blood has been nourished and the heart Yang tonified. Overall warming of the Yang while enlivening the spirit will also resolve many of the above symptoms.

Acupuncture according to the protocols below will be useful. Alternating between the following treatments, while applying even technique, will restore the Yang and help revive the patient. Renzhong (DU26), Shaoshang (LU11), Yinbai (SP1), Daling (PC7) and Fenglong (ST40) may be alternated with acupuncture at Zhongting (RN16), Dazhui (DU14), Shenzhu (DU12); Jiuwei (RN15), Fushe (RN13), Zhongwan (RN12), Fenglong (ST40); and Renzhong (DU26), Fengfu (DU16), Laogong (PC8) and Daling (PC7). Herbal formula, *Yang Xin Tang* may be prescribed to replenish qi, blood and essence. For those with severe and chronic Yang syndrome, presenting as catatonia, *Di Huang Yin Zi* or *Wen Yang Xing Fen Tang* may be administered.

Between Psychotic Episodes

Schizophrenia is characterized by alternating periods of near-normal thought and behavior interrupted by psychotic episodes of varying duration. During the remittance phase, less intensive treatment is required, and will be adjusted according to the current manifestation of symptoms. In cases of liver qi depression and constriction, a patient may present with mental, physical or emotional depression, blunted affect, limited ability or desire to engage in conversation, disjointed speech, a short temper, dark or morbid thoughts, apathy, hypochondriac pain, frequent sighing, lack of concern for food or liquids, menstrual irregularity. In more serious cases, lack of will to live, self-injurious behavior or suicidal thoughts may be present. The tongue will be dark or dusky with a thin white coat accompanied by a wiry or bowstring pulse.

Acupuncture may be administered to drain excess from the liver, move the qi and blood, and lift the spirit. An appropriate protocol may include sedating heart and liver points, such as: Taichong (LR3), Neiguan (PC6), Shenmen (HT7), Hegu (LI4), Zusanli (ST36) and Tanzhong (RN17). An herbal formula may also facilitate in draining the excess from the liver while promoting a smooth flow of qi and blood. *Chai Hu Shu Gan San Jia Wei* may be appropriate in this case: Chai Hu (12g), Xiang Fu (10g), Bai Shao (10g), Zhi Ke (10g), Chuan Xiong (6g), Yuan Zhi (10g), Su Geng (10g), Chen Xiang (6g) and Gan Cao (3g).

If the patient's condition varies, modifications can be tailored to fit the individual. When the depression is more severe, and the long-standing condition has transformed into heat, Huang Qin and Huang Lian may be added. In cases where the spleen deficiency is more severe and the patient suffers from lack of nourishment, *Xiao Yao San* can be modified to fit the specific manifestation. In cases where liver and spleen disharmony has created depressed interior heat, *Dan Zhi Xiao Yao* San or *Xiao Chai Hu Tang* may be prescribed.

Patients with Schizophrenia due to phlegm and qi stagnation may present with a combination of symptoms related to confusion and depression. Common manifestations include: physical, emotional or mental depression accompanied by lack of animation, paranoia, constant worry, incongruent speech, muttering to oneself, bouts of laughter, crying spells, frequent sighing, congestion and distention of the chest and hypochondria, no concern for food of drink, plum pit qi, excessive lung or nasal phlegm, lack of concentration, low motivation or blocked orifices. The tongue may have a thick slimy or sticky coat and the pulse may be bowstring, wiry-slippery or soft.

A patient with phlegm and qi depressed in the interior may be rectified by supporting the right qi transforming phlegm, open the orifices and moving qi and blood to alleviating depression.

An effective acupuncture protocol may include even method on points that clarify the mind while supporting the spleen's ability to transform damp, such as: Renzhong (DU26), Shenmen (HT7), Neiguan (PC6), Zhongwan (RN12), Zusanli (ST36), Xingjian (LR2) and Fenglong (ST40). Herbal formula, *Shun Qi Dao Tan Tang He Kong Xian Dan Jia Jian,* may further reinforce the treatment principles: Chen Pi (10g), Ban Xia (10g), Dan Nan Xing (10g), Fu Ling (15g), Xiang Fu (10g), Shi Chang Pu (15g), Mu Xiang (7g) with Kuan Xian Dan (2-3 pills taken with decocted herbals).

The treatment may be slightly modified for individual differences. When the chest is full, and the patient has a sense of oppression over the lungs and diaphragm, along with excessive productive phlegm or drool, *San Sheng San* may be administered as an emetic to rapidly expel the phlegm.

For patients with noticeable confusion and unclear thinking processes, blunt affect or disorganized speech, herbal formula, *Su He Xiang Wan*, may be followed by *Si Qi Tang* plus Dan Nan Xing, Yu Jin, Shi Chang Pu and Yuan Zhi. If chronic qi depression has transformed into heat; manifesting as sleeplessness and irrational fear, *Wen Dan Tang* plus Huang Lian may be combined with *Bai Jin Wan* in order to relieve stagnation, support the function of the gallbladder and clear heat. Patients whose most prominent symptoms arise from Shen disturbance, manifesting as cloudy thinking and spiritual chaos may benefit from *Zhi Bao Dan.*

When pathogenic phlegm combines with damp, obstructions of the channels, collaterals and organs may result in overall heaviness that makes movement or thinking difficult. When the accumulation has not yet transformed into heat, the condition will likely be of a cold nature. Some or all metabolic processes may slow down and the affect may be one of apathy, depression, melancholy, confusion, or blankness. Clarity of thought, purpose or behavior may be lacking, attention and focus may wane, facial expression may be lacking and fatigue and lethargy may set in. Weakness, overwhelm and a withdrawn nature may predominate. When the phlegm-damp blocks the orifices, visual, auditory and tactile hallucinations may harass the mind and vex the heart. Insomnia is also common in this case. The tongue will most likely be flabby and swollen with teeth marks and a thick, slimy white coat while the pulse may be slippery or deep and soft.

A schizophrenic patient with phlegm-damp predominating may be treated by removing the phlegm-damp accumulation, warming the Yang and tonifying the spleen's ability to transform damp and unblock the orifices. Supportive acupuncture may reinforce consciousness, clear the heart and mind, move the stagnation and tonify the spleen. Point selection may include, with even method: Renzhong (DU26), Shenmen (HT7), Neiguan (PC6), Zhongwan (RN12), Zusanli (ST36), Xingjian （LR2） and Fenglong (ST40). In conjunction, an effective herbal formula might be, *Xiang Sha Liu Jun Zi Tang He Li Zhong Tang Jia Wei:* Dang Shen (12g), Bai Zhu (10g), Fu Ling (20g), Gan Cao (10g), Mu Xiang (6g), Sha Ren (6g), Sheng Jiang (10g), Gan Jiang (10g), Chen Pi (10g), Ban Xia (10g), Cang Zhu (10g), Yuan Zhi (6g), Shi Chang Pu (10g), Huo Xiang (10g) and Pei Lan (10g). For individuals exhibiting a greater need to tonify the spleen, Huang Qi and Sheng Ma may be added. For those in greater need of Kidney tonification, Shan Yao and Bia Bian Dou may be added.

When schizophrenia erupts due to phlegm-fire harassing the heart, liver and upper orifices, the condition may be marked by strong emotions of a tense and agitated nature. The patient may be prone to tantrums, breaking items and injuring other people by using too much force. The verbiage may also be uncontrollable, leading to foul, rough, loud or blunt speech. The eyes may be red and piercing, possessing an angry or fiery look. The whole face and upper body may also be red, and veins may pulse at the sides of the head or throat. Fire may dry up fluids leading to constipation as well. Phlegm-fire tends to coincide with a red tongue, covered in a yellow slimy coat; while the corresponding pulse may be wiry, large, slippery and rapid.

In order to calm the heart, resolve phlegm, sedate the liver, drain fire and unblock the orifices; acupuncture with draining method may be applied to Guanyuan (RN14), Renzhong (DU26), Neiguan (PC6), Laogong (PC8), Fenglong (ST40) and Taichong (LR3).

Sheng Tie Luo Yin Jia Jian may provide synergistic benefit: Tie Luo (30-60g), Dan Nan Xing (10g), Bei Mu (12g), Ju Hong (12g), Shi Chang Pu (12g), Yuan Zhi (12g), Fu Shen (12g), Xuan Shen (12g), Tian Men Dong (12g), Mai Men Dong (12g), Lian Qiao (12g) and Zhu Sha (1g). When the phlegm fire is raging out of control, add *Meng Shi Shi Tan Wan.* When phlegm-fire adversely affects the heart and orifices, substitute *An Gong Niu Huang Wan.* Alternatively, when the phlegm-fire is primarily attacking the liver and gallbladder, *Dang Gui Long Hui Wan* may be prescribed. If the stomach and intestines are more affected, Da Cheng Qi Tang plus Zao Jiao and pig bile can be ingested to drain the fire and decongest phlegm stagnation. In patients who present with a clear spirit; however, insomnia and a vexed heart prevail. *Wen Dan Tang* plus *Zhu Sha An Shen Wan* may be prescribed to resolve phlegm, calm the heart and promote sleep.

Schizophrenia with deficiency of the heart and spleen may present with unsubstantial sadness and joy accompanied by scattered thoughts, appearance and demeanor. A patient exhibiting this pattern may present with lack of thought consolidation, constant worry and anxiety, dreams of disturbing or harassing entities, palpitations, fright, timidity, syncope, sensitivity, poor short-term memory, forgetfulness, poor concentration, fatigue, shortness of breath, scattered or weak speech, concerned and white or pale complexion, lack of muscular strength and reduced appetite and food intake. The tongue may be pale, enlarged with toothmarks or shaky. The pulse will likely be fine and forceless.

In order to strengthen the patient's constitution, nourish the heart and spleen, tonify qi and calm the spirit. An appropriate acupuncture protocol may include back-shu points of the heart and spleen, qi tonifying points and points that nourish the heart and calm the spirit, such as: Xinshu (BL15), Pishu (BL20), Neiguan (PC6), Shenmen (HT7), Zusanli (ST36). Herbal formula, *Gui Pi Tang,* is the classic prescription for this condition, consisting of: Dang Shen (12g), Bai Zhu (12g), Fu Shen (30g), Huang Qi (30g), Gan Cao (6g), Dang Gui (12g), Long Yan Rou (30g), Suan Zao Ren (30g), Yuan Zhi (6g), Mu Xiang (10g), Sheng Jiang (6g) and Da Zao (6 pieces). When lack of substance and spirit disturbance gives way to over-thinking, worry, anxiety, sadness, fright, constant fidgeting and unease, *Xin Tang* may be prescribed.

Schizophrenia with pronounced Yang deficiency may present in the elderly, weak or convalescent; or, when disease of the spleen has progressed, damaging the kidneys. Thinking may cause mental strain and overall sluggishness may set in. The patient may lack attentiveness, timidity, be reluctant to speak; desire for food and drink may be absent. The physicality may feel and appear feeble and empty, and the complexion may be pale, lack luster or take on a bluish hue. Loathing of cold and a cold body will be pronounced. The tongue may be pale, grey or bluish with a white coat; while the pulse may be deep, fine, weak and slow.

To enliven this patient, warming and tonifying techniques are needed. Fortifying the spleen and kidney Yang while transforming phlegm and opening the orifices will restore the foundational strength. Points may be selected that focus on tonifying the back-shu of the kidneys, spleen and stomach, while restoring ming-men fire with acupuncture and moxibustion. Point selection may include: Shenshu (BL23), Mingmen (DU4), Pishu (BL20), Weishu (BL21), Guanyuan (RN4) and Baihui (DU20). Additional benefit may be reaped through the use of herbal formula, *Wen Yang Xi Fen Tang Jia Jian:* Dang Shen (20g), Shu Di (15g), Fu Zi (10g), Rou Gui (10g), Rou Cong Rong (15g), Yin Yang Huo (15g), Gan Jiang (6g), Gui Ban (15g), Chen Pi (10g), Ba Xia (10g), Gan Cao (6g) and Fu Ling (15g). When excessive phlegm mists the mind, add Shi Chang Pu and Yuan Zhi. If blood stasis is more prominent, add Dan Pi and Yu Jin. In cases where qi is greatly depleted, Huang Qi and Shan Yao may be added.

Psychosis marked with fire due to Yin deficiency may present in those who have suffered from long-standing mania which has worsened progressively over time. The patient may be fatigued, and emaciated with a reddish hue on the cheeks, face and chest; speak in rapid bouts expressing excited or incoherent thoughts; display emotional outbursts; or be overly tense, anxious and sleep may be disturbed with vivid dreaming. The palms, soles, and chest may experience rushes of uncomfortable heat; the throat and mouth may be parched and the lips may be red, dry and cracked. The tongue will usually be red and shaky with scant or no coat and cracks; while the pulse may be fine and rapid, or floating with force at the surface with lack of force underneath.

In order to restore the Yin, quell fire and tranquilize the spirit, acupuncture may be provided at points Shenmen (HT7), Daling (PC7), Taichong (LR3) toward Yongquan (KI1) and Sanyinjiao (SP6). Synergistic aid may be received with herbal formula, *Er Yin Jian:* Sheng Di (30g), Mai Men Dong (12g), Xua Shen (12g), Fu Ling (12g), Suan Zao Ren (20g), Huang Lian (10g), Mu Tong (8g), Zhu Ye (12g), Deng Xin Cao (3g) and Gan Cao (6g). When Yin-deficient fire has led to dry stool, Huo Ma Ren, Yu Li Ren and Tao Ren may be added. When dry mouth predominates with no concern for food or drink, *San Xian* may be added. To fortify the essence and enliven the spirit, Tai Zi Ren, Huang Qi and Sheng Ma may be prescribed.

Schizophrenia due to blood stasis may present with erratic emotions and severe personality changes ranging from genuine friendliness to obsequiousness or overt hostility. A sense of oppression or constant discomfort, nausea and generalized intolerance may color daily life. When the stagnation is severe, the patient may become quite morbid. The patient may mutter quietly; the spirit may be occluded; paranoia, hallucinations and delusions may confuse the mind and the face may appear clouded and dark. Piercing pains in the head, heart or other organs may predominate. Amenorrhea or dark blood with clots may be observed in women. When the primary pattern is blood stagnation, the tongue will be dark red, purple or dusky; may display purple, raised or dark spots and the veins on the underside of the tongue may be dark and full of blood. The pulse may be wiry, irregular or choppy. In order to move the blood, dissolve blood stasis and unburden the spirit; an acupuncture protocol may include back-shu points of the heart and liver along with influential points of the blood, such as: Shenmen (HT7), Neiguan (PC6), Xuehai (SP10), Hegu (LI4), Xinshu (BL15), Geshu (BL17) and Ganshu (BL18). A concordant herbal formula for moving the blood and dissolving blood stasis, X*ue Fu Zhu Yu Tang Jia Wei,* may be taken in concert: Tao Ren (12g), Hong Hua (10g), Dang Gui (10g), Sheng Di (10g), Chuan Xiong (6g), Chi Shao (6g), Jie Geng (5g), Chuan Niu Xi (10g), Chai Hu (3g), Zhi Ke (6g), Gan Cao (6g) and Shui Zhi (6g).

If the blood stasis is accompanied by a bitter taste, dry throat, inhibited urination that is red or accompanied by heat sensations; and there is an overall feeling of internal heat, the stagnation has led to an accumulation of heat; add Mu Tong and Huang Qin. If the patient is especially excitable, restless and thoughts or movements are incessant, Mu Dan Pi and Sheng Di may be added. If the patient cannot sleep, or sleep is interrupted and restless; while mental, physical or emotional depression are accompanied by a sense of oppression and constant discomfort, He Huan Pi and Ye Jiao Teng may be added. When the patient is laconic, withdrawn, somnolescent, fatigued, lacks spirit and luster, with a demeanor possibly bordering on mutism or catatonia, add Huangqi and Dang Gui.

Classical Approaches

Yellow Emperor's Classic Approach to Schizophrenia

The following is based on Chapter 22 from the *Yellow Emperor's Classic of Medicine: Spiritual Pivot (Huang Di Nei Jing: Ling Shu)* [3].

The outer canthus, or corner, of the eye belongs to Yang, while the inner canthus belongs to Yin.

In the initial stages of mental disorders, or dian disease, a sad or melancholy affect is outwardly expressed. The patient may present with a heavy head, red eyes and a tendency to gaze blankly forward. If the condition progresses, chest oppression and restlessness may also manifest. With skillful observation of the third eye, or space between the eyebrows, early detection of onset may be predicted. The condition may be relieved by inserting acupuncture needles along the Hand Taiyang, Yangming and Taiyin meridians until the complexion normalizes.

A crying or whimpering sound is an early indication that dian disease is eminent. Contralateral acupuncture of the Hand Yangming and Taiyang channels will help prevent full manifestation of a dian disorder. Needles may be inserted on the left side if the right side is stiff, and vice versa; again, retaining needles until a healthy color returns to the face. Stiffness and rigidity of the whole body, resembling a backward-bending bow, is common at the onset of dian disease symptoms, followed by pain in the spine and back. Acupuncture may be applied to the Foot and Hand Taiyang Meridians until the complexion is restored.

To fully resolve a dian condition, inpatient observation is helpful. By observing the display of symptoms over the course of continuous time, the patient's underlying patterns may be more accurately diagnosed and the treatment approach may increase in accuracy and effectiveness. At the first sign of dian disease manifestations, blood-letting at the affected channels may be performed. According to the Yellow Emperor's Classic, if the blood is kept in a gourd, it will move during the subsequent episode; if the blood remains still during the attack, twenty moxa-cones may be applied at the tailbone, on the sacrum at Changqiang (DU1).

When a patient suffers from depressive psychosis that involves the bone; the cheeks, teeth and ren channel between the shu points may feel swollen or distended. Arthralgia, spontaneous sweating and chest tightness or oppression may also accompany. When there is vomiting of excessive saliva, it is considered an ingrained condition, and a sign that the vital energy of the kidneys is being expelled; this condition is most likely incurable.

When mental disorders affect the tendons, low energy may be accompanied by stiff or rigid muscles and a big pulse. Applying acupuncture to Dazhu (BL11), on the back of the neck, will release pathogenic wind. Again, when there is vomiting of excessive saliva, it is a serious sign indicating that the vital energy of the kidneys is escaping; the condition is likely permanent.

Falling down suddenly is a common phenomenon that may be experienced at onset of a mental disorder affecting the channel; additionally, the vessels in the four extremities will often be gorged and lack tonicity. In such cases, bloodletting may be performed to release the excess of affected vessels. Moxibustion may be applied to the Foot Taiyang Channel clipping the neck, and to acupuncture points three inches from the Girdle Channel on the waist and the shu-points of the four extremities and between the muscles. If the patient vomits abundant white foam or froth, vital energy is being expelled, and it is a sign that the disease is not curable.

When the onset of dian disease is marked by a manic episode, it will rarely by cured.

If, at onset, sadness arises prior to an initial manic episode, which is accompanied by forgetfulness, hot temper, fearfulness; and a melancholy mood and hunger tend to bring on symptoms, the Hand Taiyang and Hand Yangming Channels may be bled until the complexion is restored. The Foot Taiyin and Foot Yangming Channels may also be bled. Insomnia and lack of appetite will generally coincide during manic episodes. Delusions of grandeur are common; the patient often feeling intellectually brilliant and wise, eloquent in speech and manner, gifted and honorable. The patient may also take on an air of superiority, and regard others with a paternal or condescending tone, scolding others constantly. Acupuncture points on the Hand Yangming, Taiyang and Taiyin Channels, as well as those on the Shaoyin Channel under the tongue that are overly full may be bled in order to relieve the excess.

When mania is expressed with wild joy, severe fright, senseless laughing or unexplained giddiness, overly spontaneous actions, rash behavior, and the manic state lasts all day and night; the condition likely began with a severe and frightening shock. The Hand Yangming, Taiyang and Taiyin channels may be bled in this case. During a manic episode, a patient often will possess heightened extrasensory perception, and will often hear and see what is inaudible or unseen by the average person. Sounds, sights and sensations may also take the form of hallucinations, and the patient may scream or cry in fear, lack of spiritual grounding may be presumed. Hand Taiyang, Taiyin and Yangming channels, as well as the Foot Taiyang Channel may be bled as well as both cheeks. During a manic episode, the appetite may be voracious, and the patient may binge on all kinds of food. The patient may believe direct communication with God or demons is taking place. Bouts of strange laughing, giddiness, incoherent speech may erupt when mania leads to a lack of groundedness of spirit. The Foot Taiyin, Taiyang, and Yangming meridians should be treated first, followed by the Hand Taiyin, Taiyang, and Yangming meridians. When treating at onset, before the full manifestation of symptoms, bilateral bleeding of the vessels on either side of Ququan (LR8) may release the excess. Bleeding when the channel is abundant can expel the pathogen and cure the condition. When bleeding the vessels at the Ququan (LR8) does not resolve the condition, the above protocol may be used for dian disease, in conjunction with burning twenty moxa-cones at the sacrum.

When a patient suffers from pathogenic wind invasion that has reversed the normal flow of energy inside the body, spontaneous pain may plague the four extremities. Bouts of sudden sweating or sonorous nose-breathing due to cold may occur. The patient will generally feel irritable when hungry and restless and fidgety when full. Points that treat both the exterior and the interior of the lung and large intestine channel may be selected while also bleeding the kidney and stomach meridians. Jing-well points may also be bled on each of these channels to expel pathogenic cold from the bones.

Jueyin disease is characterized by sudden coldness in the feet, splitting sensations in the chest and extreme discomfort in the abdomen and intestines with a sensation as if the intestines are being carved out. Desire to eat is suppressed due to abdominal fullness and distention and the pulse will generally be choppy. In cases when the patient feels warm, purging techniques may be used along with bleeding points on the kidney channel; however, if the patient feels cool, methods to warm and invigorate the qi and blood are more suitable.

Abdominal distention and fullness, bowel sounds, oppression of the chest and pain on expiration, may be treated by bleeding points along the ribcage below the chest. Bleed the point most responsive while the patient coughs. The back-shu of the point that relieves cough with pressure, may also be bled. Painful urination may be treated by bleeding the kidney and urinary bladder meridians. The Changqiang point (DU1) on the sacrum may also be needled deeply. When the vital qi has been affected, the spleen and stomach meridians may be bled. When Jueni attacks with ferocity, vessels of the kidney and stomach may be bled. Spontaneous sweating, joint soreness and heavy bodily sensations accompanied by lack of desire for physical activity or speaking due to low energy requires tonifying the kidney meridian. Asthma or shortness of breath that is shallow and continuous or breathlessness upon slight exertion may be treated by tonifying the kidney meridian combined with bleeding to release the pathogen from the blood.

Sun Simiao's Approach to Schizophrenia

Sun Simiao, a respected physician during the Tang Dynasty (618-906) and author of Qian Jin Yao Fang (*Essential Formulas Worth a Thousand Pieces of Gold*); proposed a comprehensive strategy in treating psychiatric disorders. Patients with schizophrenia were treated with the thirteen-ghost point acupuncture protocol as well as with moxibustion and herbal formulas. Sun Simiao describes in full his multi-modal approach to healing patients with mental disorders. Following is a short adaptation from his renown text, *Essential Formulas Worth a Thousand Pieces of Gold* [4].

Thirteen Ghost Points

Acupuncture and Oriental medicine treat the whole person; each point or point prescription may have mental, physical or spiritual influences. The Thirteen Ghost Points have been identified as primary points through which to access a person's spiritual sense of self. Historically, unusual behavior, especially when episodic or initiating with a sudden or spontaneous onset were attributed to ghost or demonic attacks from the unseen realms as no physical cause could be found for such disturbances. Over time, the founders of Chinese medicine were able to detect the most effective and useful acupuncture points for these diseases of spirit; they termed these, "ghost points."

Sun Simiao identified the Thirteen Ghost Points spanning across the entire body. Starting at the head: traditional point, Renzhong (DU26), he named "Gui Gong," meaning ghost palace; the point is most known for revival of consciousness, or to increase conscious focus. Following, at the base of the corner of the index finger nailbed, exit point, Shaoshang (LU11), he called "Gui Xin," or Ghost Sincerity. Then, at the base of the inner nailbed of the first toe, Yinbai (SP1), he named, "Gui Lei," or, Ghost Fortress. At the midpoint of the ventral side of the wrist, Daling (PC7), he termed, "Gui Xin, meaning, Ghost Heart. Shenmai (BL62), the opening point of the Du meridian, he named, "Gui Lu," meaning, Ghost Road. On the midline of the occiput, Fengfu (DU16), he called, "Gui Zhen," translated as, Ghost Pillow. Jiache (ST6), at the corner of the jaw, he named, "Gui Chuang," or, Ghost Bed. Chengjiang (DU24), needled for many mental disorders, he termed, "Gui Shi," or, Ghost Market. Palm point of the hand, Laogong (PC8), he referred to as "Gui Ku," meaning, Ghost Cave. Another frontal lobe point, also used frequently for mental disorders, Shangxing (DU23), he called, "Gui Tang," translated as, Ghost Court. In men, he includes, Huiyin (RN1), the meeting point of the Du and Ren meridians, termed, "Gui Cang,"(men only) or Ghost Treasury. For women he includes, extra point Yumen,* "Gui Cang,"or, Ghost Treasury. On the arm near the lateral elbow crease, point Quchi (LI11), he termed, "Gui Tui," or Ghost Official. Extra point Haiquan,** he named, "Gui Feng," meaning, Ghost Seal.

*Yumen (extra) is located within the anterior vaginal fold.

**Haiquan (extra) is located in the middle of the frenum linguae underneath the tongue body.

To elaborate: Sun Simiao's Thirteen Ghost Points have regular channel functions as well as special functions regarding the spirit. Renzhong (DU26), a powerful revival point, is a place where the Du meridian meets the large intestine and stomach channels. Needling this point dredges the Yang channels, liberating them from obstructions. Shaoshang (LU11), a jing-well point, clears excess heat from the lung. Chengjiang (RN24) where the Ren meets the Du, large intestine and stomach meridians, balances Yin and Yang, clears heat and regulates qi. Laogong (PC8), a ying-spring point of the pericardium meridian, facilitates clarity of mind and heart, while expelling excess heat. Fengfu (DU16) where the bladder channel crosses the Du, is known as a sea of marrow point. Combining these five points serves to dissolve phlegm while promoting focus and clear thinking. Daling (PC7), a shu-stream and yuan-source point, nourishes the channel, clears heat and calms the spirit. Yinbai (SP1), a jing-well point of the spleen meridian. calms the mind, clears pathogenic heat, tonifies the central qi and dissolves phlegm. Extra point Haiquan, revives the mind, extinguishes fire and subdues convulsions. When used together, these three points reinforce immunity while instilling a sense of peace. Shenmai (BL62), a confluent point of the du, invigorates the vital energy and blood, thereby dissipating stasis. Quchi (LI11), a he-sea point, also invigorates qi and blood while harmonizing the wei and gu qi. Shangxing (DU23) opens the orifices, heightens the senses and clears heat, especially from the head. Jiache (ST6) expels heat and harmonizes the stomach. Together, these four points serve to invigorate the qi, resolve stasis, dissolve phlegm and remove obstructions. Huiyin (RN1), a meeting point of the ren, du and chong meridians, balances yin and yang, regulates the vital energy and blood of the chong meridian. It promotes peace of mind while renewing the spirit. It may be used to treat the local conditions such as disorders of the bowels or urogenital system, establishes grounding for those in shock and is effective in subduing convulsive disorders such as epilepsy.

Historically, many of the founders of Chinese medicine used song or prose to illustrate principles, qualities or facilitate the memorizing of specific acupuncture points, herbal formulas or conditions. Following is a short verse on the ghost points.

Sun Si Maio's Ode to Needling 13 Ghost Points

Evil spirits disturb the mind!
Thirteen ghost points treat in kind!
Make sure to needle Gui Gong first,
Although keep Gui Xin close behind.

Point by point! Thirteen in all!
Needle first the left side in man,
When treating woman start with the right.

Begin with Ren Zhong called Gui Gong.
Then treat the point at the end of the thumb,
Needle sincerely Gui Xin, or Shaoshang!

With men, start and end with the right.
For women, needle left first, remove left last
This is how it should be cast!

The third point, Yin bai, sits at the great toe.
We call it Gui Lei, needle and go!

Da Ling is the fourth, where the third finger folds in,
At the crease of the palm
Five fen does not harm
This point is also known as Gui Xin!

Three to seven quick thrusts
With a needle that's warm
On the road to Gui Lu's treatment performed!

The sixth, far above Da Zhu is Gui Zhen,
Needle into the hairline one cun.

Point seven, Gui Chuang,
Translated, Ghost Bed
Use seven-star needling
To bleed this point in the head.

The eighth point is Gui Shi, known as Shengjiang,
Found in the small dent over the chin!

Gui Ku, Ghost Cave, is the ninth part.
Where the pinky touches the palm line of the Heart!

Gui Tang is the next ghost to bring
To your needle! It's number ten, Shang Xing!

Moxa three times Gui Cang for men!
Number eleven, the point is Hui Yin!
Eleven is strangely, for women, Yu Men
Moxa this point also called, Gui Cang!

Needled warm Gui Tui,
The official twelfth ghost
Three to seven thrusts
At the least or the most!

At the tongue's base, somewhere in the middle,
The last of the ghosts, and this silly riddle,
When we needle Gui Feng
Our ghost song has been sung.

When points are paired,
As not to cause strife,
Remember to needle both husband and wife,
When the point sits alone on the line in the center,
It seems in this case; one needle is better!

All ghosts of emotions possess mortal fear
Of this ancient formula recited right here,
Just thirteen points, make all ghosts disappear!

(*One fen is equal to 1/10 cun.)
Source: adapted from Sun Si Miao's Ode to Thirteen Ghost Acupoints for the Treatment of Mental Disorders, by Ralph Alan Dale and Yan Cheng [5], American Journal of Acupuncture, Vol. 20, No. 3, 1992.

Sun Simiao's Thirteen Ghost Points alone may treat any mental, emotional or spiritual disturbance. The prescription may also be used in combination with specific pattern protocols. Shen-related disharmonies, such as depression, mania, bipolar conditions, neuroses, worry, trauma, convulsive disorders, psychotic episodes, uncontrollable weeping, lack of direction, confused states, delirium, seizures, loss of consciousness, palpitations due to fear or fright, shock, anxiety, schizophrenia and many others all may be treated with the Thirteen Ghost Points protocol.

In an attempt to gather scientific data on modern clinical applications and mechanism of action for the Thirteen Ghost Points, researchers conducted a literature review of publications spanning the past ten years. Schizophrenia, bipolar disorder, dementia, stroke, syncope, sleeping disorders, anxiety, depression and hysteria were found to respond to treatment of the Ghost Points. One theory is that the Thirteen Ghost points balance the Yin and Yang, regulate qi and blood, revive conscious awareness and calm the mind, heart and spirit; however, solid data on this is currently sparse. Researchers [6] suggest further study on the clinical applications and mechanisms by which the Ghost Points act, so as to determine their role in clinical use.

Sun Simiao's Classical Chinese Herbal Medicine Strategies

Sun Simiao presented herbal formulas that are especially useful in treating disharmonies of the mind or spirit; they have been included here. These formulas need to be further studied by researchers and clinicians [4].

Hu Jing Wan Fang

Hu Jing, Fang Feng, Qin Jiao, Fang Kui, Long Chi, Huang Qin, Xiong Huang, Fang Ji, Shan Zhu Yu, Fu Ling, Tie Jing, Gui Jiu, Ren Shen, Sheng Di Huang, Da Huang, Yin Xiao, Niu Huang, Du Huo, Yuan Zhi, Xi Xin, Guan Zhong, She Xiang, Bai Wei, Sheng Ma, Bai Xian Pi, Fu Shen, Shi Gao, Tian Xiong, Gui Jian Yu, Feng Fang, Han Shui Shi, She Tui.

Xiong Ci Wan Fang

Xiong Huang, Ci Huang, Zhen Zhu, Qian, Dan Sha.

Xu Ming Feng Yin Tang

Ma Huang, Chuang Qiong, Shi Gao, Ren Shen, Fang Feng, Gan Cao, Gui Xin, Du Huo, Fang Ji, Fu Zi, Dang Gui, Xing Ren, Gan Jiang.

Zi Shi Zhu San

Zi Shi Ying, Hua Shi, Bai Shi Zhi, Ning Shui Shi, Shi Gao, Shi Zhi, Da Huang, Long Gu, Gan Jiang, Gan Cao, Gui Xin, Mu Li.

Zhu San Fang

Zi Shi Ying, Shao Yao, Long Gu, Ma Huang, Qing Shi Zhi, Dang Gui, Gan Cao, Gui Xin, Ren Shen, Gua Lou Geng, Bai Xian Pi, Mu Li, Da Huang.

Zhi Dian Xian Jue Shi Fa Zuo Fang

Fang Kui, Dai Zhe, Ren Shen, Qian Dan, Gou Teng, Fu Shen, Lei Wan, H uGu, Yuan Zhi, Gui Xin, Fang Feng, Jiang Cab, Zhu Chi, Juan Bo, Lang Dang Zi, Guang Ming Sha, Sheng Ma, Fu Zi, Mu Dan, Long Chi, Niu Huang, Zha Chan, She Tui Pi, Bai Ma Yan Jing, Bai Lian.

Xiong Qiong Tang

Chuan Xiong, Gao Ben.

Zhi Feng Dian Fang

Ting Li Zi, Qian Dan, Guo Lou Gen, Hu Zhang, Wu Tou, Bai Zhu, Shu Jiao, Da Ji, Gan Sui, Tian Xiong, Zhi Tou, Tie Jing.

Yuan Jia Tang

Gui Jia, Gan Cao, Bai Wei, Bei Mu, Huang Qin, Fang Feng, Ma Huang, Shao Yao, Bai Zhu, Ning Shui Shi, Gui Xin, Fu Ling, Zhi Mu, Shi Gao.

Jiu Wu Niu Huang Fang

Niu Huang, Jing Shi, Zeng Qing, Yu Xiao, Xiong Huang, Kong Qing, Chi Shi Zhi, Xuan Shen, Long Gu.

Shi Huang San

Xiong Huang, Ren Shen, Huang Qin, Da Huang, Gui Xin, Huang Qi, Huang Bai, Xi Xin, Huang Lian, Huang Qi, Pu Huang, Ma Huang, Huang Huan, Ze Xie, Shan Zhu Yu.

Bie Li San

Sang Ji Sheng, Bai Zhu, Gui Xin, Yin Yu, Tian Xiong, Shi Chang Pu, Xi Xin, Qian Gen, Fu Zi, Gan Jiang.

Wu Xie Tang

Yu Yu Liang, Fang Feng, Gui Xin, Shao Yao, Yuan Zhi, Du Huo, Gan Cao, Bai Zhu, Ren Shen, Shi Gao, Mu Li, Qin Jiao, Fang Ji, Shi Chang Pu, Xiong Huang, Fu Shen, She Tui.

Fu Shen Tang

Ren Shen, Fang Feng, Wu Tou, Gan Jiang, Ze Xie, Gou Ji, Yuan Zhi, Fu Zi, Kua Lou Gen, Huang Qin, Du Huo, Qin Jiao, Mu Li, Wu Wei Zi, Qian Hu, Xi Xin, Shi Gao, Qiong Qiong, Shu Jiao, Niu Xi, Gan Cao, Shi Nan, Gui Xin, Ma Huang, Zhu Pi, Bai Zhu, Shan Zhu Yu, Ju Pi, Sang Gen Bai Pi, Fu Ling, Gui Jian, Da Zao.

Hu Jing Tang

Hu Jing, Fu Ling, Gui Xin, Fang Feng, Du Huo, Gan Cao, Ren Shen, Tian Xiong, Feng Fang, Zhi Tou, Shi Chang Sheng, Sang Ji Sheng.

Case Reports from Leading Experts on Schizophrenia

Shi Zhengxiu's Cases

Case 1. Gallbladder Deficiency [7]

A twenty-eight-year-old woman presented with dementia due to paranoid schizophrenia. The symptoms emerged after prolonged or severe terror had impaired the gallbladder. She complained of sleeplessness, difficulty being still, incoherent speech; and she seemed to have been wandering or aimless for the past two years.

The patient experienced some shock two years prior. She then became increasingly timid paranoid, suffered panic attacks and had little desire to eat. Chlorpromazine was prescribed for a period of three months, during which time she exhibited bizarre behavior, with outbursts of singing, anger or disconnected speech. She expressed grandiose ideas and delusions, claiming she could rule the country; she even bought a ticket to the moon. At her initial appointment, 300mg of chlorpromazine had been taken. She appeared normal, although she expressed being terribly scared and restless. She was able to give accurate responses when questioned; however, she denied mental illness. Her tongue lacked luster, and her pulse was tense.

A strategy to warm and restore the gallbladder and calm the Shen was adopted. Acupuncture treatment focused on Baihui (DU20), Juque (RN14) and Fengchi (GB20). Supplementary points such as: Yintang, Tanzhong (RN17), Bizhong (Extra), Tongli (HT5), Xingjian (LR2) and Jinsuo (DU8) were also reinforced. A thick needle was inserted transversely at Jinsuo (DU8) and retained for twenty-four hours. Treatments were provided daily for a course of twenty days. The patient responded well and improvement across all symptoms were obvious after eleven days.

During the course of treatment, the patient reported having a disagreement with another person. Symptoms flared-up; mania, anger and insomnia recurred. The eyes became red and a yellow tongue coating and wiry pulse were displayed. Acupuncture was applied to Liming (Extra), Taichong (LR3) penetrating Yongquan (KI1), Hegu (LI14) penetrating Laogong (PC8) and Fengyan (Extra). Twisting-rotating and lifting-thrusting methods were performed on all points. After one week of treatment, the mania subsided; and after three courses of acupuncture, all remaining symptoms were resolved, and the patient returned to normal life. At a follow-up visit eight years later, the patient reported that no relapse had occurred.

Case 2: Schizophrenic Dementia due to Liver-fire [7]

A forty-two-year-old man presented with incoherent speech, seemed insane and had been injuring others. He had a history of insomnia, a coarse demeanor and was in a constant state of agitation since an argument with a niece nine years prior. It was near that incident that he was hospitalized in a psychiatric ward three times. While hospitalized he had been given electric shock and insulin shock therapy. He did not respond to treatment; after three months, he was prescribed 1500mg chlorpromazine and released.

Upon examination, the patient seemed nervous, stared straight ahead, was rude and uncooperative. The tongue was red with a yellow coating and his pulse was wiry. According to TCM pattern differentiation he was diagnosed with dementia due to liver fire. In order to sedate the liver and extinguish fire, points for soothing the liver, grounding and releasing heat were selected, including: Dazhui (DU14), Liming (Extra), Taichong (LV3) and Yongquan (KI1). Additionally, Benshen (GB13), Fengyan (Extra), Jianshi (PC5), Zhigou (SJ6), Hegu (LI14) and Laogong (PC8) were also needled.

Treatment Procedure: Dr. Shi has developed an effective multi-point penetrating method for mania due to exuberant fire. Dr. Shi proposes that depression and mania may transform from deficiency to excess; therefore, differentiation must be applied to each case.

In the first case, above, the patient had received a western medical diagnosis of paranoid schizophrenia. Initially, she was scared and could not sleep; she became timid and easily frightened, although outwardly, she projected a sense of aloofness and arrogance. She was also restlessness, the tongue was pale and her pulse was deep, slow and tense. According to traditional Chinese medicine, she suffered from dementia as a result of weakened gallbladder function after an extreme or prolonged state of terror. Fengchi

(GB20), Xingjian (LR2) and Jinsuo (DU8) were needled in order to dissipate fright, warm the gallbladder, soothe the liver and to calm the spirit. Baihui (DU20), Yintang (Extra2), Tongli (HT5), Juque (RN14), and Bizhong (Extra32) and Tanzhong (RN17) were needled in order to quiet the mind, stabilize the heart and nourish the marrow. The patient responded well to the treatment; however, later on, liver fire seemed to be the source of the mania. The patient was angry, eyes were red and the pulse seemed wirier; indicating the internal pressure from deficiency had transformed into excess heat and fire. Multi-point penetrating technique was then employed at Liming (), to open the mind, from Taichong (LV3) to Yongquan (KI1) in order to anchor the liver yang and expelling liver wind, and from Hegu (LI14) to Laogong (PC8) and Fengyan (Extra) in order to quiet the spirit. Lifting and thrusting technique facilitated the dissipation of all manic symptoms.

In the second case report, mania was expressed through incoherent speech and rough behavior; the patient's tongue had a yellow coat and the pulse was wiry and rapid. According to TCM diagnosis, the patient suffered from Schizophrenic dementia due to exuberant liver-fire. The treatment approach adopted by Dr. Shi involved applying penetrating technique at points such as Liming (Extra), from Taichong (LR3) to Yongquan (KI1), from Jianshi (PC5) to Zhigou (TB6), and from Hegu (LI4) to Laogong (PC8). Dr. Shi also needled Dazhui (DU14) transversely, which was retained for 24 hours. The patient also took a large dose of chlorpromazine. Following the treatment, the patient began to reveal an underlying spleen deficiency, including a dull complexion, lethargy, lack of taste, and a deep pulse. In this case, the excess had transformed into deficiency as the excess liver had been imposing on the spleen. Classic spleen tonification points; Zhongwan (RN12), Zusanli (ST36) and Sanyinjiao (SP6) were needled to help restore the vital qi.

Wang Xiuzhen's Case Reports

Case 1: Schizophrenic Dementia [7]

A thirty-three-year-old woman suffered from sleeplessness for three months, which originally began with a bout of sadness. Dissatisfaction was mounting, and the insomnia was accompanied by frequent singing and spontaneous running. The patient did not seem to have concern for food, and was not aware of being either hungry or full. Paranoia manifested in fears of being killed or attacked. Hospitalization did not improve the condition, and after two months she was referred to acupuncture for bloodletting.

Her blood pressure, heart rate and lung function were normal, and she was fully conscious, and able to be still. Her appearance was not exactly neat, she was inattentive and not completely cooperative. Bloodletting was applied to Taiyang. At the second treatment, Weizhong (UB40) and Quze (PC3) were bled. Sleep improved; bouts of random singing and running diminished. Hygiene improved as well. Bloodletting was applied to Taiyang and Fenglong (ST40) at the third visit; after which, the patient felt much better. The patient was still symptom-free at a follow-up visit seven years later.

Case 2: Schizophrenic Dementia [7]

A forty-two-year-old woman presented with sleeplessness and lack of facial animation that began six months ago after an argument with a neighbor. While hospitalized for one month, she was diagnosed with schizophrenia. Lack of response to standard medical care led her to be referred to acupuncture.

Her complexion at the time lacked luster, she was unmotivated, apathetic, reluctant to speak, and denied having any mental disorder. She seemed oriented and possessed normal short-term memory. Bloodletting was performed at Taiyang which induced a sweat. Although her outlook improved, her sleep was yet disturbed. She was treated again the following week, with bloodletting at Quze (PC3) and Weizhong (UB40). Insomnia improved; she reported sleeping for four to five hours nightly. Being well-rested, her activity level improved as well. After thirteen days, bloodletting was performed at Yaoyangguan (DU3) and Taiyang; and after fourteen days, bloodletting was performed at Yangjiao (GB35). With a total of four bloodletting treatments, all symptoms improved dramatically and she was still free of symptoms after seven years.

Yi Lin Gai Cuo of Wang Qingren states, "Dementia has symptoms such as endless laughing and crying, singing and quarrying, and not recognizing family members, which are caused by the stagnation of qi and blood and disconnection between the brain qi and fu qi;" for such cases, moving the blood and eliminating stagnation are commonly applied treatment principles. Dr. Wang tends to apply bloodletting in cases of dementia. Points often included tend to be: Taiyang, Quze (PC3), Chize (LU5), Yaoyangguan (DU3), Weizhong (UB40), Weiyang (UB39), Yangjiao (GB35), and acupuncture points located on the hands and feet. The amount of blood let out depends on the temperature of the condition; hot blood tends to flow out more abundantly than cold, with manic conditions producing approximately 100ml to 200ml. A course of three treatments is generally prescribed, spaced one to two weeks apart.

Dr. Wang's treatment approach in cases of dementia is based on clinical experience as well as classic texts. She proposes that bloodletting calms the spirit, activates qi and blood, and strengthens connections between channels and collaterals. These effects suggest that bloodletting is well-suited for conditions such as schizophrenia, neurosis and insomnia.

A Case Study on Acupuncture for Schizophrenia [8]

A 63-year-old woman presented with hallucinations. The visual distortions were so realistic that she even experienced physical pain from hallucinating that a black bird was pecking at her back. Assessment and psychological testing were performed before treatment, immediately after and three months following the acupuncture treatment. After receiving a course of twelve weekly acupuncture sessions, functionality improved and she was less affected by hallucinations; even the pain associated with the hallucinations diminished. After receiving treatment for three months, symptoms were noticeably reduced. The patient immediately noticed improvements in sleep, which made daytime tasks easier to complete. A somewhat delayed improvement was also seen in depression ratings. Researchers noted that larger clinical studies on acupuncture and schizophrenia are needed to confirm results that, as this study indicates, acupuncture may be beneficial for patients with schizophrenia.

Clinical Evidence: Individual Clinical Trials

Clinical trials in acupuncture help verify the legitimacy of its role in schizophrenia. Researchers seeking to gather reliable data in a previously novel area may enroll patients in a pilot study. The first often involves gathering basic safety and efficacy data in order to apply for funding of larger scale studies.

Researchers assessed the therapeutic effect of clozapine (CZ) alone, which tends to be limited in duration, compared to clozapine with electroacupuncture (EA) in patients with schizophrenia. They randomized ninety patients into either the combined treatment group or a group receiving medication only. Researchers found treatment to be effective in 75% of patients who had received both interventions and 73% in patients receiving clozapine alone. In addition to effectively reducing symptoms; physical complaints were less prevalent among those who had received electroacupuncture. Patients receiving acupuncture also tended to follow the treatment plan more closely than those just taking medication. Researchers [9] felt that acupuncture posed potential for progressive benefit as compliance is often a prevalent issue in those during the later or more severe stages of the disorder.

Many patients with mental disorders, including schizophrenia suffer from an already compromised immune system; when hospitalized, the risk of infection increases dramatically. In addition to the added physical burden on the body, the rise of body temperature and fever often brings on or exacerbates a psychotic episode. Treatment of the infection by antibiotics can compound the problem as many with schizophrenia react negatively to antibiotics and already are carrying a heavy fungal load, which can further be aggravated by anti-biotic use. Many traditional Chinese herbs are known to have anti-infections and immune building properties; infusions and injections of which have been administered extensively in Chinese hospitals.

To determine the anti-infections and immune systems effect of injecting Huangqi at Zusanli (ST36) on hospitalized patients with schizophrenia, thirty patients were assessed. A dose of 2 mL was injected bilaterally at ST36, three times per week, for a course of eight weeks. Although there was no significant difference in terms of number of cases of infection (including sub-infection) or case-times, both were slightly lower in those who had received Huangqi compared to those who did not. Significantly, treatment duration was reduced by approximately 25%. Long-term, the group who had received Huangqi injection were infected 7.77 days/case compared to 14.08 days/case over a three-year span. Researchers [10] concluded that injection of Huangqi at Zusanli (ST36) assists the immune system in those who are hospitalized for chronic schizophrenia.

Catatonic schizophrenia can be difficult to treat as the patient is unresponsive. In order to find out how well patients with catatonic Schizophrenia respond to electroacupuncture, eighty patients were randomized into two groups, one receiving daily electroacupuncture at Baihui (DU20) and Taiyang (Extra); while the controls received modified electric convulsive therapy (MECT), every two to three days. Treatments were provided for 14 to 21 days. Researchers [11] found that effectiveness was approximately 5% greater for those receiving acupuncture; showing that electroacupuncture is at least as effective as modified electric convulsive therapy (MECT), for patients with catatonic schizophrenia.

Although the validity of sham treatment is a controversial topic; researchers used a sham electroacupuncture model to assess the effectiveness electroacupuncture in treating auditory hallucinations. Sixty hospitalized patients who had received little to no benefit from risperidone were selected for the study, a double-blind randomized controlled trial (RCT). Patients were provided 30 sham or real electroacupuncture treatments over the course of six weeks. Standardized measures revealed that patients who had received real electroacupuncture benefited to a greater extent than those who had received sham treatment. After both four and six weeks, overall scores on the Psychotic Symptom Rating Scales Auditory Hallucination Subscale improved, as did physical characteristics factor scores and the positive scores on the Positive and Negative Syndrome Scale. The study also showed that patients responded better to real acupuncture at a rate of 43.3%, versus 13.3%. Researchers [12] concluded that electroacupuncture may benefit patients with schizophrenia who are hospitalized with auditory hallucinations and may be a worthwhile course of action for those showing limited or non-responsiveness to risperidone.

To follow up on an earlier study, researchers assessed that clinical efficacy of electroacupuncture (EA) as compared with light doses of clozapine for patients with Schizophrenia. Eighty patients were randomly assigned to either a combination medication and electroacupuncture group, or a group receiving mediation only. Patients received from 50-100mg to 200-500mg of clozapine daily over a course of eight weeks. Patients receiving both interventions received three acupuncture treatments per day at Baihui (GV20) and bilateral Taiyang along with clozapine at a slightly lower upper dose maximum of 50 mg to 100-150 mg per day. Combination treatment also lasted a duration of eight weeks. Positive symptom scores and psychiatric symptoms in both the combination and clozapine only improved to a similar degree from the second week on. Starting in the fourth week, negative symptom scores also improved similarly in both groups. TESS scores showed a significant improvement in the combination group compared with the medication only group. Cure rates for the combination group were approximately 5.5%. Approximately 20% showed a dramatic improvement; while approximately 41% showed some positive benefit. Approximately 25% achieved a level of improvement less than 80%. Researchers [13] concluded that adjunct electroacupuncture may provide an additional option for those with refractory schizophrenia. Both clozapine alone and the combination of slightly lower doses of clozapine with electroacupuncture achieve similar benefits; the combination group attaining the additional benefit of a reduction in undesirable side-effects.

Differential diagnoses allow for practitioners to create patient-specific acupuncture protocols that address a unique expression of symptoms for any disease. Ronan et al. compared the results of providing individualized acupuncture as an adjunct to conventional treatment for patients with schizophrenia. To gather preliminary information, the initial evaluation was conducted through the use of case studies. Eleven patients suffering from schizophrenia were assessed across various standard measures initially, at study completion and throughout the ten-week treatment phase. Eight participants followed the course of treatment to completion; all eleven were positive regarding the acupuncture treatment. They reported reduction in negative schizophrenic symptoms, less side-effects, improved energy and more motivation. Participants also expressed positive gains in sleep, which can have a dramatic effect on psychosis. Reductions in problems related to addiction and other physical issues were also expressed. During the course of treatment, openness with providers and consistency of reports improved. Researchers felt that, overall, individualized acupuncture may provide additional benefits to patients who are receiving conventional care. Mixed research methods were recommended in order to improve accuracy of reports. They proposed that use of the Positive and Negative Syndrome Scale, the Standards for Reporting Interventions in Controlled Trials of Acupuncture and a refined self-reporting method may improve future study quality. Important factors to pay particular attention to were mentioned; such as, pharmaceutical side effects, reporting of physical activity regimen, quality of sleep and activities of daily life. Researchers [14] also requested that future studies and researchers maintain awareness of potential participant vulnerability during recovery from schizophrenia and provide a means and pathway of access to supportive care.

Plentiful complementary and alternative medicine options are now available that treat any number of conditions to varying degrees. Acupuncture continues to lead in popularity across the globe, becoming ever more familiar to diverse populations of people. More serious use for all kinds of ills, including schizophrenia, are seen in the east, with China in the heart of the epicenter. Research is accumulating to help define the role of acupuncture in Schizophrenia across cultures. To assess effectiveness among Tunisian patients, researchers conducted an inpatient clinical trial among 31 patients diagnosed with either schizophrenia or schizo-affective disorder. Each patient received either acupuncture or sham acupuncture. Ten treatments were provided, along with current medication, at a frequency of three sessions per week. Researchers [15] found standard measures, including PANSS, SAPS and SANS scores to show no significant differences between real and sham acupuncture recipients; indicating that acupuncture provided benefit equal to the placebo effect.

Depression and schizophrenia can have deleterious effects on both mood and short-term memory. Medication may be the best solution in some cases; however, differentiation of syndrome according to traditional Chinese medicine may provide insight into treatment approaches that address the underlying condition. To gather scientific data on potential benefits of acupuncture for schizophrenia and depression, researchers from conducted a clinical trial comparing acupuncture to wait-list. Researchers enrolled fifty patients each with depression or schizophrenia and twenty-five healthy controls. Participants received a twelve-week course of patient-specific acupuncture. Initially, scores on the Beck's Depression Inventory were lowest in patients experiencing depression, followed by those with schizophrenia; healthy individuals scored the highest. Digit span tests scores were similar between patients with schizophrenia and controls; however, patients with schizophrenia scored lowest of all three groups on letter-number sequencing tasks. Researchers [16] found that depression inventory scores improved after acupuncture in those experiencing depression. Digit span and letter-number sequencing performance were not affected in patients with schizophrenia or depression.

Clinical Evidence: Systematic Reviews and Meta-analysis

To compile the accumulated research on a given topic, researchers often conduct systemic literature reviews and meta-analysis. The standards maintain that a thorough literature search of stated valid databases is preliminary. Articles are collected within a specific topic; those that meet the specific study criteria are then selected. Methodological of each study is rated to indicate quality of information and any bias is noted. Study results can be pooled, which may reveal common conclusions or conflicting results of the collective data over numerous studies. Total effects and benefits then carry more weight than the results of a single study. The methods by which review was carried out are included in the meta-analysis report as well as sample size needed to show relevance. Studies are coded; heterogenicity of populations, differences between subgroups, meta-regression, bias and standards are also explicit.

A systemic review [17] was conducted in order to gather collective data on acupuncture's role in schizophrenia. Researchers searched for RCTs including acupuncture, electroacupuncture or moxibustion and schizophrenia in relevant databases through May 2009 across all languages. Interestingly, only thirteen studies, all from China, met the specific study criteria. Researchers reported that one trial reported a significant reduction of positive symptoms and benefit from electroacupuncture for patients experiencing auditory hallucinations, when compared with a combination of sham electroacupuncture and pharmaceutical intervention. Four trials noted a significantly improved rate of response rate over those taking antipsychotic medicines. Seven trials reported significant improvements in rate of response when acupuncture was provided as an adjunct to antipsychotic medications compared to those who only received mediation. One trial showed that laser acupuncture was beneficial for patients experiencing hallucinations and another revealed significant improvement in response rate, Brief Psychiatric Ratings and clinical symptoms compared to sham laser treatments. Unfortunately, methodology was not exemplary, in fact, quality was quite poor. Although results were not overwhelmingly compelling, the lack of quality data available suggests that higher quality studies with larger populations may yield more accurate indications of the true benefit of acupuncture in different types of schizophrenia.

Acupuncture modalities including traditional acupuncture, electroacupuncture, laser acupuncture, and acupoint injection, have been proven safe with adverse effects rare or of a mild nature. Widely accessible and affordable in China, acupuncture and related modalities are often included in the treatment of psychosis. Researchers compiled data on the efficacy of acupuncture in schizophrenia and related psychosis. Thirty studies were selected through 2012. Researchers found that patients who received acupuncture in addition to conventional antipsychotic intervention compared to conventional medicine alone showed some improvement more often. Specifically, overall state of mind improved and length of hospital stay was reduced. Adverse effects were also diminished in those who had received acupuncture. Acupuncture in conjunction with low dose antipsychotics produced a reduced rate of relapse when compared to those who had received standard dose antipsychotic medications without acupuncture; although similar rates of ineffectiveness were seen. Extrapyramidal symptoms were also reduced in those who had received acupuncture with a lower dose of medication. Researchers [18] also found that applying acupuncture together with traditional Chinese herbal formulas was more effective than herbal treatments given without acupuncture; however, short-term benefits of acupuncture compared with Chinese herbal formulas were similar. Studies also showed that the global state of electroacupuncture recipients was less likely to deteriorate. For the most part, study completion rates were high. Researchers concluded that acupuncture may improve global index scores and state of mind while producing minimal adverse effects in those suffering from schizophrenia and related psychosis. They recommended higher quality studies with larger populations in order to better elucidate the potential role of acupuncture in those suffering from schizophrenia.

Another acupuncture review [19] gathered the cumulative data on depression while attempting to discover the mechanisms by which acupuncture works. Reputable databases through mid-March, 2014 were searched; systematic reviews, meta-analyses, randomized controlled trials and case studies were included. Researchers found some benefit for depression. Limited benefits were found for schizophrenia, such as in terms of quality of life and sleep; of no little importance as sleep especially can dramatically affect some of the most deleterious symptoms of psychosis and schizophrenia. Although the mechanisms by which acupuncture produces specific or global effects remains a bit mysterious some brain research has indicated that acupuncture modulates and balances the neurochemistry via the limbic-paralimbic-neocortical network (LPNN). Acupuncture's powerful influence over sleep and mood may be attributed to the close association the LPNN has with both sleep and emotional response. Researchers found that the accumulated data to date shows that acupuncture shows promise as an adjunct to conventional care for those with depression. Some benefits may also be gained by those with Schizophrenia; researchers recommended larger studies to further assess general and specific potential benefits.

CHAPTER NINE

ACUPUNCTURE FOR DYSMENORRHEA

A Patient History

This patient history comes from a case that one of the authors treated several years ago. A 28-year-old female insurance agent with a 10-year history of menstrual pain came in for an acupuncture consultation and treatment. She was referred by her family physician. To control her pain, she was using over-the-counter pain pills and non-steroidal anti-inflammatory drugs, as well as the oral contraceptive pills. When she presented at the clinic, she complained of menstrual pain worsening over the preceding months, with little to no relief from the analgesics. She had severe distending pain in the lower abdomen 3-5 days before her periods and the first day of menses, with blood clots in the menstrual discharge. She also had severe pre-menstrual breast tenderness. Her periods were regular, with a 30-day cycle and 5-day duration. The pain disappeared when menstruation was over. Her tongue was red with a thin white coating; her pulse was wiry and slightly rapid. She rated her pain as a "9" on a scale of 1 – 10, with "1" representing the least pain and "10" the worst. This patient's clinical manifestations were differentiated in Chinese medicine terms as Qi stagnation and blood stasis. Acupuncture treatment was used to regulate Qi, move blood, disperse blood stasis, and stop pain. The acupuncture points selected include Guilai (ST29), Zhongji (RN3), Diji (SP8), Sanyinjiao (SP6), Taichong (LR3), Hegu (LI4), and Xuehai (SP10). All the points were punctured with even reinforcing-reducing manipulation by lifting-thrusting. The needles were retained for 30 minutes. The treatment was given twice per week. After three months, this patient's menstrual pain was reduced by 90%, with results exceeding her expectations.

The Clinical Problem

Dysmenorrhea is the occurrence of painful menstrual-related cramping of the uterus during, before and/or after menstrual periods. It refers to the pain in the lower abdomen, lower back and/or sacral region occurring in relation to menstrual periods. In severe cases, it may be accompanied with nausea, vomiting, cold perspiration, or even fainting, which affects a patient's work or daily life.

Primary dysmenorrhea is the most common gynecologic problem in menstruating women. It has been reported that the prevalence rate of primary dysmenorrhea is as high as 90 percent. A prospective study of college students found that 72 percent of monitored periods were painful, most commonly during the first day of menses. Sixty percent of the women studied reported at least one episode of severe pain [1]. In a study on the prevalence of dysmenorrhea on Italian women, menstrual pain was reported by 84.1% of women, with 43.1% reporting that pain occurred during every period, and 41% reporting that pain occurred during some periods [2]. Dysmenorrhea is prevalent among college students. In a study obtained from menstruation-related diary data from 2640 female college students in North Sichuan Medical College, menstrual pain occurred in 56.4% of students; 6.5% suffered from "hard to bear" (unbearable) menstrual pain, and 6.5% had pre-menstrual dysmenorrhea. Menstrual pain occurred on 37% of the menstrual dates on average. The percentages of students taking medicine to manage mild, moderate and unbearable dysmenorrhea were 4.0%, 13.3% and 23.7%, respectively [3]. In another study among college students conducted in Hong Kong, the prevalence of dysmenorrhea was 80%. Dysmenorrhea affected their daily life, such as reduced ability to concentrate and/or disturbance of their ability to study (75%), and changes in normal physical activity (60%). The surveyed students used both pharmacological and non-pharmacological means to relieve pain which included non-steroidal anti-inflammatory drugs (100%), traditional Chinese medicine (93%), and dietary/nutritional supplements (92%) [4].

In Chinese medicine theory, emotional factors are very important etiological factors for dysmenorrhea. Depression, anger, frustration, and resentment could all lead to liver qi stagnation. liver qi stagnation causes blood stasis in the uterus which leads to dysmenorrhea. Qi stagnation and blood stasis are the most important pattern(s) of dysmenorrhea. Invasion of exogenous cold/dampness pathogens can cause obstruction of the Chong and Ren meridians, qi stagnation and blood stasis marked by painful periods. With a condition of qi and blood deficiency or liver and kidney deficiency, the uterus lacks nourishment, manifesting as painful periods. Deficiency conditions lead to proper circulation of qi and blood, causing stagnation leading to painful periods. Acupuncture can not only reduce the pain, but can also resolve the underlying imbalance in the body which causes the painful periods.

The Clinical Treatment

For dysmenorrhea, the most critical differentiation is between excess and deficiency. When painful periods mostly occur before a menstrual period or on the first or the second day of the menstrual period, it indicates an excessive condition. It is caused by obstruction of qi and blood due to qi stagnation, blood stagnation or attack by cold. After the menstrual blood is discharged, the obstruction is removed, so painful periods will disappear after the menstrual period.

If painful periods occur towards the end of the menstrual period or after the menstrual period, it indicates a deficient type. This kind of pain is caused by loss of nourishment to the uterus due to deficiency of blood or deficiency of the liver and kidney. When there is an original deficiency of qi and blood, the uterine collaterals will lose nourishment as a result of discharge of the menstrual blood, resulting in painful periods. The basic therapeutic principle is to regulate qi and blood in the Chong and Ren Meridians and relieve pain. The main acupuncture prescription includes acupuncture points Guilai (ST29), Zhongji (RN3), Diji (SP8), and Sanyinjiao (SP6). Depending on the pattern differentiations, the above general prescription can be modified in the following ways: for qi stagnation, add Taichong (LR3) and Hegu (LI4); for blood stasis, add Xuehai (SP10); for cold accumulation, add Guanyuan (RN4), and Jinsuo (DU8) with moxabustion; for blood deficiency, add Zusanli (ST36); for liver and kidney deficiency, add Guanyuan (RN4), Taixi (KI3), and Taichong (LR3). To obtain the optimal therapeutic effect of acupuncture treatment, the acupuncture points in the prescription are needled in the following way: Zhongji (RN3) is inserted toward the pubic bone at a 30-degree angle to a depth of 1.0-1.2 cun. Guilai (ST29) is punctured perpendicularly with a depth of 0.5-1.5 cun. Sanyinjiao (SP6) is inserted perpendicularly to a depth of 0.5-1.2 cun along the posterior border of the tibia. Diji (SP8) is punctured perpendicularly to a depth of 1-1.5 cun. All these points are punctured with even reinforcing-reducing manipulation by lifting-thrusting. The needles are retained for 30 minutes. The treatment is started at least two weeks before the onset of menstruation and performed twice per week.

In the main acupuncture prescription, Zhongji (RN3) and Guilai (ST29) can regulate local qi and blood, benefit menstruation and stop pain. Sanyinjiao (SP6), a crossing point of the spleen, liver and kidney meridians, is an essential point for gynecologic issues. Needling Sanyinjiao (SP6) can tonify the liver and kidney, nourish blood and essence, and regulate menstruation. Diji (SP8), the xi-cleft point where the qi and blood of the meridian are deeply converged, is used for acute painful symptoms. The combination of all these points has a good function to regulate menstruation and stop pain.

A clarification of nomenclature is appropriate at this point: in discussions of Chinese medicine, "acupuncture" is used as a generic term for a collection of treatment procedures including acupuncture itself, acupressure, electroacupuncture, auricular acupuncture, moxibustion, acupuncture point injection, hand acupuncture, ankle acupuncture, transcutaneous electrical nerve stimulation (TENS), laser acupuncture, and many other acupuncture-related techniques. In clinical practice, these acupuncture modalities are all used by practitioners to a varying degree, depending on their training and their choice. The following clinical trials and systematic reviews, however, tend to focus specifically on acupuncture, electroacupuncture and acupressure.

Clinical Evidence: Individual Clinical Trials

Researchers have generated an increasing amount of data on the application of acupuncture to dysmenorrhea. We have selected six clinical trials in this section to illustrate the multi-faceted nature of the research data, and its increasing refinement. Acupressure and transcutaneous electrical nerve stimulation (TENS) were proven to be effective therapies in the first and second trials discussed below. Obtaining qi sensation is a critical factor for optimal effect in the third trial. Needling a single acupuncture point – Shiqizhui (Extra) – proved to be a powerful acupuncture treatment in the fourth trial. The fifth trial highlights the importance of pattern differentiation. The last trial discussed here compares acupuncture treatment with the use of a non-steroidal anti-inflammatory drug (NSAID) for dysmenorrhea.

Acupressure is a very non-invasive acupuncture approach to treat dysmenorrhea. In acupressure, physical pressure by finger, hand, elbow or various devices is applied to acupuncture points with the aim of clearing blockages in the meridians and stopping pain. A research study [5] conducted in Department of Midwifery at Tarbiat Modares University, Tehran, Iran, showed that applying acupressure to acupoint Taichong (LR3) can effectively decrease the severity of dysmenorrhea. In this single-blind clinical trial, 194 female students with dysmenorrhea were recruited to participate in the study. They were randomized to receive acupressure five days before menstruation for three months on either Taichong (LR3) or a placebo point. The severity of dysmenorrhea was assessed in the first and last of the four study cycles using the Andersch and Milsom scale. The difference in pain severity between the acupressure group and placebo group was not significant in the first cycle, but it was significant in the fourth cycle ($P<0.001$), and the decrease in dysmenorrhea severity was also significant in the study group ($P<0.05$).

Transcutaneous electrical nerve stimulation (TENS) is another non-invasive acupuncture approach to treat dysmenorrhea. TENS is a treatment that has been shown to be effective for pain relief in a variety of conditions. When using TENS, electrodes are placed on the skin and electric current applied at different frequencies and intensities is used to stimulate these areas so as to provide pain relief. In dysmenorrhea, TENS works by means of altering the body's ability to receive or perceive pain signals, rather than by having a direct effect on uterine contractions. A study [6] was to investigate whether TENS with medium-level frequency (1000 Hz-10,000 Hz) electric waves applied at both Hegu (LI4) and Sanyinjiao (SP6) could mitigate dysmenorrheal pain. Sixty-six patients with primary dysmenorrhea were randomly assigned to an experimental group (n=34) and control group (n=32). Main outcomes were measured by the McGill Questionnaire Short-form and a numerical rating scale for pain intensity. TENS was applied to Hegu (LI4) and Sanyinjiao (SP6) in the experimental group twice weekly for eight weeks; it was applied to non-acupuncture points in the control group. Pre- and post-intervention results were recorded and compared. No significant differences were found in pain scale and pain intensity between the experimental and control groups before TENS intervention. Average pain score in the experimental group was significantly lower than in the control group after TENS intervention (experimental group 2.9 ± 1.2, control group 5.4 ± 2.2; $p<0.001$). Significant differences were observed between the experimental and control groups in average change in pain scores between pre- and post-intervention (experimental group 4.5 ± 1.9, control group 1.39 ± 2.0; $p<0.001$). Significant difference in pain intensity between groups was also observed at post-intervention ($p<0.001$).

A study [7] investigated what role obtaining qi sensation (de-qi) during acupuncture treatment played in relieving menstrual pain. De-qi can be understood as "needle sensation," "arrival of qi" or "needling response," and is associated with sensations felt by the patients during acupuncture treatment. Needling sensation is the subjective feelings and perceived responses of patients and acupuncturists. Arrival of qi is a healing process, which activates the anti-pathogenic qi to expel the pathogens. De-qi experienced by patients is described as aching or soreness, numbness or tingling, fullness, distention, or pressure, and heaviness. A patient's de-qi as felt by a practitioner when grasping the needle is often described as tense, tight, and full. It is believed that de-qi is an important factor in acupuncture theory and practice. One hundred thirty-one patients with primary dysmenorrhea were randomly assigned to an acupuncture group with manual manipulation (n=67) and an acupuncture group without manipulation (n=64). Pain intensity and pain duration were measured to evaluate the therapeutic effect of acupuncture treatment. Qi sensation (de-qi) was scored on a 4-point scale by the patients. Psychological factors, including belief in acupuncture, the level of nervousness, anxiety, and depression, were also assessed. One hundred-twenty patients, sixty patients in each group, completed the study and their data was obtained. The study revealed the following: statistically significant differences in pain intensity ($P<0.01$) and pain duration ($P<0.01$) between the two groups were demonstrated. The number of de-qi acupoints ($P<0.01$) and the average intensity of de-qi ($P<0.01$) were significantly higher in the manipulation group as compared with the non-manipulation group. The correlation between de-qi and the therapeutic effect of acupuncture was much stronger than that between psychological factors and therapeutic effect. The authors concluded that compared with the psychological factors, de-qi is critical for achieving therapeutic effect and contributed more to the pain-relieving effect of acupuncture in subjects with primary dysmenorrhea.

In acupuncture theory and practice, a multiple-point prescription is an essential component of an effective acupuncture treatment. In some cases, only one point constitutes this prescription. Shiqizhui (EX-B8) is such a prescription for dysmenorrhea. A study [8] conducted at the Medical School at Shandong University of Traditional Chinese Medicine, Jinan, China investigated the clinical therapeutic effect of acupuncture at single point Shiqizhui (EX-B8) and multi-points in time-varying treatment for primary dysmenorrhea. Six hundred patients with primary dysmenorrhea were recruited and randomly assigned to: the single point group (n=200) including group A (treating before the menstruation, n=100) and group B (immediately treating as soon as pain occurred, n=100); the multi-point group (n=200) including group C (treating before the menstruation, n=100) and group D (immediately treating as soon as pain occurrence, n=100); or the control group, group E (n=200, no treatment). The therapeutic effects were measured and analyzed after treatment during three menstrual cycles and patients interviewed for three follow-up periods. The study obtained the following results: acupuncture could effectively relieve menstrual pain for primary dysmenorrhea compared with the control group ($P<0.05$, $P<0.01$); immediate pain relief occurred following acupuncture within 5 minutes in group B ($P<0.01$) and group D ($P<0.01$); and the two groups obviously relieved menstrual pain for VAS scores. Both group A and group C obviously relieved menstrual pain ($P<0.01$), and group C was better than group A ($P<0.05$). Compared with group D, Group C was much better for

CMSS scores in cycle 1. The authors concluded that multi-point acupuncture before menstruation was more effective than immediate acupuncture when pain occurred in improving symptoms of dysmenorrhea. And, further, that single-point acupuncture was better used at pain occurrence than multi-point acupuncture. The trial suggested that Shiqizhui (EX-B8) should be chosen as a convenient point.

A fundamental concept in traditional Chinese medicine (TCM) is pattern differentiation, *i.e.* assessing a patient's signs and symptoms and ascribing them to a specific TCM pattern. Chinese medicine treatment, including acupuncture, is pattern-based, with different treatment applied to different patterns. Testing pattern-based treatment is challenging. Liu *et al.* [9] from the School of Acupuncture-Moxibustion and Tuina, Beijing University of Chinese Medicine, Beijing, China, attempted to conduct a TCM pattern subdivision analysis of the first intervention data from a multicenter, randomized, controlled trial. This trial recruited patients from six hospitals in three provinces in China. Five hundred and one patients with primary dysmenorrhea were recruited to the trial. Patients were randomly and equally assigned into three groups: Sanyinjiao (SP6) group; Xuanzhong (GB39) group; and an adjacent non-acupoint group. For each group, bilateral electroacupuncture at the site was performed. Patients were differentiated with TCM patterns before treatment. The intervention was carried out when the visual analogue scale (VAS) score of a participant's menstrual pain was $\geq$ 40 mm on the first day of menstruation and lasted for 30 minutes. The immediate improvement of pain was measured with a 100-mm VAS before the intervention, at 5 minutes, 10 minutes, and 30 minutes during the intervention, and at 30 minutes after the completion of this intervention. Three TCM patterns (n=320) were eligible for analysis: Cold and Dampness Stagnation pattern (n=184); Qi and Blood Stagnation pattern (n=84); and Qi and Blood Deficiency pattern (n=52). For the Cold and Dampness Stagnation pattern, the Sanyinjiao (SP6) group had a significant reduction in VAS scores compared with the Xuanzhong (GB39) group (mean difference -7.6 mm) and the non-acupoint group (mean difference -8.2 mm), respectively. There was no significant difference between the latter two groups. There were no significant differences in VAS scores in the other two patterns. The study suggests that TCM pattern might affect acupoint specific effect on the immediate pain relief obtained for patients with primary dysmenorrhea.

Nonsteroidal anti-inflammatory drugs (NSAIDs) and the oral contraceptive pill are two common medical therapies for dysmenorrhea, both of which work by reducing myometrial (uterine muscle) activity. However, both treatments are accompanied by a number of side effects, making an effective non-pharmacological method of treating dysmenorrhea of potential value. A study [10] from the Kahramanmaras Sutcu Imam University School of Medicine, Department of Obstetrics and Gynecology, Kahramanmaras, Turkey, was conducted to compare the therapeutic effect of acupuncture and NSAID therapy in primary dysmenorrhea patients. Thirty-five young women with a diagnosis of primary dysmenorrhea participated in the study. Their dysmenorrheal pain intensity was rated by visual analog scale (VAS) immediately prior to entry into the study. They were randomly assigned into two groups: NSAID group (n=24) or acupuncture group (n=11). Pain intensity was rated again with VAS during menstruation in both groups. The study found that after one month's treatment, pain scores were significantly lower in both groups ($p<0.05$). Mean pain scores decreased by 52.2% in the NSAID group and 69.5% in acupuncture group, respectively. These results revealed that acupuncture was as effective as NSAID therapy for patients with primary dysmenorrhea.

A study [11] conducted by Liu et al. revealed that deqi (obtaining qi sensation) at different acupuncture or nonacupoint or even the point locations is not that essential to managing menstrual pain. Their results were obtained from a larger randomized controlled trial (RCT). This study enrolled 501 primary dysmenorrhea patients and they were randomly assigned to one of three treatment groups: Acupuncture at Sanyinjiao (SP 6) Group, Acupuncture at Xuanzhong (GB39) Group or Acupuncture at Nonacupoint Group. Sanyinjiao (SP6) is the primary choice for treating menstrual pain. Xuanzhong (GB39) is unrelated to treating menstrual pain. Patients received three sessions with electro-acupuncture at a Sanyinjiao (SP6), or Xuanzhong (GB39), or a nonacupoint, respectively. The deqi sensations during acupuncture was measured by the Massachusetts General Hospital acupuncture sensation scales (MASS). The outcomes were measured by a 100-mm visual analogue scale (VAS) before and after acupuncture. They were measured at 0, 5, 10, 30, and 60 minutes following the first treatment. Patients experienced sharp pain, heaviness and dull pain at Sanyinjiao (SP 6) and Xuanzhong (GB39) and sharp pain, heaviness, numbness at the nonacupoint. The study showed that VAS scores following the first treatment demonstrated that Sanyinjiao (SP6) group was more effective than Xuanzhong (GB39) (-4.0 mm, 95% CI -7.1 to -0.9, $P = 0.010$) and nonacupoint (-4.0 mm, 95% CI -7.0 to -0.9, $P = 0.012$) groups. VAS scores of pain after acupuncture were significantly decreased after acupuncture treatment in all three groups, but no clinically significant differences were found among three groups at the baseline and the end of acupuncture treatment.

Deqi (qi sensation) and pattern differentiation are two fundamental concepts of acupuncture and Chinese medicine. Zhao et al. [12] conducted a multicenter randomized controlled trial to test how much *deqi* contribute to the immediate analgesic effect of acupuncture in patients with primary dysmenorrhea for patients with a specific pattern diagnosis of *cold and dampness stagnation*.

The study [12] enrolled eighty-eight primary dysmenorrhea patients with *cold and dampness stagnation*. They were randomly assigned to *deqi* group (n=43) or no *deqi* group (n=45). Acupuncture treatment on Sanyinjiao (SP6) was performed for 30 minutes. Deep needling at Sanyinjiao (SP6) with manipulation using thick needles was offered to the de qi group; Shallow needling with no manipulation using thin needles was given to the no *deqi* group. A visual analogue scale for pain (VAS-P) and the acupuncture *deqi* clinical assessment scale (ADCAS) were used to evaluate the pain scores and actual *deqi* sensation. The study showed reductions in VAS-P in both groups, but with no significant differences between groups, although ADCAS scores indicated significant differences in *deqi* and no *deqi* groups.

Gao et al. [13] conducted a randomized double blind clinical trial of crossover design to investigate the effect of moxibustion on alleviating menstrual pain and relieving the symptoms of dysmenorrhea. This two-phase study was performed in a cohort of 56 young nursing students with menstrual pain in Guangzhou University of Chinese Medicine. The trial randomly allocated participants into Group A (n=28) who received moxibustion therapy from five days before the menstrual period to the onset through a specific heating box in which burning moxa stick was fixed, and Group B (n=28) who received the same heating box but with a paper-wrapped stick incense fixed inside (placebo therapy) during the same intervention period. Moxibustion and placebo were applied to Guanyuan (CV4) and Shenque (CV8). The intervention was stopped for three menstrual after the first treatment phase for two menstrual cycles. The intervention of two groups were switched in the second treatment phase in which Group A received the placebo therapy and Group B received moxibustion therapy. The outcome measurements included NRS, VRS, PRI, VAS and BRS-6 at the baseline and after each treatment phase.

Trial results included that the score of BRS-6 has significant differences between two groups at the first menstrual cycle ($p<0.05$) after the first treatment phase; the score of VAS, BRS-6, sensory of PRI, affective dimension of PR and total score of PRI in Group A were much lower than Group B ($p<0.05$) at the second menstrual cycle; NRS and VRS had significant differences between two groups after the first treatment phase ($p<0.05$); the score of VAS, BRS-6, PRI, total score of PRI and VRS had significant differences between two groups after the second treatment phase ($p<0.01$); the severity rating of abdominal pain, weakness, leg aches, dizziness, nervousness and the total score had significant differences between two groups after the second treatment phase ($p<0.05$). The study suggested that moxibustion therapy was effective for alleviating menstrual pain and symptoms of young female university students in China and the operation is easy for the young females themselves to administer it.

Acupuncture point injection is a subfield of acupuncture practiced in China and is allowed to practice in certain states in the United States. A double-blind randomly controlled clinical trial [14] comparing vitamin K3 acupuncture point injection to saline acupuncture point injection and vitamin K3 deep muscle injection was conducted to determine if injection of vitamin K3 in an acupuncture point is optimal for the treatment of primary dysmenorrhea, when compared with 2 other injection treatments. This trial was performed in a Menstrual Disorder Centre at a public hospital in Shanghai, China. The study recruited participants 80 patients with primary dysmenorrhea, aged 14-25 years with severe primary dysmenorrhea for at least 6 months and no relief by any other treatment. Participants in each group received 3 injections at a single treatment visit.

The study used an 11 unit Numeric Rating Scale (NRS) as primary outcome and Cox Pain Intensity and Duration scales as secondary measurement and the consumption of analgesic tablets before and after treatment and during the 6 following cycles. The trial showed that patients experienced pain relief from the injection treatments in all three groups and the differences between the treatment group and both active control groups (1.11, CI 0.45 to 1.78) and (1.82, CI 1.45 to 2.49) were statistically significant. The study validified that acupuncture point injection of vitamin K3 relieves menstrual pain rapidly and is a useful treatment option.

An Antipodes study [15] was published to investigate the impact of self-care advice on primary dysmenorrhea and to test that an acupuncture treatment consisted of "more than needles" for both practitioners and participants. 19 TCM acupuncture practitioners from New Zealand or Australia and 12 New Zealand women who had recently undergone acupuncture treatment for primary dysmenorrhea as part of a randomized controlled trial were involved in this qualitative, pragmatic study. Data were collected from focus groups and semi-structured interviews. Both the practitioners and participants discussed the partnership they engaged in during treatment. Participants felt that the TCM self-care advice was a positive factor for the outcomes of their dysmenorrhea relief and improved their menstrual symptoms.

Yang *et al.* [16] conducted a pragmatic, randomized, conventional drug controlled, open-labeled clinical trial to investigate the therapeutic effect of moxibustion. The trial recruited 152 eligible participants who were randomly assigned into moxibustion group and conventional drug group, both groups received three-month treatments. Pain relief measured by the Visual Analogue Scale was the primary outcome.

The results of the study showed that both the menstrual pain intensity in moxibustion group and drug group was reduced significantly after treatment relative to baseline, but the pain reduction was not significantly different between these two groups. But three months after treatment, the effect with moxibustion sustained and showed superior to the drug's effect. Additional analysis on the serum levels of pain mediators such as PGF2α, OT, vWF, β-EP, PGE2 demonstrated that moxibustion was as effective as drugs in alleviating menstrual pain-related symptoms. Moxibustion is an option for menstrual pain relief.

Cha *et al.* [17] conducted a randomized controlled trial to examine the effect of auricular acupressure therapy on primary dysmenorrhea among female high school students in South Korea. The study recruited 91 female high school students with average age of 16.7 years, with 45 participants in the experimental group and 46 in the control group. The experimental group received auricular acupressure therapy was applied on the ear's Jagung, Sinmun, Gyogam, and Naebunbi for 3 days during periods of extreme primary dysmenorrhea. For the control group, only the skin paper tape without an auricular acupressure needle was applied on the same acupoints. Menstrual Distress Questionnaire was used to assess primary dysmenorrhea, and the visual analog scale to assess abdominal and back pain of participants.

Results showed that auricular acupressure therapy decreased abdominal pain, back pain, and primary dysmenorrhea of female high school students in South Korea, and the differences on abdominal pain ($t = 24.594$, $p < .001$), back pain ($t = 22.661$, $p < .001$), and primary dysmenorrhea ($t = 32.187$, $p < .001$) were significant between the two groups.

Armour *et al.* [18] conducted a randomized controlled trial with four arms to examine the effect of changing treatment timing and the use of manual, electro acupuncture on the symptoms of primary dysmenorrhea. A total of 74 women were randomly assigned to one of the four groups: low frequency manual acupuncture (LF-MA), high frequency manual acupuncture (HF-MA), low frequency electro acupuncture (LF-EA) and high frequency electro acupuncture (HF-EA). Over three menstrual cycles, twelve treatments were offered, either once per week (LF groups) or three times in the week prior to menses (HF groups). A treatment was performed in the first 48 hours of menses for all groups. The reduction in peak menstrual pain at 12 months from trial entry was the primary outcome.

The results of the study showed that statistically significant ($p < .001$) reductions in peak and average menstrual pain compared to baseline during the treatment period and nine-month follow-up for all groups, but there were no differences between groups ($p > 0.05$). Other results included health related quality of life increased significantly in six domains in groups having high frequency of treatment compared to two domains in low frequency groups; manual acupuncture groups required less analgesic medication than electro-acupuncture groups ($p = 0.02$); and manual acupuncture was most effective in reducing secondary menstrual symptoms compared to both-EA groups ($p<0.05$). The study demonstrated that changing mode of stimulation or frequency of treatment on menstrual pain was not significant.

Bazarganipour *et al.* [19] reported a randomized, single blinded clinical trial to assess a simple acupressure protocol in Taichong (LR3) and Hegu (LI4) for women with primary dysmenorrhea. The trial recruited 90 young women with dysmenorrhea and they were randomly assigned three groups to receive 20min acupressure every day in either Taichong (LR3) or Hegu (LI4), or placebo points. Acupressure was performed five days before menstruation for three successive menstrual cycles. The outcome was measured by the Wong Baker faces pain scale, and the quality-of-life short form-12 (QOL SF-12) on menstruation.

Results showed that the intensity and duration of pain among the three groups in the second and third cycles during the intervention ($p<0.05$) differed significantly; and significant differences were observed in all domains of QOL except for mental health ($p=0.4$), general health ($p=0.7$) and mental subscale component ($p=0.12$) in the second cycle, and mental health ($p=0.9$), and mental subscale component ($p=0.14$) in the third cycle. The trial demonstrated that even a simple acupressure protocol is effective to decrease the intensity and duration of dysmenorrhea and improve the QOL.

Gaubeca-Gilarranz *et al.* [20] performed a randomized, single blind, parallel-group trial to compare the effectiveness of trigger point dry needling (TrP-DN) versus placebo needling, relative to an untreated control group, on pain and quality of life in primary dysmenorrhea. The study recruited 56 females with primary dysmenorrhea and they were randomly allocated to TrP-DN group (n=19), placebo needling group (n=18) or no treatment group (n=19). The TrP-DN group received a single session of TrP-DN to trigger points (TrPs) in the rectus abdominis, and the placebo group received placebo needling. All participants were directed for stretching at each session. The pain intensity (visual analogue scale) was chosen as the primary outcome. The quality of life, use of non-steroidal anti-inflammatory drugs, the number of days with pain, and self-perceived improvement, measured using a Global Rate of Change were the secondary outcomes. At baseline, and 1 and 2 months after the treatment, the outcomes were measured.

Results showed that the patients receiving TrP-DN exhibited greater decreases ($P<0.001$) in pain than those receiving placebo (1 month: Δ-19.8 mm, 25.9 to -13.7; 2 months: Δ-26.0 mm, -33.1 to -18.9) or those in the untreated control group (1 month: Δ-26.0mm, -32.5 to -19.5; 2 months: Δ-20.1 mm, -26.4 to -13.8); the TrP-DN group also exhibited a greater decrease in the amount of medications ($P<0.001$), but no differences in the number of days with pain or quality of life were observed (all $P>0.1$). The study demonstrated that a single session of TrP-DN of the rectus abdominis combined with stretching was more effective than placebo needling and stretching alone at reducing pain and the amount of medication used in primary dysmenorrhea.

Clinical Evidence: Systematic Reviews and Meta-analysis

A systematic review is a critical assessment and evaluation of all clinical trials that address a particular clinical issue such as acupuncture intervention dysmenorrhea. The researchers use an organized method of locating, assembling, and evaluating a body of literature on the subject under investigation using a set of specific criteria. A systematic review typically includes a description of the findings of the collection of research studies. The systematic review, including a quantitative pooling of data from all the individual studies, is called a meta-analysis. Five systematic reviews in this section illustrate the increasing evidence for applying acupuncture, acupressure, and electro-acupuncture to dysmenorrhea. These reviews not only reflect the evolution of clinical research on acupuncture for dysmenorrheal pain, but also investigate nuanced aspects of this clinical application, such as the study comparing Sanyinjiao (SP6) vs. Xuanzhong (GB9) cited in the final paragraph of this section.

One early systematic review by Proctor, *et al.* [21] in the Department of Obstetrics and Gynecology, National Women's Hospital, Claude Road, Epsom, Auckland, New Zealand, was conducted to determine the effectiveness of high and low frequency transcutaneous electrical nerve stimulation (TENS) and acupuncture when compared to each other, placebo, no treatment, or medical treatment for primary dysmenorrhea. Nine randomized controlled trials of transcutaneous electrical nerve stimulation and acupuncture that compared these treatments to each other, placebo, no treatment, or medical treatment for primary dysmenorrhea were included. Mild, infrequent or secondary dysmenorrhea and dysmenorrhea associated with an IUD were excluded. Among the nine RCTs included for this review, seven involved TENS, one acupuncture, and one both treatments. Meta analysis was performed using odds ratios for dichotomous outcomes and weighted mean differences for continuous outcomes. The outcome measures were pain relief, adverse effects, use of analgesics additional to treatment and absence from work or school. The review found that high frequency TENS was more effective for pain relief than placebo TENS; low frequency TENS was no more effective in reducing pain than placebo TENS.

In a 2008 systematic review [22] to evaluate the effects of acupuncture-related therapies for treating primary dysmenorrhea, thirty randomized controlled trails (RCTs) and two controlled clinical trials (CCTs) were identified. Low methodologic quality of these trials and small sample size revealed conflicting results regarding whether acupuncture-related therapies were more effective than control treatments, although some small, methodologically sound trials of acupuncture suggested that acupuncture was more effective than control groups. The survey highlighted an urgent need for randomized, blinded, placebo-controlled trials to assess the effects of acupuncture.

In a 2010 systematic review [23] to assess the effectiveness of acupuncture for the symptomatic treatment of primary dysmenorrhea, nineteen electronic databases, including English, Korean, Japanese and Chinese databases, were systematically searched for RCTs investigating acupuncture for primary dysmenorrheal. All RCTs which evaluated the effects of acupuncture compared with controls were included, but moxibustion or acupressure studies for dysmenorrheal pain were excluded. Nine of the twenty-seven systematically reviewed RCTs clearly described their methods of randomization. The review found that compared with pharmacological treatment or herbal medicine, acupuncture was associated with a significant reduction in pain. This review found promising evidence for the use of acupuncture in the treatment of primary dysmenorrhea compared with pharmacological treatment or herbal medicine. But the evidence for the effectiveness of acupuncture for the treatment of primary dysmenorrhea was not convincing when compared with sham acupuncture.

A 2011 systematic review [24] examined the then-available evidence supporting the use of acupuncture to treat primary dysmenorrhea to determine the efficacy and safety of acupuncture in the treatment of primary dysmenorrhea when compared with a placebo, no treatment, or conventional medical treatment such as oral contraceptives and NSAIDs. Extensive databases were searched to include all published and unpublished randomized controlled trials comparing acupuncture, electro-acupuncture, and acupressure with placebo control, usual care, and pharmacological treatment. Patients in the trials were women of reproductive age with primary dysmenorrhea during the majority of their menstrual cycles or for three consecutive menstrual cycles, and with moderate to severe symptoms. The study performed meta-analyses with odds ratios (OR) for dichotomous outcomes and mean differences or standard mean differences (SMD) for continuous outcomes, with 95% confidence intervals (CI). Pain relief and improved menstrual symptoms, measured by self-rating scales were the primary outcomes. Ten trials were included in the review with data reporting on 944 participants, among which six trials reported on acupuncture ($n = 673$) and four trials ($n = 271$) reported on acupressure. The study showed that there was an improvement in pain relief from acupuncture compared with a placebo control (OR 9.5, 95% CI [21.17, 51.8]), NSAIDs (SMD -0.70, 95% CI [-1.08, -0.32]) and Chinese herbs (SMD -1.34, 95% CI [-1.74, -0.95]). There was an improvement in pain relief from acupressure compared with a placebo control (SMD -0.99, 95% CI [-1.48, -0.49]). The authors concluded that acupuncture and acupressure reduced menstrual-related pain.

In a 2012 systematic review [25] to investigate the effectiveness of acupoint stimulation for primary dysmenorrhea, thirty randomized controlled trials comparing acupoint stimulation with non-acupoint-related stimulation or medication were included, twenty-five of which reported sufficient data for pooling. Cure rate, total effective rate, pain intensity, menstrual pain, plasma PGF(2α)/PGE(2) ratio, and adverse events were the main outcomes to be assessed. Dichotomous variables were described by odds ratios with 95% confidence intervals, and continuous variables were expressed as mean±standard deviation, depending on the outcome measures being discrete or continuous. Meta-analysis for twenty-five RCTs with a total of over 3000 patients was performed by fixed-effects models. The results showed that acupuncture has significant effects when compared with non-acupoint-related stimulation or medication. Although both invasive and noninvasive acupuncture was effective, the latter was more effective. The authors concluded that acupuncture, especially non-invasive acupoint stimulation, had good short-term effects on pain of primary dysmenorrhea.

In a 2013 meta-analysis [26] evaluating the effectiveness of acupuncture or acupressure at Sanyinjiao (SP6) in relieving pain associated with primary dysmenorrhea, seven randomized controlled trials (three acupuncture and four acupressure trials) were identified. The visual analogue scale (VAS) pain score was the primary outcome. For the acupuncture analysis, no significant difference in the mean VAS score reduction between the Sanyinjiao (SP6) group and the control Xuanzhong (GB39) group (-4.935; 95% CI [-15.757, 5.887]; P = 0.371) was discovered. For the acupressure analysis, there was a significant difference in the mean VAS score after intervention between the Sanyinjiao (SP6) group with acupressure and the control group with rest/light touch at Sanyinjiao (SP6), or the non-acupoint acupressure groups, which favored the Sanyinjiao (SP6) acupressure group (-1.011; 95% CI [-1.622, -0.400]; P = 0.001). Good reliability of the meta-analysis findings was demonstrated by sensitivity analyses. The study suggested that acupuncture at Sanyinjiao (SP6) is not more effective than acupuncture at a control point Xunazhong (GB39) in relieving pain from primary dysmenorrhea, but acupressure at Sanyinjiao (SP6) may be effective in the relief of primary dysmenorrheal pain.

In a study [27] intended to compare the effectiveness of acupuncture related techniques such as sandwiched moxibustion, moxibustion, acupuncture, floating needle, and acupoint application-with other therapeutic methods for the treatment of primary dysmenorrhea, Xu *et al.* conducted a meta-analysis of randomized, controlled trials from six electronic databases (PubMed, Web of Science, the Chinese Biomedical Literature Database (CBM), the Chinese Journal Full-text Database (CNKI), the Chinese Science and Technology Journal Full-text Database (VIP), and Chinese Wanfang Data) covering from inception to December, 2012. The selected RCTs were grouped into two types of primary dysmenorrhea based on the participants being undifferentiated type group (UTG) and the cold-damp stagnation type group (CDSTG). The outcomes were measured by total effective rate, symptom score, and variation of peripheral blood prostaglandin F2α (PGF2α).

With 20 RCTs of 2134 participants, the meta-analysis showed that the total efficacy for the two studied interventions was statistically significantly different from that of the control methods for the CDSTG; the studied interventions were statistically significantly different in relieving the severity of symptoms of primary dysmenorrhea; and no statistical difference was found between the intervention and control groups in the reduction of the level of peripheral blood PGF2α.

This early meta-analysis demonstrated that acupuncture related techniques can relieve pain effectively for individuals with primary dysmenorrhea, but more large, multicenter studies may warrant that the conclusion is substantiated.

The number on clinical trials has been increased significantly, but the quality of those trials and reporting, consistency have been challenged. A Cochrane study by Smith *et al.* [28] was conducted to determine the effectiveness and safety of acupuncture and acupressure in the treatment of primary dysmenorrhea when compared with a placebo, no treatment, or conventional medical treatment. Published and unpublished randomized controlled trials comparing acupuncture with sham acupuncture or placebo control, usual care, pharmacological treatment or no treatment were extracted from the following databases: the Cochrane Menstrual Disorders and Subfertility Group Trials Register (to September 2015), Cochrane Central Register of Controlled Trials (CENTRAL) (the Cochrane Library), MEDLINE, EMBASE, PsycINFO, CINAHL and Chinese databases including Chinese Biomedical Literature Database (CBM), China National Knowledge Infrastructure (CNKI), VIP database and registers of ongoing trials. Treatment modalities included acupuncture, electro-acupuncture, and acupressure.

Odds ratios (ORs) for dichotomous outcomes and mean differences (MDs) or standardized mean differences (SMDs) for continuous outcomes, with 95% confidence intervals (CIs) were calculated, with pain as the primary outcome and menstrual symptoms, quality of life, and adverse effects as the secondary outcomes. 42 RCTs with 4640 women were included, in which acupuncture or acupressure was compared with a sham/placebo group, medication, no treatment or other treatment.

Smith et al. pointed out the insufficient evidence and limitations on risk of bias, poor reporting, inconsistency and risk of publication bias to demonstrate whether or not acupuncture or acupressure are effective in treating primary dysmenorrhea, by dividing the 42 RCTs into multiple categories: acupuncture versus sham or placebo control; acupuncture versus NSAIDs; acupuncture versus no treatment; acupressure versus sham or placebo control; acupressure versus NSAIDs; acupressure versus no treatment.

Sanyinjiao (SP6) is an essential point for acupuncture and acupressure to treat primary dysmenorrhea. Abaraogu *et al.* [29] conducted a review for the evidence of Sanyinjiao (SP6) acupressure for the relief of primary dysmenorrhea symptoms, and patients' experiences of this intervention. The authors extracted data from six relevant databases and gray literature for publications dated up to March 2016. Six out of 72 potential studies, with a total of 461 participants, were included in the study. The review used pain intensity as the primary outcome. Although the Cochrane criteria applied to the data demonstrated that the included studies were generally of low quality with a high risk of bias, but the review showed that Sanyinjiao (SP6) acupressure delivered by trained personnel significantly decreased pain intensity immediately after the intervention (effect size = -0.718; CI = -0.951 to -0.585; p = 0.000), and pain relief remained up to 3 h after the intervention (effect size = -0.979; CI = -1.296 to 0.662; p = 0.000) and promise for the alleviation of primary dysmenorrhea symptoms from self-administered acupressure.

Acupuncture dose including number of needles, retention time and mode of stimulation, number of treatments and frequency of treatments, needle location and treatment timing are important parameters for acupuncture intervention and outcomes. Armour *et al.* [30] conducted a systematic review of clinical trials to determine the effectiveness or efficacy of acupuncture in primary dysmenorrhea.

The study extracted eight databases for locating trials examining penetrating body acupuncture for primary dysmenorrhea published in English up to September 2015. Eleven trials with well reported acupuncture dose components were included. Results showed that the relationship between needle location and menstrual pain demonstrated conflicting results; acupuncture before menses produced greater reductions in pain than treatment starting at the onset of menses; a single needle during menses provided greater pain reduction compared to multiple needles; multiple needles before menses were superior to a single needle; electroacupuncture provided more rapid pain reduction compared to manual acupuncture, but didn't have a significantly different effect on overall menstrual pain; needle location, number of needles used and frequency of treatment showed clear dose-response relationships with menstrual pain outcomes.

Xu *et al.* [31] conducted a systematic review and meta-analysis to compare the effectiveness of acupuncture with Non-Steroidal Anti-Inflammatory Drugs (NASIDs) in the treatment of primary dysmenorrhea. The authors extracted six databases to include sixteen randomized controlled trials involving 1679 primary dysmenorrhea patients. Clinical effectiveness rate, symptom score, visual analogue score, variation in peripheral blood prostaglandin F2α (PGF2α) and side effects were assessed as the main outcomes. The study found that the total efficacy of acupuncture intervention was better than control group; the acupuncture intervention was superior in relieving the severity of primary dysmenorrhea symptoms; no statistical difference was proved between two groups in terms of reduction in the VAS; the acupuncture intervention on the variation in peripheral blood PGF2α between two groups was positive; the side effects of control groups was more severe than the acupuncture groups.

A Scientific Explanation

The clinical trials, systematic reviews and meta-analyses cited above have shown acupuncture to be a useful, non-pharmacological method for treating dysmenorrheal pain. Scientific exploration of the mechanisms by which acupuncture produces analgesic effects has been going on for decades and is well-documented. There is strong consensus on the following scientific explanations of how and why acupuncture alleviates or eliminates pain. Studies show that acupuncture can raise the pain tolerance threshold, and reduce the emotional response to pain. Acupuncture blocks pain impulses by exciting receptors or nerve fibers, precipitating complicated interactions with neurotransmitters or neuropeptides such as serotonin and endorphins. Acupuncture can increase the release of brain opioid peptides, including β-endorphin and enkephalin which have a strong analgesic effect.

Enkephalin and dynorphin released by acupuncture produce an analgesic effect in the spinal cord. Acupuncture stimulates nerve fibers in the muscle, which then send impulses to the spinal cord and activate three neurological centers (spinal cord, midbrain, and hypothalamus-pituitary) to cause analgesia. In the spinal cord, enkephalin and dynorphin are mobilized to block incoming pain messages. In the midbrain, enkephalin is activated to stimulate the raphe descending system, which inhibits spinal cord pain transmission by a synergistic effect on monoamines, serotonin, and norepinephrine. In the hypothalamus-pituitary, β-endorphin is released into the blood and cerebrospinal fluid (CSF) to cause analgesia [32].

CHAPTER TEN

MOXIBUSTION ON ZHIYIN (BL67) FOR BREECH PRESENTATION

Summary

- Moxibustion is a modality of Chinese medicine which involves burning a preparation of the herb *artemesia vulgaris* (moxa) close to acupuncture points on the skin. This article considers the application of moxa to the acupuncture point Zhiyin (BL67), which is located at the tip of the fifth toe. Applying moxa to Zhiyin (BL67) has been practiced as a way of correcting breech presentation of a fetus for at least a thousand years in China.
- In conventional medicine, caesarean section is often performed when there is breech presentation of a fetus to avoid potential complications during labor. The optimal solution would be to reposition the fetus before labor starts. This article examines the effectiveness and safety of moxibustion at Zhiyin (BL67) to rectify a fetus in breech position as an alternative approach to caesarean section.
- Four observational studies establish the correlation between moxibustion at Zhiyin (BL67) and the outcome of correcting breech presentation.
- Ten clinical trials conducted in different countries provide supportive evidence for the effectiveness and safety of moxibustion at Zhiyin (BL67) for breech presentation.
- Four clinical trials provide indeterminate or non-supportive evidence for the application of moxibustion at Zhiyin (BL67) to breech presentation.
- Three systematic reviews provide fairly strong evidence on the effectiveness of applying moxibustion at Zhiyin (BL67) to breech presentation.
- Three meta-analysis studies indicate that moxibustion at Zhiyin (BL67) results in fewer births by caesarean section and is an effective treatment for the correction of nonvertex presentation. The

meta-analyses further indicate that moxibustion might reduce the need for administration of oxytocin.

- A cost-effectiveness study with a modeling approach suggested that the rectification of a fetus in breech presentation in women at 33 weeks' gestation with acupuncture-type interventions at Zhiyin (BL67) was less costly when compared to expectant management, including external cephalic versions.
- Studies provide explanations of how moxibustion intervention works to correct breech presentation. Moxibustion at Zhiyin (BL67) causes adrenocortical stimulation, leading to increased placental estrogens and changes in prostaglandin levels. Estrogens increase myometrial sensitivity, which results in increased contractility. This stimulates fetal movements. The increase in fetal movements (monitored by fetal heart rate) is a striking effect of moxibustion on breech presentation, with the stimulating effects persisting even after the end of direct stimulation.

Introduction

Moxibustion is an integral treatment modality of traditional Chinese medicine. In the Chinese language, traditional Chinese medicine is called *zhenjiu*. This word consists of two parts: *zhen* and *jiu*, which are united in the naming of this medicine. *Zhen* means "acupuncture" or "needles," and *jiu* is moxibustion. While acupuncture is now popular and widely used around the world, moxibustion is less well-known. Moxibustion therapeutically utilizes the heat generated by burning herbal preparations of the artemisia plant, which is also called mugwort. The word *moxa* is derived from the Japanese word *moekusa,* which means "burning herb." Moxibustion technique consists of lighting a moxa stick (compressed moxa) and bringing it close to the skin until it produces hyperemia due to local vasodilatation. It is used to stimulate acupuncture points on the skin. According to the theory of traditional Chinese medicine, heat generated from moxibustion is typically applied to acupuncture points to treat diseases by regulating the function of meridians and visceral organs. A classical explanation for how moxibustion works says that the heat stimulates acupuncture points, which increases qi circulation, eliminates pathological cold, and relieves qi stagnation, leading to an improved disease state. Moxibustion uses heat stimulation at various temperature levels, ranging from mild skin warming to tissue damage from burning. This heat stimulation can yield inflammatory responses and induce vascular changes. In most cases, the intensity of moxibustion stimulation is kept just below the threshold of an individual's ability to tolerate it.

Breech presentation occurs when the fetus presents "bottom-down" in the uterus. Three types of breech presentation are categorized: breech with extended legs (frank); breech with fully flexed legs (complete); and footling (incomplete) with one or both thighs extended. The association of breech presentation with higher prenatal mortality and morbidity when compared to cephalic presentations is a significant concern. This could be due to one the following factors: pre-existing congenital malformation, increased incidence of breech in premature deliveries and increased risk of intrapartum trauma or asphyxia.

Caesarean section is the conventional mode of delivery for term breech presentations, as it is believed that this procedure reduces the risk of birth-related complications [1]. In the USA, over 85% of all breech presentations are now delivered by caesarean section. This is a significant increase from 14% in 1970 [2]. Intrapartum and neonatal deaths associated with breech presentation have been declining: one study based on Scottish births between 1985 and 2004 demonstrated a 75% decrease in deaths; but the increased application of planned caesarean section only provided a partial explanation [3]. A study from the Royal College of Obstetricians and Gynecologists reported that the proportion of babies in the breech position declines as gestation progresses: 20% at 28 weeks, 15% between 29-32 weeks, and only 3-4% of these presentations will stay in this position until labor begins. By the 36th week, the majority of fetuses turn spontaneously, adopting the 'best fit' position that a normal gravid uterus provides. [4].

Vaginal birth for a breech baby has become more and more uncommon as the midwifery skills to assist women have been lost, with most doctors recommending a caesarean birth for breech presentations. Finding an effective way of turning a breech fetus quickly and safely to the physiologically optimum head down position is very desirable. Moxibustion on Zhiyin (BL67) is such an option.

Moxibustion for Breech Presentation

Moxibustion for breech presentation is almost always taken to specifically mean applying moxibustion at acupuncture point Zhiyin (BL67). Occasionally, practitioners apply moxibustion on other acupuncture points instead of, or in addition to, Zhiyin (BL67). This review focuses solely on moxibustion at Zhiyin (BL67), or protocols containing moxibustion at Zhiyin (BL67).

Acupuncture Point Zhiyin (BL 67)

Acupuncture point Zhiyin (BL67), the end point of the bladder meridian, is located in the vicinity of the outer proximal corner of the toenail of the fifth toe. Moxibustion at acupuncture point Zhiyin (BL 67) is a classical Chinese medicine method of obtaining the revision of abnormal presentation of the fetus during the last three months of pregnancy. In classical acupuncture theory, Zhiyin (BL 67) acts to expel wind, clear the head and eyes, turn the fetus and facilitate labor. It is the jing-well and metal point of the bladder meridian. This point appeared in the first classical Chinese medicine text: *The Yellow Emperor's Classic of Medicine, The Spiritual Pivot*. The *Spiritual Pivot* states "For diseases of the head, select points from the feet." The *Song to Keep Up Your Sleeve* says that Zhiyin (BL67) is indicated for "disorders of the face and head." Zhiyin (BL67) is indicated for vertex headache, occipital headache, heaviness of the head, neck pain, nasal congestion, nosebleed, and eye pain, pain of the inner canthus, superficial visual obstruction, deafness and tinnitus. Zhiyin (BL67) is particularly applicable for vertex and occipital headache, whether due to exterior pathogens or to internal disharmony, as well as for disorders of the neck, eyes, nose and ears. Zhiyin (BL67) is a distal point on the bladder meridian indicated for disorders of urination, including painful urinary dysfunction and difficult urination. Other indications include seminal emission, cold malaria, wind cold starting from the little toe, absence of sweating, heat in the soles of the feet, cramps, spasm, and swelling of the knees.

Zhiyin (BL67) is most impressive in clinical practice when it is applied to the treatment of malposition of the fetus, for which it has attracted the most attention to this remarkable acupuncture point. According to the theory of yin yang, "yang is activity, yin is quiescence; yang brings forth and yin develops" and "when yin reaches its maximum it will necessarily transform into yang." In Chinese medicine theory, the kidney and urinary bladder are yin/yang paired and interior/exterior connected. Kidney yin nourishes and dominates the development and growth of the fetus during pregnancy. As labor approaches and yin reaches its zenith, yang begins to grow in order to turn the fetus and prepare for the intense activity of birth. If there is insufficient yang activity in the uterus at the time of delivery, due either to deficiency or stagnation, then yang must be stimulated from the outside. Moxibustion on Zhiyin (BL67) serves this purpose. Zhiyin (BL67) is the terminal point of the yang bladder meridian, where the qi changes polarity and enters its paired yin kidney meridian. The Chinese name of the acupuncture point, Zhiyin, "reaching yin" reflects this dynamic and transformative process. Clinical experiences and historical records indicate that Zhiyin (BL67) is the most dynamic point to activate the uterus and turn the fetus and promote and facilitate labor. It accomplishes this when Zhiyin (BL67) is stimulated by the yang heat of moxibustion. The effect of Zhiyin (BL67) on the uterus extends further to inducing delayed labor, hastening delivery once labor has commenced, and promoting the expulsion of the placenta after childbirth.

Procedure for Correcting Breech Presentation with Moxibustion

Moxibustion for breech presentation is performed by acupuncture practitioners, midwives or other practitioners who are licensed to practice moxibustion. When moxibustion is performed by one of these practitioners, the following procedures are generally followed. The patient is placed in a comfortable sitting position for treatment, with her legs raised. It is advised for the patient to wear loose clothing, especially over her abdomen. Two moxa-sticks, 1.5 cm in diameter by 20 cm length approximately, are lit by the practitioner and held over the Zhiyin (BL67) points of both feet at the same time. Moxa sticks are held still, maintaining a required distance of 1.5 to 2.5 centimeters between the burning moxa and the acupuncture points. Ideally, they are close enough for the patient to feel pleasantly warm, but not uncomfortable. Each treatment session lasts 15-20 minutes, once or twice daily for 10 treatments. Once the moxa sticks are applied, the patient may feel the baby start to move. If significant movements are felt, the practitioner stops the treatment and checks the baby's position. Because moxa ignites very easily, precautions should be taken to put it out after use.

Moxibustion for breech presentation can be performed by pregnant women themselves at home. In that case, the following procedures are recommended, preferably conducted in a well-ventilated room. A woman should empty the bladder, sit in a comfortable semi-reclining position, loosen tight clothing, and relax the abdominal muscles. The woman then removes half a centimeter of wrapping paper from the tips of the moxa sticks, lights the ends and extinguishes the flame – the tips will now be smoking and burning. Heat is directed towards the Zhiyin (BL67) point on both toes, holding the sticks about a half a centimeter away from the skin so that it feels comfortably warm but not excessively hot. Hot moxa sticks should never touch the skin. The recommendation is for two 15-minute sessions per day, up to a maximum of ten treatments. The fetus may be more active than usual during or just after the treatment. To stop the sticks from burning further, they should be gently knocked against a sink or metal bin so that the ash falls off. If it seems that the fetus has turned, or there are any concerns, the woman should stop the treatment and contact her practitioner to check the fetus' position. Best results are achieved if this treatment is started in the 34th week. It is important to note that once the fetus has turned, moxibustion should be stopped, otherwise further malposition may be induced.

Stakeholders in Moxibustion for Breech Presentation

Before we move into reviewing the clinical observations, clinical trials and systematic reviews and meta-analysis on moxibustion for breech presentation, we will consider the experiences and opinions of those people who are most directly concerned in the process. In moxibustion for breech presentation, the stakeholders are obviously acupuncturists or practitioners who practice moxibustion, and pregnant women. What are their experiences in applying moxibustion to breech presentation? What are their opinions on moxibustion for breech presentation? The following three studies address these questions and provide some answers.

A very interesting study [5] was conducted with the objective of estimating the efficacy of moxibustion to facilitate the cephalic version of fetuses in breech presentation and the acceptability of moxibustion by pregnant women in a Swiss university hospital maternity unit. This was a randomized controlled trial. Moxibustion was applied to Zhiyin (BL67) daily for two weeks for 212 consenting women between 34 and 36 weeks of gestation, with a single fetus in breech presentation. The moxibustion intervention was performed three times weekly in the hospital, and participants were given a teaching session and information leaflet on the technique for additional daily therapy at home. Expectant management care was offered to the control group. The external cephalic version was still available for both groups. Comparison of the proportion of women with cephalic presentation at delivery was the main outcome measure. The results showed that the percentage of versions was similar between the two groups: 18% in the moxibustion group compared with 16% in the control group (relative risk 1.12, 95% confidence interval 0.62 to 2.03). The frequency of cesarean delivery was similar (64% compared with 58% in the moxibustion group and the control group, respectively). Women were very accepting of the intervention, and they had very favorable perceptions. Although this study didn't show any significant beneficial effect of moxibustion to facilitate the cephalic version of fetuses in breech presentation, women had positive opinions on the intervention.

A research study [6] was conducted to explore women's feelings and experiences of using moxibustion for cephalic version in breech presentation at the University of the West of England, United Kingdom. Eight women with an uncomplicated breech presentation at term participated in the study and were offered moxibustion. The study used the following patient pool and moxibustion protocol: Women must have a confirmed breech presentation, no contraindications, and be no less than 33 weeks' gestation. Women and their partners were taught how to use moxibustion, with assessment of competence in lighting the moxibustion sticks, conducting the treatment, and extinguishing the moxa. Women were supplied with moxa sticks, a fire blanket and extinguishing material. The treatment required the partner to light the moxibustion sticks and hold them over the acupuncture points Zhiyin (BL67) on both feet for a 15-minute session. This procedure was carried out twice a day for a total for 7 days. Continuing support was offered for the duration of the treatment. A repeat ultrasound was carried out to confirm fetal presentation. If the moxibustion was unsuccessful, an ECV was offered and mode of delivery discussed. The authors conducted in-depth interviews with the participants before and after the treatment, and participants were requested to complete daily logs of their experiences. Anxieties about the implications of breech presentation and the options offered to them were experienced by all the participating women. The treatment was performed for all women successfully, and they reported a positive experience. All the patients were very compliant, and few negative effects were reported. The cooperation between patients and practitioners was important to ensure that the procedure was carried out effectively and safely. The authors interviewed both the patients and the practitioners to determine their views on incorporating moxibustion into the maternity services. All participants felt that moxibustion had the potential to, at minimum, confer benefits to women in terms of increased choices. The need for research evidence of effectiveness was revealed as a priority. From the key-stakeholders perspective, before moxibustion therapy could be accepted and established in the British National Health System (NHS), evidence of effectiveness and cost efficiency would need to be demonstrated.

Another relevant study [7] examined the perspective of acupuncture practitioners. It attempted to investigate what experienced acupuncture practitioners and researchers considered key aspects of treatment to promote cephalic version for women with a breech presentation, and to establish a treatment protocol through consensus to guide the self-administration of moxa by pregnant women. Sixteen Australian and New Zealand acupuncturists working in the field of pregnancy were invited to participate in the study. An online survey was conducted among the participants, and their views were sought on treatment parameters guiding the intervention of breech presentation within a research setting. Two rounds of the Delphi process seeking the opinions of key informants were undertaken: twelve participants completed round one, and ten completed round two. The results showed that eighty percent of acupuncturists agreed that moxa therapy should commence between 34 and 35 weeks' gestation; ninety percent agreed to self-administration of moxa by the woman, and use of smokeless moxas; seventy percent agreed moxa should be applied for a minimum of 10 days, and be applied once a day for 30 minutes; ninety percent agreed that study clinical outcomes should assess side effects including burns, and maternal and foetal outcomes. This study promoted the clinical validity of moxibustion for breech presentation for a future research protocol, and highlighted the essential elements to evaluate the role of acupuncture and moxibustion with normalizing birth.

Twenty Studies Concerning Moxibustion on Zhiyin (BL67)

Twenty clinical studies are collected and reviewed in this literature review. They are grouped into four categories: observational studies, clinical trials, systematic reviews, and meta-analysis. Unlike acupuncture treatment for other conditions, the prescription for breach presentation is unique: moxibustion application on Zhiyin (BL67). This paper serves acupuncture practitioners and Chinese medicine students as a learning tool for different levels of evidence-based medicine in regard to our specific and unique case: moxibustion application on Zhiyin (BL67).

Observational Studies

An observational study draws inferences about the possible effect(s) of a treatment such as moxibustion for breech presentation on subjects, in cases where the assignment of subjects into a treatment group or a control group is outside the control of the researchers. In an observational study, investigators observe subjects and measure the outcomes of studies for which they had no direct input. Cohort studies, case-control studies and cross-sectional studies are three types of observational studies.

In observational studies, the investigators can only observe associations between intervention treatments such as moxibustion received by the subjects and their subsequent health status (correlations). They cannot infer causality relationship between the intervention and the outcome. Therefore, observational studies provide less compelling evidence than the randomized controlled trials discussed in the next section.

The following observational studies are selected from the early literature on acupuncture and moxibustion for correcting breech presentations. These observational studies established the correlations between acupuncture/moxibustion at Zhiyin (BL67) and the clinical results of correcting breech presentations.

In an early study, Cardini *et al.* [8] reviewed the Chinese references on the subject of moxibustion for breech presentation and stressed the importance of parity and gestational age in testing the efficacy of this therapy. Preliminary results are described and compared with those reported in Chinese articles. Success rates in fetal version by moxibustion versus spontaneous version are also compared. Engel *et al.* [9] reported a case which raised the concern of safety. In a primigravida with a fundal/anterior wall placenta, a successful cephalic version was noted at 39 weeks after repeated moxibustion at Zhiyin (BL67). Since routine fetal heart rate monitoring showed a sinusoidal pattern with severe decelerations in this case, immediate Caesarean section was performed. Fetomaternal macrotransfusion of about 300 ml of blood was found. Because of this complication, the authors recommended that moxibustion was not suitable as self-therapy without close medical follow-up. In a study, Cardini *et al.* [10] treated a group of women during pregnancy by moxibustion at Zhiyin (BL 67), to obtain inversion of fetuses in breech presentation. Comparison was made with a control group drawn retrospectively from clinical files at a regional hospital. This study attempted to identify the ideal population (in terms of parity and gestational age) to be included in a randomized controlled trial. Li *et al.* [11] followed forty-eight cases of malposition of fetus treated by electro-acupuncture at Zhiyin (BL67) points. They reported that 39 cases were corrected with a rate of 81.3%. The average sessions of treatment were 1.41.

Clinical Trials

Clinical trials are the process by which a product or procedure's safety and effectiveness are tested – in this case, moxibustion for breech presentation. Clinical trials are prospective medical research studies on human subjects that are designed to answer specific questions about procedures or interventions from which safety and efficacy data are generated. Clinical trials are designed experimental studies in which researchers apply the designated intervention and study the effects. Most experimental studies are randomized, meaning the research subjects are assigned into different groups with equal probability. All randomized trials are controlled, although not all controlled studies are randomized. In randomized controlled trials (RCT), eligible subjects are randomly assigned to treatment or control groups. The treatment group receives the actual intervention, while the control group receives nothing or an inactive placebo. The researchers then investigate what happens to the subjects in each group. In well-designed randomized controlled clinical trials, any difference in outcomes can then be linked to the intervention which is being studied. In controlled clinical trial (CCT), the procedure is similar to an RCT, except that subjects are not randomly assigned to the treatment or control groups. This potentially produces a "bias," in that people with similar qualities may be intentionally assigned to one group or another, which could influence the final outcome of the study.

Clinical trial size varies, and can involve a single research entity or multiple entities. Because the number of patients is a strong limiting factor for the size of a clinical trial, researchers initially enroll patients into small pilot studies. Once positive safety and efficacy data are generated, progressively larger scale comparative studies are conducted with large number of patients. The highest-standard trials are designed as randomized, double-blind, and placebo-controlled: each study subject is randomly assigned to receive either the intervention or a placebo (random); neither the research subjects nor the researchers involved in the study know which intervention (real intervention or placebo) a subject is receiving: this prevents researchers from treating the two groups differently (double-blind); the use of a placebo allows the researchers to isolate the effect of the study intervention from the placebo effect (placebo-controlled).

Rigorously designed randomized controlled trials can provide the most compelling evidence that the study intervention causes an effect on the subjects.

Clinical Trials with Positive Results

Among the clinical trials which aimed to assess the effectiveness of moxibustion for breech presentation, we found ten of them to be supportive, meaning that these trials provide evidence that moxibustion is an effective option for breech presentation, and is furthermore a safe procedure.

The first randomized, controlled, open clinical trial on moxibustion for breech presentation [11] was conducted in the outpatient departments of the Women's Hospital of Jiangxi Province, Nanchang, and Jiujiang Women's and Children's Hospital in the People's Republic of China. This research was a joint effort between Chinese and Italian researchers. This landmark study was published in the *Journal of American Medical Association (JAMA)*. The study was designed to evaluate the efficacy and safety of moxibustion at Zhiyin (BL67) to correct breech presentation. Participants were randomly assigned into two groups: the treatment group consisted of 130 women having their first baby (primigravidas), who received moxibustion at Zhiyin (BL67) at 33 weeks' gestation. The control group of 130 women, also primigravidas, received no intervention. Moxibustion treatment was performed for 7 days, at which point the subjects were assessed. If the fetal position had not been corrected, they received an additional 7 days of moxibustion treatment. Outcome measures included fetal movements, as counted by the mother for one hour each day for one week, and the number of cephalic presentations both at 35 weeks' gestation and at delivery. At 35 weeks' gestation, 75.4% of participants in the intervention group *vs*. 47.7% in the control group exhibited cephalic presentation. Participants in both groups then had the option of external cephalic version (ECV). One woman in the intervention group and 24 in the control group took this option. At delivery the presentation of 75.4% of the intervention group *vs*. 62.3% in the control group were cephalic. The presentation did not change in either group after 35 weeks, except in those undergoing ECV. In terms of fetal movement, the moxibustion group experienced a greater number of movements (a mean of 48.45 *vs*. 35.35 in the control group).

The study also assessed whether or not there was a difference in delivering moxibustion sessions once or twice a day. Among the women in the treatment group, 87 used moxibustion once a day for a total of 30 minutes (15 minutes to each point), while 43 women used moxibustion in the same way, but received treatment twice a day. At the end of the first week, 79% of the cephalic versions were obtained in the women using moxibustion twice a day compared to 55.2% in the daily treatment subgroup. But by the end of the second week, 15 additional cephalic versions were obtained in the group having moxibustion treatment once a day, and only one additional version was obtained in the group using moxibustion twice a day. This showed that at 35 weeks, the resulting differences between these two groups were not significant (72.4% in the once-a-day moxibustion subgroup *vs.* 81% in the twice-a-day moxibustion subgroup). The study demonstrated that there were no adverse events (such as intrauterine death or placental detachment) in the treatment group. It was noted that while the incidence of premature rupture of membranes was similar in both groups, the number of premature births was lower in the intervention group, and that the use of oxytocin, before or during labor, was also reduced in the moxibustion group.

Kanakura *et al.* [12] demonstrated that breech presentation was successfully corrected by stimulating acupuncture points with moxibustion or low-frequency electrical current. The study only admitted patients with breech pregnancies at the 28th week or later. Moxibustion was provided daily for thirty minutes until the breech presentation was corrected, or no further response was induced by moxibustion. BL67 (Zhiyin), SP6 (Sanyinjiao), and KI1 (Yongquan) were the points on which low-frequency percutaneous acupuncture or moxibustion was performed. Results showed that, with moxibustion treatment, the control group had a spontaneous correction rate of 165/224 (73.66%), and the treatment group had a correction rate of 123/133 (92.48%) ($P<0.0001$). With low-frequency percutaneous electrical stimulation, the correction rate was 20/941 (83.87%) in the control group and 171/191 (89.52%) in the treatment group ($P=0.094$). In the study, the controls in the moxibustion study did no exercises and received no external manipulation to correct breech presentation, whereas those in the electrical stimulation study experienced both. Acupuncture stimulation, especially with moxibustion, is expected to serve as a safe and effective modality in the management of breech presentation in a clinical setting.

Neri, *et al.* [13] conducted a single-blind trial to assess fetal heart variability and activity using a computerized non-stress test (NST) during acupuncture plus moxibustion at acupuncture point Zhiyin (BL67). They compared the changes for both true acupuncture/moxibustion and placebo acupuncture (minimal acupuncture) in the same subjects. They enrolled twelve pregnant women who were in the 33rd week of gestation, carrying singletons in the breech presentation. Each woman received a first session of minimal acupuncture followed 1-2 days later by true acupuncture. During all these sessions, women were monitored using computerized non-stress testing starting 20 minutes before acupuncture stimulation and continuing for 20 minutes after treatment. During true acupuncture, a significant reduction in fetal baseline heart rate, and more accelerations and movement were observed. During placebo minimal acupuncture, there were no significant changes in these variables. No fetal distress or changes in short- or long-term variability were observed, and no uterine contractions were noted. The study showed that application of acupuncture plus moxibustion did not cause fetal distress as assessed by either fetal heart rate decelerations or changes in either short- or long-term variability. This small trial demonstrated that acupuncture/moxibustion stimulation related to the modification of fetal movement and heart rate occurred in true acupuncture, but not during minimal acupuncture.

Habek et al. [14] conducted a randomized prospective controlled clinical study to assess the value of acupuncture in the conversion of fetal breech presentation into vertex presentation. The study included 67 pregnant women with fetal breech presentation: 34 women with singleton pregnancies treated with manual acupuncture at Zhiyin (BL67) and a control group which included 33 women with singleton pregnancies without acupuncture treatment. The acupuncture treatment lasted 30 minutes a day, and was conducted during and after the 34th week of pregnancy with simultaneous cardiotocography. The study showed that the success rate of the acupuncture correction of fetal breech presentation was 76.4% (26/34), and spontaneous conversion without acupuncture in vertex presentation was 45.4% (15/33) ($p<0.001$). This study demonstrated that acupuncture correction of fetal breech presentation is a relatively simple, efficacious and inexpensive approach associated with a lower percentage of operatively completed deliveries, which definitely reflects in improved parameters of vital and perinatal statistics.

Neri *et al.* [15] conducted a randomized, controlled trial addressing stimulation of Zhiyin (BL67) by moxibustion, acupuncture, or both as an alternative to Cesarean section on pregnant Italian women at 33-35 weeks of gestation who were carrying a fetus in breech presentation. The study randomized a total of 240 women to receive active treatment (acupuncture plus moxibustion) or to be assigned to an observation group. For the treatment group, bilateral acupuncture plus moxibustion was applied at Zhiyin (BL67). The primary outcome measure was fetal presentation at delivery. 226 cases finished the study (14 cases dropped out): 114 in the observation group, and 112 in the acupuncture plus moxibustion group. Results showed that the proportion of cephalic version was lower in the observation group (36.7%) than in the treatment group (53.6 %) ($p = 0.01$) at delivery. The proportion of Cesarean sections indicated for breech presentation was significantly lower in the treatment group than in the observation group (52.3% vs. 66.7%, $p = 0.03$). Acupuncture plus moxibustion was demonstrated as more effective than observation in repositioning fetuses in breech presentation. Acupuncture/moxibustion provided a valid option for women willing to experience a natural birth.

Manyande, *et al.* [16] conducted a prospective study over a two-year time period from February 2004 until January 2006 to explore the effects of moxibustion treatment: specifically, to examine the predictors of its use in causing a breech presentation to spontaneously change to a cephalic presentation, resulting in a vaginal birth. Researchers also offered external cephalic version (ECV) subsequently after moxibustion treatment when the fetus remained in a breech presentation. The study recruited 76 pregnant women from different acupuncture clinics in the UK, who exhibited a third-trimester breech presentation. In the study, the acupuncture practitioners taught the women how to apply moxibustion treatment at home by stimulating Zhiyin (BL67) for seven days twice a day (morning and afternoon). If the breech presentation persisted after treatments, ECV was carried out by the obstetricians during the routine antenatal hospital visits towards the end of the pregnancy. The results showed that after receiving treatments with moxibustion, 40.8% (31/76) of the breech presentations spontaneously turned to cephalic presentations, and a further 43.4% (33/76) of breech presentations were turned by ECV. The study also reported that women who involved other people in the administration of moxibustion were twice as likely to be successful; and multiparous women were also 16% more likely than primiparous women to succeed in achieving a spontaneous version with the use of moxibustion. Among the women who were successful in turning their babies using moxibustion, 88% had a normal birth and 12% had a caesarean section. This study demonstrates that moxibustion treatment also significantly increases version from a breech presentation to a cephalic presentation. The study recommended that moxibustion treatment should be offered to all women with a breech presentation because it is non-invasive and can be self-administered by the woman.

Do *et al.* [17] undertook a pilot study to assess the feasibility of conducting a randomized controlled trial of moxibustion plus usual care, compared with usual care alone, to promote cephalic version in women with a breech presentation; and furthermore, examined the views of women and health care providers towards implementing a trial within an Australian context. The study was performed at a public hospital in Newcastle, New South Wales, Australia. Twenty women at 34-36.5 weeks of gestation with a singleton breech presentation which was confirmed by ultrasound were randomized to two groups: moxibustion plus usual care or usual care alone. The intervention was administered over ten days. Outcome measures included: cephalic presentation at birth, the need for ECV, mode of birth; perinatal morbidity and mortality, and maternal complications. Feasibility outcomes included: recruitment rate, acceptability, compliance, and a sample size for a future study. Interviews were conducted with 19 midwives and obstetricians to examine the acceptability of moxibustion, as well as their views on the trial. Results showed that 51% of women approached accepted randomization to the trial. An increase in cephalic version at delivery (RR 5.0; 95% CI 0.7-35.5) was found for women receiving moxibustion compared with usual care. Compliance with the moxibustion protocol was acceptable, and no side effects were reported. From the interviews, clinicians expressed the need for research to establish the safety and efficacy of moxibustion, and gave support for the intervention as a way to increase women's choices and explore options to normalize birth. This study also estimated that the sample size for a future trial should be 381 women. The increased rate of correcting breech presentation and the acceptance of moxibustion by women and health professionals warranted future research.

Vas, *et al.* [18] performed a multicenter randomized controlled trial to compare the effectiveness of additional moxibustion at Zhiyin (BL67) with moxibustion at a non-specific acupuncture point, and with usual care alone to correct non-vertex presentation. The study recruited pregnant women from a primary-care health center, and enrolled 406 low-risk pregnant women with a fetus in ultrasound breech presentation, at a gestational age of 33-35 weeks. The women were randomly assigned to one of the three arms: true moxibustion at Zhiyin (BL67) plus usual care; moxibustion at Yinbai (SP1), a non-specific acupuncture point (sham moxibustion) plus usual care; or usual care alone. Cephalic presentation at birth was the primary outcome measure. Results showed that in the true moxibustion group, 58.1% of the full-term presentations were cephalic, compared with 43.4% in the sham moxibustion group (RR 1.34, 95% CI 1.05 to 1.70), and 44.8% in the usual care group (RR 1.29, 95% CI 1.02 to 1.64). The reduction in RR of the primary outcome in women allocated to the true moxibustion group compared with the usual care group was 29.7% (95% CI 3.1% to 55.2%), which was significant. The study reported no severe adverse effects during the treatment. Moxibustion represents an effective treatment option for achieving version of the non-vertex fetus. The authors concluded that moxibustion at Zhiyin (BL67) is effective and safe to correct non-vertex presentation when used between 32 and 34 weeks of gestation. They also note that moxibustion is well-accepted by women and represents an effective treatment option for achieving version of the non-vertex fetus.

Because of the lack of clinical studies on the safety of moxibustion, Guittier *et al.* [19] conducted a randomized controlled trial to detect any side-effects and acceptability of moxibustion intervention. In the trial to evaluate the efficacy of moxibustion for breech version, the first twelve participants randomized in the moxibustion group had additional fetal surveillance by electronic monitoring. The authors performed a cardiotocogram 10 minutes before, 20 minutes during, and 10 minutes after each session. A maximum of nine sessions of moxibustion were scheduled every other day, and stopped when cephalic version was diagnosed. Fetal well-being was evaluated by the cardiotocogram; effect on the mother was evaluated by blood pressure recorded before and after each session. Maternal views, contractions, and perceived changes in fetal movements were assessed with a questionnaire. A total of 65 cardiotocograms were analyzed by the readers. Results showed that all scores were normal, with no significant maternal or fetal side-effects discovered. The study concluded that no alterations of fetal and maternal well-being or other side-effects associated with moxibustion applied to Zhiyin (BL67) for cephalic version of breech presentations were detected. It also concluded that moxibustion is safe for both the mother and the fetus.

Clinical Trials with Indeterminate or Negative Results

In clinical trials aimed to assess effectiveness of moxibustion for breech presentation, we found four of them to be indeterminate or non-supportive, meaning that these trials provide no evidence that moxibustion is effective for correcting breech presentation.

Cardini *et al.* [20] conducted a single-blind randomized controlled trial (RCT) in six obstetric departments in Italy to evaluate the efficacy of moxibustion for the correction of fetal breech presentation in a non-Chinese population. They recruited healthy non-Chinese nulliparous pregnant women at 32 to 33 weeks (+3 days) of gestational age with the fetus in breech presentation. Participants were randomly assigned to a treatment group or an observation group. Moxibustion at Zhiyin (BL67) for one or two weeks was performed on the treatment group. Each participant was subjected to an ultrasonic examination of the fetal presentation two weeks after recruitment. The number of participants with cephalic presentation in the 35th week was the outcome measure. When 123 participants had been recruited (46% of the planned number), the study was interrupted. The authors analyzed the available data and found that no difference in cephalic presentation in the 35th week (treatment group: 22/65, 34%; observation group: 21/58, 36%; RR 0.95; 99% CI 0.59-1.5). The study did not draw any conclusion to support either the effectiveness or the ineffectiveness of moxibustion in correcting fetal breech presentation.

In a three-arm clinical trial, Neri *et al.* [21] evaluated cardiovascular effects and fetal behavior during three different methods of stimulation (moxibustion, acupuncture, and acupuncture plus moxibustion) applied to Zhiyin (BL67) in women with fetal breech presentation. During the stimulation at Zhiyin (BL67) which lasted 20 minutes twice a week, the participants were submitted to a computerized non-stress test. Fourteen cases were treated by both acupuncture and moxibustion; 15 cases by moxibustion only; and 10 cases by acupuncture only. In 56% of cases, fetal position was converted from breech position to cephalic position: the success rate was 80% for moxibustion, 28% for acupuncture, 57% for acupuncture plus moxibustion. The conversion, on average, was achieved after three sessions. Statistical analysis indicated that acupuncture plus moxibustion was able to reduce fetal heart rate during the application of stimulation, while acupuncture and moxibustion separately did not affect such a parameter. Moreover, moxibustion and acupuncture with moxibustion reduced fetal movements, while acupuncture alone appeared ineffective. This study demonstrated that fetal movements were reduced by both acupuncture plus moxibustion and moxibustion, and that fetal heart rate was only reduced by use of acupuncture plus moxibustion. The study claimed these preliminary reports mainly investigated the impact of different methods of stimulation on Zhiyin (BL67), and did not draw any conclusion about the effectiveness of the different treatments.

Millereau *et al.*, [22] conducted the first French randomized clinical trial to investigate whether acupuncture, or more exactly, moxibustion, at the 34th week of gestation with breech presentation can increase the rate of fetal reverse. Sixty-eight pregnant women whose fetus was in breech presentation at the eighth month were recruited. They were randomly assigned into a treatment group or a no-treatment group. Results showed that the rate of fetal reverse was not statistically higher with moxibustion for the primipara (7/19 versus 6/19) and for the multipara (9/14 versus 11/19). No positive effect on moxibustion for the fetal rate reverse was found.

In a randomized placebo-controlled single-blind trial, Coulon *et al.*, [23] attempted to assess the efficacy of moxibustion with acupuncture for version of breech presentations after 33 4/7 weeks of gestation to reduce their rate at 37 weeks of gestation and at delivery. The study included 328 pregnant women recruited from a university hospital center between 33 4/7 and 35 4/7 weeks of gestation. They were randomized into two groups: moxibustion with acupuncture (n=164); or placebo (n=164). Moxibustion with acupuncture or inactivated laser (placebo) treatment was applied to

Zhiyin (BL 67) for six sessions. The outcome measure was the percentage of fetuses in breech presentation at 37 2/7 weeks of gestation. The results showed that the percentage of fetuses in breech presentation at 37 2/7 weeks of gestation was not significantly different in both groups (72.0% in the moxibustion with acupuncture group vs 63.4% in the placebo group, relative risk 1.13, 95% confidence interval 0.98-1.32, P=.10). The study concluded that treatment by moxibustion with acupuncture was not effective in correcting breech presentation in the third trimester of pregnancy.

Systematic Reviews

A systematic review is a summary of the clinical literature with critical assessment and evaluation of all research studies that address a particular clinical issue such as the effectiveness of moxibustion to breech presentation. A systematic review aims to sum up the best available studies on a clinical issue such as moxibustion to breech presentation. A systematic review is accomplished by synthesizing the results of multiple studies.

A systematic review uses an organized method of finding, assembling, synthesizing and evaluating the clinical studies on moxibustion for breech presentation using a set of specific criteria. Systematic reviews include the following steps and components: thorough search of the literature for relevant studies with an explicit search strategy; listing the databases and citation indexes; presenting explicit inclusion/ exclusion criteria; checking the titles and the abstracts of the identified articles against pre-determined criteria for eligibility and relevance; assigning each included study an objective assessment of methodological quality; an objective and transparent approach for research synthesis with the aim of minimizing bias; and systematic coding and analysis of included studies. Systematic reviews seek to identify all relevant published and unpublished evidence; select studies or reports for inclusion; assess the quality of each study or report; synthesize the findings from individual studies or reports in an unbiased way; interpret the findings; and present a balanced and impartial summary of the findings with due consideration of any flaws in the evidence. In the *Cochrane Handbook*, eight steps are considered essential for a systematic review:

1. Defining the review question(s) and developing criteria for including studies
2. Searching for studies
3. Selecting studies and collecting data
4. Assessing risk of bias in included studies
5. Analyzing data

6. Addressing reporting biases
7. Presenting results and "summary of findings" tables
8. Interpreting results and drawing conclusions

Coyle *et al.* [24] conducted a systematic review to examine the effectiveness and safety of moxibustion for changing the presentation of a fetus in the breech position, the need for external cephalic version (ECV), mode of birth, and perinatal morbidity and mortality for breech presentation. The authors searched the Cochrane Pregnancy and Childbirth Group trials register, the Cochrane Central Register of Controlled Trials, MEDLINE, EMBASE, CINAHL, MIDIRS, CISCOM and bibliographies of relevant papers, and included three trials involving a total of 597 women. Published and unpublished randomized controlled trials comparing moxibustion (either alone or in combination with acupuncture) with a control group (no moxibustion), or other methods (e.g. external cephalic version, acupuncture) in women with a singleton breech presentation was the inclusion criteria. The eligibility and quality of trials were assessed by the authors independently. The baby's presentation at birth, need for external cephalic version, mode of birth, perinatal morbidity and mortality, maternal complications and maternal satisfaction, and adverse events were the outcome measures. No meta-analysis for the main outcome was performed due to differences in interventions and sample size. The review showed that moxibustion reduced the need for ECV (relative risk (RR) 0.47, 95% confidence interval (CI) 0.33 to 0.66), and resulted in decreased use of oxytocin before or during labor for women who had vaginal deliveries (RR 0.28, 95% CI 0.13 to 0.60). The review concluded that moxibustion may be beneficial in reducing the need for ECV and decreasing the use of ocytocin. However, the review also noted that there is a need for well-designed randomized controlled trials to assess moxibustion for breech presentation which report on clinically relevant outcomes as well as the safety of the intervention.

Berg, *et al.*, [25] conducted a systematic review to assess the effectiveness of acupuncture-type interventions (moxibustion, acupuncture, or electro-acupuncture) at acupuncture point Zhiyin (BL67) to correct breech presentation compared to expectant management, based on controlled trials. They collected controlled trials published from 1980 to May, 2007 in the databases Medline, EMBASE, the Cochrane Central Register of Controlled Trials, AMED, NCCAM, Midirs and reference lists. Only original randomized controlled trials (RCT) or controlled cohort studies were included. The included studies dealt with acupuncture-type intervention at Zhiyin (BL67) compared with expectant management; ultrasound-confirmed breech presentation and ultrasound-confirmed position of the fetus after treatment; position at delivery; and/or the proportion of caesarean sections reported. Of 65 retrieved studies, six RCT's and three cohort studies met the inclusion criteria. Random-effects models were used to pool the data. In the RCT's the pooled proportion of breech presentations was 34% (95% CI: 20-49%) following treatment versus 66% (95% CI: 55-77%) in the control group (OR 0.25 95% CI: 0.11-0.58). In the cohort studies, the pooled proportion of breech presentations was 15% (95% CI: 1-28%) following treatment versus 36% (95% CI: 14-58%) in the control group (OR 0.29, 95% CI: 0.19-0.43). In all studies, the pooled proportion was 28% (95% CI: 16-40%) versus 56% (95% CI: 43-70%) (OR 0.27, 95% CI: 0.15-0.46). The systematic review showed that acupuncture-type interventions at Zhiyin (BL67) were effective in correcting breech presentation compared to expectant management.

Vas *et al*. [26] conducted a systematic review for randomized controlled trials, comparing moxibustion with a non-moxibustion control group, or other methods such as external cephalic version, postural methods, and acupuncture. Their data came from both Western and Chinese sources up to June 2007. Six studies, including 1087 subjects with a high degree of heterogeneity, were selected to compare moxibustion *vs*. observation or postural methods. The results showed a rate of cephalic version among the moxibustion group of 72.5% *vs*. 53.2% in the control group (relative risk, 1.36; 95% confidence interval, 1.17-1.58); and the number of times needed to treat was five (95% confidence interval, 4-7). No significant differences on safety were found in the comparison of moxibustion with other techniques. The study demonstrated that moxibustion at Zhiyin (BL67) had produced a positive effect, whether used alone or in combination with acupuncture or postural measures, in comparison with observation or postural methods alone, for the correction of nonvertex presentation. Because of a considerable heterogeneity among studies, the results in this review should be interpreted with caution.

Meta-Analysis

It is common to find that several clinical trials have attempted to answer the same questions about clinical effectiveness. For example: does moxibustion intervention for breech presentation confer significant benefits compared with the conventional treatment? Individual trials often fail to demonstrate a statistically significant difference between the treatment and control groups. Meta-analysis provides a tool to address these issues. Meta-analysis is a statistical process for pooling data from many clinical trials to obtain a clear answer. It is an analytical method that uses statistical techniques to combine results from different studies and obtain an estimate of the overall effect of a particular intervention on a defined outcome. Meta-analysis produces a stronger conclusion than a series of individual studies. This approach strengthens the result generated from the systematic review by increasing the power of the analysis, and improves the precision of the estimates of treatment effect. It is essential to the validity of the result of a meta-analysis for the compilers to make a decision as to whether or not the results of individual studies are similar enough to be combined in a meta-analysis. Meta-analysis is not simply adding up individual participants across studies: it considers the participants in all the studies as if they were part of one big study.

As a hallmark of evidence-based medicine, meta-analysis carries out a rigorous systematic review and offers an unbiased synthesis of the empirical data. In the meta-analysis, systematic review presents a balanced and impartial summary of the existing research, enabling decisions on effectiveness to be based on all relevant studies (published and unpublished) of adequate quality. A quantitative (statistical) estimate of net benefit aggregated over all the included studies is generated from such systematic reviews. In a meta-analysis, the following steps are essential:

1. Systematic review methods
2. Calculating effect size
3. Coding individual studies
4. Aggregating effect sizes
5. Analyzing heterogeneity
6. Subgroup analysis
7. Conducting meta-regression
8. Assessing publication bias
9. Reporting standards

Following these standards, three systematic reviews with meta-analysis were published in regard to evaluating moxibustion for breech presentation.

In a systematic review with meta-analysis to evaluate the efficacy and safety of moxibustion and other acupuncture point stimulations to treat breech presentation, Li, *et al.* [27] included randomized controlled trials (RCTs) and controlled clinical trials (CCTs) on moxibustion, acupuncture or any other acupoint stimulating methods for breech presentation in pregnant women. They searched clinical trials from PubMed, the Cochrane Library,

China National Knowledge Information (CNKI), Chinese Scientific Journal Database (VIP) and WanFang Database up to July 2008. Ten RCTs including 2090 participants and seven CCTs including 1409 participants were included in the study. Meta-analysis showed significant differences between moxibustion and no treatment (RR 1.35, 95% CI 1.20 to 1.51; 3 RCTs). No significant difference between moxibustion and knee-chest position was found (RR 1.30, 95% CI 0.95 to 1.79; 3 RCTs). Moxibustion plus other therapeutic methods showed significant beneficial effects (RR 1.36, 95% CI 1.21 to 1.54; 2 RCTs). Laser stimulation was more effective than assuming the knee-chest position plus pelvis rotating. Moxibustion was more effective than no treatment (RR 1.29, 95% CI 1.17 to 1.42; 2 CCTs) but was not more effective than the knee-chest position treatment (RR 1.22, 95% CI 1.11 to 1.34; 2 CCTs). Laser stimulation at Zhiyin (BL67) was more effective than the knee-chest position treatment (RR 1.30, 95% CI 1.10 to 1.54; 2 CCTs). This review concluded that moxibustion, acupuncture and laser acupoint stimulation were effective in the correction of breech presentation.

In 2012, Coyle *et al.* [28] published a meta-analysis of eight randomized trials of moxibustion application on breech presentation in 1346 patients, to examine the effectiveness and safety of moxibustion on changing the presentation of an unborn baby in the breech position, the need for external cephalic version (ECV), mode of birth, and perinatal morbidity and mortality for breech presentation. The authors searched the Cochrane Pregnancy and Childbirth Group's Trials Register (26 March 2012), MEDLINE (1966 to 1 August 2011), EMBASE (1980 to August 2011), CINAHL (1982 to 1 August 2011), MIDIRS (1982 to 1 August 2011) and AMED (1985 to 1 August 2011). Both published and unpublished randomized controlled trials comparing moxibustion (either alone or in combination with acupuncture or postural techniques) with a control group (no moxibustion), or other methods such as external cephalic version, acupuncture, postural techniques in women with a singleton breech presentation were included. The baby's presentation at birth, need for external cephalic version, mode of birth, perinatal morbidity and mortality, maternal complications and maternal satisfaction, and adverse events were the outcome measures. This meta-analysis was an updated version of a previous systematic review with six new trials added. The results showed that moxibustion was not found to reduce the number of non-cephalic presentations at birth compared with no treatment (P = 0.45), but moxibustion resulted in decreased use of oxytocin before or during labor for women who had vaginal deliveries compared with no treatment (risk ratio (RR) 0.28, 95% confidence interval (CI) 0.13 to 0.60). Moxibustion application resulted in fewer non-cephalic presentations at birth compared with acupuncture (RR 0.25, 95% CI 0.09 to 0.72). Further, moxibustion combined with acupuncture resulted in fewer non-cephalic presentations at birth (RR 0.73, 95% CI 0.57 to 0.94), and fewer births by caesarean section (RR 0.79, 95% CI 0.64 to 0.98) compared with no treatment. Moxibustion combined with a postural technique resulted in fewer non-cephalic presentations at birth compared with the postural technique alone (RR 0.26, 95% CI 0.12 to 0.56). This review found evidence to suggest that the use of moxibustion may reduce the need for oxytocin, but not sufficient evidence to support the use of moxibustion for correcting breech presentation. Moxibustion combined with acupuncture resulted in fewer births by caesarean section; and Moxibustion combined with postural management techniques reduced the number of non-cephalic presentations at birth. The study called for well-designed randomized controlled trials to evaluate moxibustion for breech presentation which report on clinically relevant outcomes as well as the safety of the intervention.

The above meta-analysis demonstrated some value of moxibustion application for breach presentation. The noted limitation of the moxibustion value may be due to the narrower scope of the clinical trials. In 2013, Zhang *et al.* [29] expanded the scope of clinical trials without any language restrictions. They searched all randomized controlled trials (RCTs) done up to February 2013 which compared moxibustion with other therapies in women with a singleton nonvertex presentation. Methodological quality of the trials was assessed with the Cochrane risk of bias criteria. Only seven of 392 potentially relevant studies met the inclusion criteria. A meta-analysis revealed a significant difference in favor of moxibustion on the correction of nonvertex presentation at delivery (risk ratio (RR) 1.29, 95% confidence interval (CI) 1.12 to 1.49, and $I^2 = 0$) when moxibustion was compared with other interventions. The same findings applied to cephalic presentation after cessation of treatment (RR 1.36, 95% CI 1.08 to 1.71, and $I^2 = 80\%$). This systematic review with meta-analysis suggested that moxibustion is an effective treatment for the correction of nonvertex presentation. Moxibustion therapy resulted in decreased use of oxytocin, which increased safety.

Cost Effectiveness

With clinical effectiveness of moxibustion for breech presentation established through clinical trials, systematic review and meta-analysis, the next step is to inform patients, health systems and insurance companies about the cost effectiveness of moxibustion intervention in reversing breech presentation and reducing the number of caesarean sections at term, compared with expected management including associated procedures such as external cephalic version. In 2010, Berg *et al.* [30] demonstrated the cost effectiveness of acupuncture-type interventions at Zhiyin (BL 67) with a modeling approach.

Their study was designed to assess the effectiveness and costs of addressing breech version with acupuncture-type interventions at Zhiyin (BL67), including moxibustion, compared to expectant management for women with a fetal breech presentation at 33 weeks' gestation. In their study, a decision tree was developed to predict the number of caesarean sections prevented by acupuncture-type interventions at Zhiyin (BL67) compared to expectant management to rectify breech presentation. The model accounted for external cephalic versions (ECV), treatment compliance, and costs for 10,000 simulated breech presentations at 33 weeks gestational age. Event rates were taken from Dutch population data and international literature, and the relative effectiveness of acupuncture-type interventions at Zhiyin (BL67) was based on a specific meta-analysis. The robustness of the results was evaluated through sensitivity analysis. The authors calculated percentages of breech presentations at term, caesarean sections, and costs from the third-party payer perspective. Odds ratios (OR) and cost differences of acupuncture-type interventions at Zhiyin (BL67), versus expectant management were calculated. Sensitivity analysis and expected value of perfect information analysis were performed. The simulated outcomes demonstrated 32% breech presentations after acupuncture-type interventions on Zhiyin (BL67), versus 53% with expectant management (OR 0.61, 95% CI 0.43, 0.83). The percentage for caesarean section was 37% after acupuncture-type interventions at Zhiyin (BL67), versus 50% with expectant management (OR 0.73, 95% CI 0.59, 0.88). The mean cost-savings per woman was euro 451 (95% CI euro 109, euro 775; p=0.005) using moxibustion. Sensitivity analysis showed that if 16% or more of women who were offered moxibustion complied, it would be more effective and less costly than expectant management. To prevent one caesarean section, seven women had to use acupuncture-type interventions at Zhiyin (BL67). The expected value of perfect information from further research was euro 0.32 per woman. The results of this modeling analysis suggested that for the rectification of a fetus in breech presentation in women at 33 weeks' gestation, acupuncture-type interventions at Zhiyin (BL67) reduced the number of breech presentations at term, the number of caesarean sections, and was less costly when compared to expectant management, including ECV.

Mechanism of Action of Moxibustion at Zhiyin (BL67)

The mechanism of stimulation of Zhiyin (BL67) has been scientifically investigated, although the mechanism of action of moxibustion at Zhiyin (BL67) for its widely indicated conditions generally, and breech presentation specifically, has not been completely understood. Fetal participation theory and endogenous opioid theory are two of the mechanisms which have been explored. The mechanism of action of moxibustion at Zhiyin (BL67) definitely warrants further research.

One study [31] of the morphological basis and relationship between Zhiyin (BL67) and the viscera showed that seven segments (L2-S1) of the uterus innervation and the sensory innervation of Zhiyin (BL67) overlap. It [32] has been reported that moxibustion at Zhiyin (BL67) causes adrenocortical stimulation, which results in increased placental estrogens and changes in prostaglandin (PG) levels. Increased estrogen levels escalate myometrial sensitivity, which results in increased contractility in response to placental growth factor (PGF). These actions stimulate fetal movements and make version more likely. The increase in fetal movements (verified by monitoring fetal heart rate) is a striking effect of moxibustion therapy which is perceived by almost all women towards the second half of the stimulation period. This effect persists even after the end of stimulation. For cases of intra-uterine fetal death, stimulation failed to produce version. This finding demonstrates that this type of version relies on active fetal participation, and that any other explanation based purely on segmental reflex action must be considered less likely. Naloxone, a chemical antagonist of endogenous opioid peptides, has been reported to increase fetal movements, heart rate accelerations and breathing movements. Endogenous opioids exert a tonic inhibition of fetal movements. Acupuncture application has been demonstrated to stimulate central and peripheral endorphins. These facts indicate an explanation for the effect of acupuncture on fetal behavior [33].

REFERENCES

Preface

1. Morey SS. 1998. NIH Issues Consensus Statement on Acupuncture. *Am Fam Physician*. 57(10):2545-6.
2. Zhang YQ, Jiao RM, Witt CM, Lao LX, Liu JP , Thabane L, Sherman KJ, Cummings M, Richards DP, Kim EA, Kim TH, Lee MS, Wechsler ME, Brinkhaus B, Mao JJ, Smith CA, Gang WJ, Liu BY, Liu ZS, Liu Y, Zheng H, Wu JN, Carrasco-Labra A, Bhandari M, Devereaux PJ, Jing XH, Guyatt G. 2022. How to design high quality acupuncture trials-a consensus informed by evidence. *BMJ.* 376:e067476.
3. Lu LM, Zhang YQ, Tang XR, Ge SQ, Wen H, Zeng JC, Wang L, Zeng Z, Rada G, Ávila C, Vergara C, Tang YY, Zhang PM, Chen RH, Dong Y, Wei XJ, Luo W, Wang L, Guyatt G, Tang CZ, Xu NG. 2022. Evidence on acupuncture therapies is underused in clinical practice and health policy. *BMJ*. 376:e067475.
4. Zhang YQ, Lu LM, Xu NG, Tang XR, Shi XS, Carrasco-Labra A, Schünemann H, Chen YL, Xia J, Chen G, Liu JP, Liu BY, Wang JY, Qaseem A, Jing XH, Guyatt G, Zhao H. 2022. Increasing the usefulness of acupuncture guideline recommendations. *BMJ*. 376:e070533.

Chapter One

1. Wang HT. 2004. *Huang Di Nei Jing Su Wen*. Beijing: People's Hygiene Press.
2. Hu H. 2001. *Chinese Medicine Clinicians: Yang Jiasan*. Beijing: China Chinese Medicine Press.
3. Chen YB. and Deng LY. 1987. *Essentials of Comtempory Chinese Acupuncturists' Clinical Experiences. Tianjin:* Tianjin Science and Technology Press.
4. Zhu B and Wang, HC. 2009. *Case Studies from Medical Records of Leading Chinese Acupuncture Experts*. Beijing: People's Military Medical Press.
5. Wang JY. 2014. *Lectures of Wang Juyi's Acupuncture Cases*. Beijing: China Chinese Medicine Press.

6. Peng JS and Fei JZ. 1985. *Acupuncture Secretive Experience and Absolute Skills*. Shenyang: Liaoning Science and Technology Press.
7. Zhou SD and Zhou MS. 1982. *The Poetry of Golden Needle Plum Flower*. Hefei: Anhui Science and Technology Press.
8. Gao LS. 1985. *Heart Reflection on Acupuncture*. Beijing: People's Hygiene Press.
9. Pach D, Yang-Strobel X, Lüdtke R, Roll S, Icke K, Brinkhaus B, Witt CM. 2013. Standardized versus Individualized Acupuncture for Chronic Low Back Pain: A Randomized Controlled Trial. *Evid Based Complement Alternat Med*. 2013:125937.
10. Hasegawa TM, Baptista AS, de Souza MC, Yoshizumi AM, Natour J. 2014. Acupuncture for acute non-specific low back pain: a randomized, controlled, double-blind, placebo trial. *Acupunct Med.* 32(2):109-15.
11. Huang T, Han B, Tian YY, Wang GJ, Jia SY, Zhang WB. 2014. Low back pain of cold-damp pattern treated with electric-thermal Bian-stone therapy and traditional moxibustion: a randomized controlled trial. *Zhongguo Zhen Jiu*. 34(6):585-9.
12. Akbarzadeh M, Ghaemmaghami M, Yazdanpanahi Z, Zare N, Azizi A, Mohagheghzadeh A. 2014. The Effect Dry Cupping Therapy at Acupoint BL23 on the Intensity of Postpartum Low Back Pain in Primiparous Women Based on Two Types of Questionnaires, 2012; A Randomized Clinical Trial. *Int J Community Based Nurs Midwifery*. 2(2):112-20.
13. Cevik C, Anil A, Işeri SO. 2015. Effective chronic low back pain and knee pain treatment with acupuncture in geriatric patients. *J Back Musculoskelet Rehabil*. 28(3):517-20.
14. Kim SY, Lee H, Lee H, Park JY, Park SK, Park HJ. 2015. An observational study on the costs and consequences of acupuncture for the management of chronic low back pain in Korean patients. *Acupunct Med.* 33(2):148-53.
15. Xuan C, Xiaoran Y, Suying G, Zhifang Y, Xiaoqing H. 2015. Frequency steps and compositions determine properties of needling sensation during electroacupuncture. *J Tradit Chin Med*. 35(2):154-9.
16. AlBedah A, Khalil M, Elolemy A, Hussein AA, AlQaed M, Al Mudaiheem A, Abutalib RA, Bazaid FM, Bafail AS, Essa A, Bakrain MY. 2015. The Use of Wet Cupping for Persistent Nonspecific Low Back Pain: Randomized Controlled Clinical Trial. *J Altern Complement Med.* 21(8):504-8.
17. Liu YT, Chiu CW, Chang CF, Lee TC, Chen CY, Chang SC, Lee CY, Lo LC. 2015. Efficacy and Safety of Acupuncture for Acute Low Back

Pain in Emergency Department: A Pilot Cohort Study. *Evid Based Complement Alternat Med.* 2015:179731.
18. Koppenhaver SL, Walker MJ, Smith RW, Booker JM, Walkup ID, Su J, Hebert JJ, Flynn T. 2015. Baseline Examination Factors Associated with Clinical Improvement After Dry Needling in Individuals With Low Back Pain. *J Orthop Sports Phys Ther.*45(8):604-12.
19. Chen LC, Cheng LJ, Zhang Y, He X, Knaggs RD. 2015. Acupuncture or low frequency infrared treatment for low back pain in Chinese patients: a discrete choice experiment. *PLoS One.* 10(5):e0126912.
20. Shi Y, Liu Z, Zhang S, Li Q, Guo S, Yang J, Wu W. 2015. Brain Network Response to Acupuncture Stimuli in Experimental Acute Low Back Pain: An fMRI Study. *Evid Based Complement Alternat Med.* 2015:210120.
21. Stomski NJ, Mackintosh SF, Stanley M. 2014, The experience of acupuncture care from the perspective of people with chronic low back pain: a grounded theory study. *Acupunct Med.* 32(4):333-9.
22. Taylor P, Pezzullo L, Grant SJ, Bensoussan A. 2014. Cost-effectiveness of Acupuncture for Chronic Nonspecific Low Back Pain. *Pain Pract.* 14(7):599-606.
23. Kim SY, Lee H, Lee H, Park JY, Park SK, Park HJ. 2015. An observational study on the costs and consequences of acupuncture for the management of chronic low back pain in Korean patients. *Acupunct Med.* 33(2):148-53.
24. Hutchinson AJ, Ball S, Andrews JC, Jones GG. 2012. The effectiveness of acupuncture in treating chronic non-specific low back pain: a systematic review of the literature. *J Orthop Surg Res.* Oct 30;7:36.
25. Kong LJ, Fang M, Zhan HS, Yuan WA, Pu JH, Cheng YW, Chen B. 2012. Tuina-focused integrative Chinese medical therapies for inpatients with low back pain: a systematic review and meta-analysis. *Evid Based Complement Alternat Med.* 2012:578305.
26. Huang CY, Choong MY, Li TS. 2013. Effectiveness of cupping therapy for low back pain: a systematic review. *Acupunct Med.* 31(3):336-7.
27. Pennick V, Liddle SD. 2013. Interventions for preventing and treating pelvic and back pain in pregnancy. *Cochrane Database Syst Rev.* Aug 1;8:CD001139.
28. Lam M, Galvin R, Curry P. 2013. Effectiveness of acupuncture for nonspecific chronic low back pain: a systematic review and meta-analysis. *Spine (Phila Pa 1976).* 38(24):2124-38.
29. Lee JH, Choi TY, Lee MS, Lee H, Shin BC, Lee H. 2013. Acupuncture for acute low back pain: a systematic review. *Clin J Pain.* 29(2):172-85.

30. Cho HW, Hwang EH, Lim B, Heo KH, Liu JP, Tsutani K, Lee MS, Shin BC. 2014. How current Clinical Practice Guidelines for low back pain reflect Traditional Medicine in East Asian Countries: a systematic review of Clinical Practice Guidelines and systematic reviews. *PLoS One*. 9(2):e88027.
31. Yuan QL, Guo TM, Liu L, Sun F, Zhang YG. 2015. Traditional Chinese medicine for neck pain and low back pain: a systematic review and meta-analysis. *PLoS One*. 10(2):e0117146.
32. Liu L, Skinner M, McDonough S, Mabire L, Baxter GD. 2015. Acupuncture for low back pain: an overview of systematic reviews. *Evid Based Complement Alternat Med*. 2015:328196.
33. Lin X, Li R. 2014. Comparative literature study between investigations in foreign Science Citation Index journals and Chinese core domestic journals in the treatment of low back pain with acupuncture. *J Tradit Chin Med*. 34(3):373-80.

Chapter Two

1. Mei ZG, Cheng CG, Zheng JF. 2011. Observations on curative effect of high-frequency electric stimulation and point-injection therapy on knee osteoarthritis. *J Tradit Chin Med*. 31(4):311-5.
2. Ren XM, Cao JJ, Shen XY, Wang LZ, Zhao L, Wu F, Zhang HM. 2011. Knee osteoarthritis treated with moxibustion: a randomized controlled trial. *Zhongguo Zhen Jiu*. 31(12):1057-61.
3. Son HM, Kim DH, Kim E, Jung SY, Kim AR, Kim TH. 2013. Qualitative study of the experiences of patients with knee osteoarthritis undergoing moxibustion. *Acupunct Med*. 31(1):39-44.
4. Zhao L, Cheng K, Wang L, Wu F, Deng H, Tan M, Lao L, Shen X. 2014. Effectiveness of moxibustion treatment as adjunctive therapy in osteoarthritis of the knee: a randomized, double-blinded, placebo-controlled clinical trial. *Arthritis Res Ther*. 16(3):R133.
5. Kim TH, Kim KH, Kang JW, Lee M, Kang KW, Kim JE, Kim JH, Lee S, Shin MS, Jung SY, Kim AR, Park HJ, Jung HJ, Song HS, Kim HJ, Choi JB, Hong KE, Choi SM. 2014. Moxibustion treatment for knee osteoarthritis: a multi-centre, non-blinded, randomised controlled trial on the effectiveness and safety of the moxibustion treatment versus usual care in knee osteoarthritis patients. *PLoS One*. 9(7):e101973.
6. Fu MY, Zhang ZL. 2011. Knee osteoarthritis treated with acupuncture at the points selected according to syndrome differentiation: a randomized controlled trial. *Zhongguo Zhen Jiu*. 31(12):1062-6.

7. Gao J, Ouyang BS, Zhang Y, Li J, Yang HZ, Ji LL, Wu YJ, Wang W. 2012. Comparison of the clinical therapeutic effects between electroacupuncture and warming needle moxibustion for knee osteoarthritis of kidney deficiency and marrow insufficiency pattern/syndrome. *Zhongguo Zhen Jiu.* 32(5):395-8.
8. Mavrommatis CI, Argyra E, Vadalouka A, Vasilakos DG. 2012. Acupuncture as an adjunctive therapy to pharmacological treatment in patients with chronic pain due to osteoarthritis of the knee: a 3-armed, randomized, placebo-controlled trial. *Pain.* 153(8):1720-6.
9. Soni A, Joshi A, Mudge N, Wyatt M, Williamson L. 2012. Supervised exercise plus acupuncture for moderate to severe knee osteoarthritis: a small randomized controlled trial. *Acupunct Med.* 30(3):176-81.
10. Yang XC, He SF, Wang RC, Zhou YM. 2012. Observation on curative effect of thermal acupuncture needle muscular stimulation therapy for knee osteoarthritis patients. *Zhen Ci Yan Jiu.* 37(3):237-41.
11. Liu MR, Li L, He ZW. 2012. Efficacy observation on osteoarthritis of the knee treated with the ultrastructural acupotomy therapy at the counter-Ashi points. *Zhongguo Zhen Jiu.* 32(7):621-4.
12. Dai Z, Liu Q, Bai W, Liu HS, Yang JY, Wang SJ. 2012. Efficacy observation of knee osteoarthritis treated with acupuncture. *Zhongguo Zhen Jiu.* 32(9):785-8.
13. Hong KD, Li L, Li XH. 2012. Clinical observation of warm needling therapy for treating knee osteoarthritis of different Chinese medical syndrome types. *Zhongguo Zhong Xi Yi Jie He Za Zhi.* 32(11):1466-9.
14. Karner M, Brazkiewicz F, Remppis A, Fischer J, Gerlach O, Stremmel W, Subramanian SV, Greten HJ. 2013. Objectifying specific and nonspecific effects of acupuncture: a double-blinded randomized trial in osteoarthritis of the knee. *Evid Based Complement Alternat Med.* 2013:427265.
15. Horng HC, Kuo CP, Cherng CH, Yeh CC, Wang TC, Liaw WJ, Ko SC, Wong CS. 2013. The effects of collateral meridian therapy for knee osteoarthritis pain management: a pilot study. *J Manipulative Physiol Ther.* 36(1):51-6.
16. Bao F, Zhang Y, Wu ZH, Wang Y, Sheng M, Hu N, Feng F, Wang DH, Zhang YX, Li T, Sun H. 2013. Efficacy observation on knee osteoarthritis treated with electroacupuncture and its influence on articular cartilage with T2 mapping. *Zhongguo Zhen Jiu.* 33(3):193-7.
17. Qiu L, Kan JW, Zheng X, Zhang M, Zhang J. 2013. Observation on the long-term efficacy of knee osteoarthritis treated with warm needling and rehabilitation training. *Zhongguo Zhen Jiu.* 33(3):199-202.

18. Saleki M, Ahadi T, Razi M, Raeisi GR, Forough B, Ali MK. 2013. Comparison of the effects of acupuncture and isometric exercises on symptom of knee osteoarthritis. *Int J Prev Med.* 4(Suppl 1):S73-7.
19. Liu K, Tian LF. 2013. Knee osteoarthritis treated with acupuncture at Neiguan (PC 6) and Taichong (LR 3). *Zhongguo Zhen Jiu.* 33(2):105-8.
20. Xie H, Xu F, Chen R, Luo T, Chen M, Fang W, Lü F, Wu F, Song Y, Xiong J. 2013. Image formation of brain function in patients suffering from knee osteoarthritis treated with moxibustion. *J Tradit Chin Med.* 33(2):181-6.
21. Qin WK, Zhao Y, Zhang K, Gu LJ, Fang W, Liu CY. 2013. Clinical evaluation of stiletto needle for pain of knee osteoarthritis. *Zhongguo Zhen Jiu.* 33(4):347-9.
22. Wei S, Chen ZH, Sun WF, Zhang GP, Li XH, Hou CF, Lu LD, Zhang L. 2013. Evaluating meridian-sinew release therapy for the treatment of knee osteoarthritis. *Evid Based Complement Alternat Med.* 2013:182528.
23. Spaeth RB, Camhi S, Hashmi JA, Vangel M, Wasan AD, Edwards RR, Gollub RL, Kong J. 2013. A longitudinal study of the reliability of acupuncture deqi sensations in knee osteoarthritis. *Evid Based Complement Alternat Med.* 2013:204259.
24. Chen LX, Mao JJ, Fernandes S, Galantino ML, Guo W, Lariccia P, Teal VL, Bowman MA, Schumacher HR, Farrar JT. 2013. Integrating acupuncture with exercise-based physical therapy for knee osteoarthritis: a randomized controlled trial. *J Clin Rheumatol.* 19(6):308-16.
25. Cheng Y, Wu K, Cheng Z, Zhu Y, Yang ZG, Ma H, Wang SW, Jiang ZL. 2013. Randomized controlled study on the treatment of knee osteoarthritis with different acupuncture methods at different stages. *Zhongguo Zhen Jiu.* 33(6):508-12.
26. Chen R, Chen M, Xiong J, Su T, Zhou M, Sun J, Chi Z, Zhang B, Xie D. 2013. Comparative effectiveness of the deqi sensation and non-deqi by moxibustion stimulation: a multicenter prospective cohort study in the treatment of knee osteoarthritis. *Evid Based Complement Alternat Med.* 2013:906947.
27. Wang L, Wu F, Zhao L, Zhang H, Shen X, Huang Y, Lao L. 2013. Patterns of traditional Chinese medicine diagnosis in thermal laser acupuncture treatment of knee osteoarthritis. *Evid Based Complement Alternat Med.* 2013:870305.
28. Weiner DK, Moore CG, Morone NE, Lee ES, Kent Kwoh C. 2013. Efficacy of periosteal stimulation for chronic pain associated with

advanced knee osteoarthritis: a randomized, controlled clinical trial. *Clin Ther.* 35(11):1703-20.e5.
29. Xu L, Jing L, He K, Wang JL, Wang Y. 2013. Treatment of knee osteoarthritis with acupuncture and moxibustion: a randomized controlled trial. *Zhongguo Zhen Jiu.* 33(10):871-6.
30. Gao YL, Yao JH, Guo JX. 2013. Clinical observation on fire needles at bones combined with cupping and Tuina for knee osteoarthritis. *Zhongguo Zhen Jiu.* 33(8):697-9.
31. Cai GW, Li J, Xu XJ, Xue YZ, Li G, Wu M, Li PF. 2013. Effect of acupoint heat-sensitive moxibustion intervention on serum osteopontin and matrix metalloproteinase-3 in patients with acute knee pain. *Zhen Ci Yan Jiu.* 38(6):488-92.
32. Yu D, Xie HW, Zhang B, Wen HJ, Chen RX. 2013. Observation on clinical effects of moxibustion stimulation of different sensitive status acupoints for knee osteoarthritis. *Zhen Ci Yan Jiu.* 38(6):497-501.
33. Martins F, Kaster T, Schützler L, Witt CM. 2014. Factors influencing further acupuncture usage and a more positive outcome in patients with osteoarthritis of the knee and the hip: a 3-year follow-up of a randomized pragmatic trial. *Clin J Pain.* 30(11):953-9.
34. Plaster R, Vieira WB, Alencar FA, Nakano EY, Liebano RE. 2014. Immediate effects of electroacupuncture and manual acupuncture on pain, mobility and muscle strength in patients with knee osteoarthritis: a randomized controlled trial. *Acupunct Med.* 32(3):236-41.
35. Ashraf A, Zarei F, Hadianfard MJ, Kazemi B, Mohammadi S, Naseri M, Nasseri A. 2014. Khodadadi M, Sayadi M. Comparison the effect of lateral wedge insole and acupuncture in medial compartment knee osteoarthritis: a randomized controlled trial. *Knee.* 21(2):439-44.
36. Al Rashoud AS, Abboud RJ, Wang W, Wigderowitz C. 2014. Efficacy of low-level laser therapy applied at acupuncture points in knee osteoarthritis: a randomized double-blind comparative trial. *Physiotherapy.* 100(3):242-8.
37. Lin M, Li X, Liang W, Liu J, Guo J, Zheng J, Liu X. 2014. Needle-knife therapy improves the clinical symptoms of knee osteoarthritis by inhibiting the expression of inflammatory cytokines. *Exp Ther Med.* 7(4):835-842.
38. Allam H, Mohammed NH. 2013. The Role of Scalp Acupuncture for Relieving the Chronic Pain of Degenerative Osteoarthritis: A Pilot Study of Egyptian Women. *Med Acupunct.* 25(3):216-220.
39. Cheng G, Cheng W, Jiang YG. 2014. Controlled observation of clinical efficacy on knee osteoarthritis treated with auricular electroacupuncture

and the isolated moxibustion with Lingxian herbal paste. *Zhongguo Zhen Jiu.*;34(3):230-4.

40. Yin Y, Zhao Y. 2014. Case-controlled study on the synergistic effects of electroacupuncture on knee osteoarthritis after arthroscopic debridement. *Zhongguo Gu Shang.* 27(4):287-90.
41. Chen X, Spaeth RB, Retzepi K, Ott D, Kong J. 2014. Acupuncture modulates cortical thickness and functional connectivity in knee osteoarthritis patients. *Sci Rep.* Sep 26;4:6482.
42. Hinman RS, McCrory P, Pirotta M, Relf I, Forbes A, Crossley KM, Williamson E, Kyriakides M, Novy K, Metcalf BR, Harris A, Reddy P, Conaghan PG, Bennell KL. 2014. Acupuncture for chronic knee pain: a randomized clinical trial. *JAMA.* 312(13):1313-22.
43. Yu H, Wang Y, Guo Y, Wang H, Chen B, Zhao X. 2014. Quality assessment of randomized controlled trials reporting on knee osteoarthritis treated with warming needle moxibustion. *J Tradit Chin Med.* 34(5):621-6.
44. Xie XJ, Jiao L, Fu Y, Zhang B, Xiong J, Chen RX, He L, Qian HL, Luo XJ. 2014. Clinical effect of different schemes of mild moxibustion for treatment of knee osteoarthritis. *Zhen Ci Yan Jiu.* 39(6):496-9.
45. Ren X, Yao C, Wu F, Li Z, Xing J, Zhang H. 2015. Effectiveness of moxibustion treatment in quality of life in patients with knee osteoarthritis: a randomized, double-blinded, placebo-controlled trial. *Evid Based Complement Alternat Med.* 2015:569523.
46. Chen R, Chen M, Su T, Zhou M, Sun J, Xiong J, Chi Z, Xie D, Zhang B. 2015. Heat-sensitive moxibustion in patients with osteoarthritis of the knee: a three-armed multicentre randomised active control trial. *Acupunct Med.* 33(4):262-9.
47. Chen X, Spaeth RB, Freeman SG, Scarborough DM, Hashmi JA, Wey HY, Egorova N, Vangel M, Mao J, Wasan AD, Edwards RR, Gollub RL, Kong J. 2015. The modulation effect of longitudinal acupuncture on resting state functional connectivity in knee osteoarthritis patients. *Mol Pain.* 11(1):67.
48. Li JW, Zheng SJ, Zhang JC, Huang JJ, Liu XG. 2015. Effect of Acupuncture plus Different Frequency Shock-wave Interventions on Pain Reactions and Motor Function in Knee Osteoarthritis Patients. *Zhen Ci Yan Jiu.* 40(4):300-3.
49. Egorova N, Gollub RL, Kong J. 2015. Repeated verum but not placebo acupuncture normalizes connectivity in brain regions dysregulated in chronic pain. *Neuroimage Clin.* 9:430-5.

50. Cao L, Zhang XL, Gao YS, Jiang Y. 2012. Needle acupuncture for osteoarthritis of the knee. A systematic review and updated meta-analysis. *Saudi Med J.* 33(5):526-32.
51. Choi TY, Choi J, Kim KH, Lee MS. 2012. Moxibustion for the treatment of osteoarthritis: a systematic review and meta-analysis. *Rheumatol Int.* 32(10):2969-78.
52. Cao H, Bourchier S, Liu J. 2012. Does Syndrome Differentiation Matter? A Meta-Analysis of Randomized Controlled Trials in Cochrane Reviews of Acupuncture. *Med Acupunct.* 24(2):68-76.
53. Purepong N, Jitvimonrat A, Sitthipornvorakul E, Eksakulkla S, Janwantanakul P. 2012. External validity in randomised controlled trials of acupuncture for osteoarthritis knee pain. *Acupunct Med.* 30(3):187-94.
54. Ambrósio EM, Bloor K, MacPherson H. 2012. Costs and consequences of acupuncture as a treatment for chronic pain: a systematic review of economic evaluations conducted alongside randomised controlled trials. *Complement Ther Med.* 20(5):364-74.
55. Kim SY, Lee H, Chae Y, Park HJ, Lee H. 2012. A systematic review of cost-effectiveness analyses alongside randomised controlled trials of acupuncture. *Acupunct Med.* 30(4):273-85.
56. Vickers AJ, Cronin AM, Maschino AC, Lewith G, MacPherson H, Foster NE, Sherman KJ, Witt CM, Linde K; Acupuncture Trialists' Collaboration. 2012. Acupuncture for chronic pain: individual patient data meta-analysis. *Arch Intern Med.* 172(19):1444-53.
57. Corbett MS, Rice SJ, Madurasinghe V, Slack R, Fayter DA, Harden M, Sutton AJ, Macpherson H, Woolacott NF. 2013. Acupuncture and other physical treatments for the relief of pain due to osteoarthritis of the knee: network meta-analysis. *Osteoarthritis Cartilage.* 21(9):1290-8.
58. MacPherson H, Vertosick E, Lewith G, Linde K, Sherman KJ, Witt CM, Vickers AJ, 2014. Acupuncture Trialists' Collaboration. Influence of control group on effect size in trials of acupuncture for chronic pain: a secondary analysis of an individual patient data meta-analysis. *PLoS One.* 9(4):e93739.
59. Manyanga T, Froese M, Zarychanski R, Abou-Setta A, Friesen C, Tennenhouse M, Shay BL. 2014. Pain management with acupuncture in osteoarthritis: a systematic review and meta-analysis. *BMC Complement Altern Med.* 14:312.

Chapter Three

1. Paulus WE, Zhang M, Strehler E, El-Danasouri I, Sterzik K. 2002. Influence of acupuncture on the pregnancy rate in patients who undergo assisted reproduction therapy. *Fertil Steril.* 77(4):721-4.
2. Cahill DJ, Wardle PG. 2002. Management of infertility. *BMJ* 325:28–32.
3. Magarelli P and Cridennda D. The Evolution of a Revolution: How Traditional Chinese Medicine Brings IVF into Modern Times. *Fertility Nurses First*, Issue 34. Walgreens.
4. Nygren KG, Sullivan E, Zegers-Hochschild F, Mansour R, Ishihara O, Adamson GD, de Mouzon J. 2011. International Committee for Monitoring Assisted Reproductive Technology (ICMART) world report: assisted reproductive technology 2003. *Fertil Steril.* 95(7):2209-22, 2222.e1-17.
5. Abdalla HI. 2010. Are US results for assisted reproduction better than the rest? Is it a question of competence or policies? *Reprod Biomed Online*. 21:624–630.
6. Dieterle S, Ying G, Hatzmann W, Neuer A. 2006. Effect of acupuncture on the outcome of *in vitro* fertilization and intracytoplasmic sperm injection: a randomized, prospective, controlled clinical study. *Fertil Steril.* 85(5):1347-51.
7. Westergaard LG, Mao Q, Krogslund M, Sandrini S, Lenz S, Grinsted J. 2006. Acupuncture on the day of embryo transfer significantly improves the reproductive outcome in infertile women: a prospective, randomized trial. *Fertil Steril.* 85(5):1341-6.
8. Craig LB, Criniti AR, Hansen KR, et al. 2007. Acupuncture lowers pregnancy rates when performed before and after embryo transfer. *Fertil Steril*. 88:S40.
9. Hullender Rubin LE, Opsahl MS, Taylor-Swanson L, Ackerman DL. 2013. Acupuncture and in vitro fertilization: a retrospective chart review. *J Altern Complement Med.* 19(7):637-43.
10. Manheimer E, Zhang G, Udoff L, Haramati A, Langenberg P, Berman BM, Bouter LM. 2008. Effects of acupuncture on rates of pregnancy and live birth among women undergoing *in vitro* fertilisation: systematic review and meta-analysis. *BMJ.* 336(7643):545-9.
11. Ng EH, So WS, Gao J, Wong YY, Ho PC. 2008. The role of acupuncture in the management of subfertility. *Fertil Steril*. 90:1–13.
12. Cheong YC, Hung Yu Ng E, Ledger WL. 2009. Acupuncture and assisted conception. *Cochrane Database Syst Rev*. 4:CD006920.

13. El-Toukhy T, Sunkara SK, Khairy M, Dyer R, Khalaf Y, Coomarasamy A. 2008. A systematic review and meta-analysis of acupuncture in *in vitro* fertilisation. *BJOG*. 115:1203–13.
14. Cheong Y, Nardo LG, Rutherford T, Ledger W. 2010. Acupuncture and herbal medicine in *in vitro* fertilisation: a review of the evidence for clinical practice. *Hum Fertil (Camb)*. 13:3–12.
15. El-Toukhy T, Khalaf Y. 2009. The impact of acupuncture on assisted reproductive technology outcome. *Curr Opin Obstet Gynecol*. 21:240–6.
16. Sunkara SK, Coomarasamy A, Khalaf Y, El-Toukhy T. 2009. Acupuncture and in vitro fertilization: updated meta-analysis. *Hum Reprod*. 24: 2047–8.
17. Anderson BJ, Haimovici F, Ginsburg ES, Schust DJ, Wayne PM. 2007. In vitro fertilization and acupuncture: clinical efficacy and mechanistic basis. *Altern Ther Health Med.* 13(3):38-48.
18. So EW, Ng EH, Wong YY, Lau EY, Yeung WS, Ho PC. 2009. A randomized double blind comparison of real and placebo acupuncture in IVF treatment. *Hum Reprod*. 24(2):341-8.
19. Streitberger K, Kleinhenz J. 1998. Introducing a placebo needle into acupuncture research. *Lancet*. 352(9125):364-5.
20. Zhu D, Gao Y, Chang JL, and Kong J. 2013. Placebo Acupuncture Devices: Considerations for Acupuncture Research. *Evidence-Based Complementary and Alternative Medicine,* 2013:628907.
21. Domar AD, Meshay I, Kelliher J, Alper M, Powers RD. 2009. The impact of acupuncture on in vitro fertilization outcome. *Fertil Steril.* 91(3):723-6.
22. Magarelli PC, Cridennda DK, Cohen M. 2009. Changes in serum cortisol and prolactin associated with acupuncture during controlled ovarian hyperstimulation in women undergoing in vitro fertilization-embryo transfer treatment. *Fertil Steril.* 92(6):1870-9.
23. Stener-Victorin E, Waldenström U, Andersson SA, Wikland M. 1996. Reduction of blood flow impedance in the uterine arteries of infertile women with electro-acupuncture. *Hum Reprod.* 11(6):1314-7.
24. de Lacey S, Smith CA, Paterson C. 2009. Building resilience: a preliminary exploration of women's perceptions of the use of acupuncture as an adjunct to In Vitro Fertilisation. *BMC Complement Altern Med.* 12;9:50.
25. Balk J, Catov J, Horn B, Gecsi K, Wakim A. 2010. The relationship between perceived stress, acupuncture, and pregnancy rates among IVF patients: A pilot study. *Complementary Therapies in Clinical Practice.* 16:154-7.

26. Zhang R, Feng XJ, Guan Q, Cui W, Zheng Y, Sun W, Han JS. 2011. Increase of success rate for women undergoing embryo transfer by transcutaneous electrical acupoint stimulation: a prospective randomized placebo-controlled study. *Fertil Steril.* 96(4):912-6.
27. Moy I, Milad MP, Barnes R, Confino E, Kazer RR, Zhang X. 2011. Randomized controlled trial: effects of acupuncture on pregnancy rates in women undergoing in vitro fertilization. *Fertil Steril.* 95(2):583-7.
28. Manheimer E. 2011. Selecting a control for in vitro fertilization and acupuncture randomized controlled trials (RCTs): how sham controls may unnecessarily complicate the RCT evidence base. *Fertil Steril.* 95(8):2456-61.
29. Villahermosa DI, Santos LG, Nogueira MB, Vilarino FL, Barbosa CP. 2013. Influence of acupuncture on the outcomes of in vitro fertilisation when embryo implantation has failed: a prospective randomised controlled clinical trial. *Acupunct Med.* 31(2):157-61.
30. Zheng CH, Huang GY, Zhang MM, Wang W. 2012. Effects of acupuncture on pregnancy rates in women undergoing *in vitro* fertilization: a systematic review and meta-analysis. *Fertil Steril.* 97(3):599-611.
31. Qu F, Zhou J, Ren RX. 2012. Effects of acupuncture on the outcomes of in vitro fertilization: a systematic review and meta-analysis. *J Altern Complement Med.* 18(5):429-39.
32. Manheimer E, van der Windt D, Cheng K, Stafford K, Liu J, Tierney J, Lao L, Berman BM, Langenberg P, Bouter LM. 2013. The effects of acupuncture on rates of clinical pregnancy among women undergoing in vitro fertilization: a systematic review and meta-analysis. *Hum Reprod* Update. 19(6):696-713.
33. Shen C, Wu M, Shu D, Zhao X, Gao Y. 2015 The Role of Acupuncture in *in vitro* Fertilization: A Systematic Review and Meta-Analysis. *Gynecol Obstet Invest.* 79(1):1-12.
34. Ho M *et al.* 2009. Electroacupuncture Reduces Uterine Artery Blood Flow Impedance in Infertile Women. *Taiwanese Journal of Obstetrics and Gynecology* 48:148-51.
35. Liu XY *et al.* 2007. Preliminary study on the mechanisms of acupuncture in promoting embryo implantation in rats. *Zhongguo Zhong Xi Yi Jie He Za Zhi* 27:633-6.
36. Jin CL *et al.* 2009. Increased Oocyte Production after Acupuncture Treatment during Superovulation Process in Mice. *Journal of Reproduction and Contraception*. 20:35-44.

37. Chen J *et al.* 2009. Effects of electroacupuncture on *in vitro* fertilization-embryo transfer (IVF-ET) of patients with poor ovarian response. *Zhongguo Zhenjiu*. 29:775-9.
38. Huang HDJ, Zhang MM. 2009. Effects of acupuncture on the luteal function of rats with dysfunctional embryo implantation. *Zhongguo Zhen jiu* 29:910-3.
39. Huang DM, Huang GY, Lu FE, Stefan D, Andreas N, Robert G. 2011. Acupuncture for infertility: is it an effective therapy? *Chin J Integr Med.* 17(5):386-95.

Chapter Four

1. Gardani G, Cerrone R, Biella C, Mancini L, Proserpio E, Casiraghi M, Travisi O, Meregalli M, Trabattoni P, Colombo L, Giani L, Vaghi M, Lissoni P. 2006. Effect of acupressure on nausea and vomiting induced by chemotherapy in cancer patients. *Minerva Med.* 97(5):391-4.
2. Streitberger K, Ezzo J, Schneider A. 2006. Acupuncture for nausea and vomiting: an update of clinical and experimental studies. *Auton Neurosci.* 129(1-2):107-17.
3. Gottschling S, Reindl TK, Meyer S, Berrang J, Henze G, Graeber S, Ong MF, Graf N. 2008. Acupuncture to alleviate chemotherapy-induced nausea and vomiting in pediatric oncology - a randomized multicenter crossover pilot trial. *Klin Padiatr*. 220(6):365-70.
4. Nystrom E, Ridderstrom G, Leffler AS. 2008. Manual acupuncture as an adjunctive treatment of nausea in patients with cancer in palliative care—a prospective, observational pilot study. *Acupunct Med.* 26(1):27-32.
5. You Q, Yu H, Wu D, Zhang Y, Zheng J, Peng C. 2009. Vitamin B6 points PC6 injection during acupuncture can relieve nausea and vomiting in patients with ovarian cancer. *Int J Gynecol Cancer*. 19(4):567-71.
6. Taspinar A, Sirin A. 2010. Effect of acupressure on chemotherapy-induced nausea and vomiting in gynecologic cancer patients in Turkey. *Eur J Oncol Nurs.* 14(1):49-54.
7. Genç F, Tan M. 2015. The effect of acupressure application on chemotherapy-induced nausea, vomiting, and anxiety in patients with breast cancer. *Palliat Support Care.* 13(2):275-84.
8. Avc HS, Ovayolu N, Ovayolu Ö. 2016. Effect of Acupressure on Nausea-Vomiting in Patients with Acute Myeloblastic Leukemia. *Holist Nurs Pract*. 30(5):257-62.

9. Yang Y, Zhang Y, Jing NC, Lu Y, Xiao HY, Xu GL, Wang XG, Wang LM, Zhang YM, Zhang DJ, Duan QL. 2009. Electroacupuncture at Zusanli (ST 36) for treatment of nausea and vomiting caused by the chemotherapy of the malignant tumor: a multicentral randomized controlled trial. *Zhongguo Zhen Jiu.* 29(12):955-8.
10. Enblom A, Lekander M, Hammar M, Johnsson A, Onelöv E, Ingvar M, Steineck G, Börjeson S. 2011. Getting the grip on nonspecific treatment effects: emesis in patients randomized to acupuncture or sham compared to patients receiving standard care. *PLoS One.* 6(3):e14766.
11. Enblom A, Tomasson A, Hammar M, Steineck G, Börjeson S. 2011. Pilot testing of methods for evaluation of acupuncture for emesis during radiotherapy: a randomised single subject experimental design. *Acupunct Med.* 29(2):94-102.
12. Enblom A, Johnsson A, Hammar M, Onelöv E, Steineck G, Börjeson S. 2012. Acupuncture compared with placebo acupuncture in radiotherapy-induced nausea--a randomized controlled study. *Ann Oncol.* 23(5):1353-61.
13. Yeh CH, Chien LC, Chiang YC, Lin SW, Huang CK, Ren D. 2012. Reduction in nausea and vomiting in children undergoing cancer chemotherapy by either appropriate or sham auricular acupuncture points with standard care. *J Altern Complement Med.* 18(4):334-40.
14. D'Alessandro E, de Brito C, Cecatto R, Saul M, Atta JA, Lin CA. 2013. Evaluation of acupuncture for cancer symptoms in a cancer institute in Brazil. *Acupunct Med.* 31(1):23-6.
15. Zhang X, Fan YH. 2014. Effects of electroacupuncture on chemotherapy-induced nausea and vomiting and its mechanism. *Zhongguo Zhen Jiu.* 34(11):1061-4.
16. Tas D, Uncu D, Sendur MA, Koca N, Zengin N. 2014. Acupuncture as a complementary treatment for cancer patients receiving chemotherapy. *Asian Pac J Cancer Prev.* 15(7):3139-44.
17. Shen Y, Liu L, Chiang JS, Meng Z, Garcia MK, Chen Z, Peng H, Bei W, Zhao Q, Spelman AR, Cohen L. 2015. Randomized, placebo-controlled trial of K1 acupoint acustimulation to prevent cisplatin-induced or oxaliplatin-induced nausea. *Cancer.* 121(1):84-92.
18. Rithirangsriroj K, Manchana T, Akkayagorn L. 2015. Efficacy of acupuncture in prevention of delayed chemotherapy induced nausea and vomiting in gynecologic cancer patients. *Gynecol Oncol.* 136(1):82-6.
19. Liu YQ, Sun S, Dong HJ, Zhai DX, Zhang DY, Shen W, Bai LL, Yu J, Zhou LH, Yu CQ. 2015. Wrist-ankle acupuncture and ginger

moxibustion for preventing gastrointestinal reactions to chemotherapy: A randomized controlled trial. *Chin J Integr Med.* 21(9):697-702.
20. McKeon C, Smith CA, Gibbons K, Hardy J. 2015. EA versus sham acupuncture and no acupuncture for the control of acute and delayed chemotherapy-induced nausea and vomiting: a pilot study. *Acupunct Med.* 33(4):277-83.
21. Eghbali M, Yekaninejad MS, Varaei S, Jalalinia SF, Samimi MA, Sa'atchi K. 2016. The effect of auricular acupressure on nausea and vomiting caused by chemotherapy among breast cancer patients. *Complement Ther Clin Pract.* 24:189-94.
22. Ezzo J, Streitberger K, Schneider A. 2006. Cochrane systematic reviews examine P6 acupuncture-point stimulation for nausea and vomiting. *J Altern Complement Med.* 12(5):489-95.
23. Chao LF, Zhang AL, Liu HE, Cheng MH, Lam HB, Lo SK. 2009. The efficacy of acupoint stimulation for the management of therapy-related adverse events in patients with breast cancer: a systematic review. *Breast Cancer Res Treat.* 118(2):255-67.
24. O'Regan D, Filshie J. 2010. Acupuncture and cancer. *Auton Neurosci.* 157(1-2):96-100.
25. Garcia MK, McQuade J, Haddad R, Patel S, Lee R, Yang P, Palmer JL, Cohen L. 2013. Systematic review of acupuncture in cancer care: a synthesis of the evidence. *J Clin Oncol.* 31(7):952-60.
26. Towler P, Molassiotis A, Brearley SG. 2013. What is the evidence for the use of acupuncture as an intervention for symptom management in cancer supportive and palliative care: an integrative overview of reviews. *Support Care Cancer.* 21(10):2913-23.
27. Chien TJ, Liu CY, Hsu CH. 2013. Integrating acupuncture into cancer care. *J Tradit Complement Med.* 3(4):234-9.
28. Cheon S, Zhang X, Lee IS, Cho SH, Chae Y, Lee H. 2014. Pharmacopuncture for cancer care: a systematic review. *Evid Based Complement Alternat Med.* 2014:804746.
29. Wu X, Chung VC, Hui EP, Ziea ET, Ng BF, Ho RS, Tsoi KK, Wong SY, Wu JC. 2015. Effectiveness of acupuncture and related therapies for palliative care of cancer: overview of systematic reviews. *Sci Rep.* 5:16776.

Chapter Five

1. Maciocia G. 2007. *The Practice of Chinese Medicine: The Treatment of Diseases with Acupuncture and Chinese Herbs,* 2nd Edition, Churchill Livingstone,

2. Lu SY and Zhu RG. 2009. *Case Histories from Lu Shouyan and Zhu Rugong*. Beijing: People's Military Press.
3. Zhao JX, Yu YF and Huang M. 2007. Selected readings of Case Histories of Famous Acupuncturists, Beijing: People's Military Press.
4. Chen QX. 2004. *Chen Quanxin's Acupuncture Clinical Experience*. Beijing: People's Hygiene Press.
5. Yang JS. 2001. *China Hundred Years Hundred Chinese Medicine Series: Yang Jiasan*. Beijing: China Chinese Medicine Press.
6. Iseki C, Furuta T, Suzuki M, Koyama S, Suzuki K, Suzuki T, Kaneko A, Mitsuma T. 2014. Acupuncture Alleviated the Nonmotor Symptoms of Parkinson's Disease including Pain, Depression, and Autonomic Symptoms. *Case Rep Neurol Med*. 2014:953109.
7. Wang Y, Xie CL, Wang WW, Lu L, Fu DL, Wang XT, Zheng GQ. 2013. Epidemiology of complementary and alternative medicine use in patients with Parkinson's disease. *J Clin Neurosci.* 20(8):1062-7.
8. Joh TH, Park HJ, Kim SN, Lee H. 2010. Recent development of acupuncture on Parkinson's disease. *Neurol Res.* 32 Suppl 1:5-9.
9. Pecci C, Rivas MJ, Moretti CM, Raina G, Ramirez CZ, Díaz S, Uribe Roca C, Micheli FE. 2010. Use of complementary and alternative therapies in outpatients with Parkinson's disease in Argentina. *Mov Disord*. 25(13):2094-8.
10. Eng ML, Lyons KE, Greene MS, Pahwa R. 2006. Open-label trial regarding the use of acupuncture and yin tui na in Parkinson's disease outpatients: a pilot study on efficacy, tolerability, and quality of life. *J Altern Complement Med.* 12(4):395-9.
11. Chen XH, Li Y, Kui Y. 2007. Clinical observation on abdominal acupuncture plus Madopa for treatment of Parkinson's disease. *Zhongguo Zhen Jiu.* 27(8):562-4.
12. Ren XM. 2008. Fifty cases of Parkinson's disease treated by acupuncture combined with madopar. *J Tradit Chin Med.* 28(4):255-7.
13. Dong J, Cui HS. 2014. Clinical experience of Qin's eight scalp needles for treatment of Parkinson's disease. *Zhongguo Zhen Jiu*. 34(5):491-4.
14. Fukuda S, Kuriyama N, Tsuru H, Egawa M. 2015. Immediate effects of acupuncture on tongue pressure including swallowing reflex latency in Parkinson's disease. *Acupunct Med*. 34(1):59-61.
15. Fukuda S, Kuriyama N, Egawa M. 2015. Acupuncture for Gait Disturbance in Parkinson's Disease: Immediate Effects of Acupuncture Treatment. *J Am Geriatr Soc.* 63(10):2189-90.
16. Doo KH, Lee JH, Cho SY, Jung WS, Moon SK, Park JM, Ko CN, Kim H, Park HJ, Park SU. 2015. A Prospective Open-Label Study of Combined Treatment for Idiopathic Parkinson's Disease Using

Acupuncture and Bee Venom Acupuncture as an Adjunctive Treatment. *J Altern Complement Med.* 21(10):598-603.

17. Cho SY, Shim SR, Rhee HY, Park HJ, Jung WS, Moon SK, Park JM, Ko CN, Cho KH, Park SU. 2012. Effectiveness of acupuncture and bee venom acupuncture in idiopathic Parkinson's disease. *Parkinsonism Relat Disord.* 18(8):948-52.
18. Yeo S, Lim S, Choe IH, Choi YG, Chung KC, Jahng GH, Kim SH. 2012. Acupuncture stimulation on GB34 activates neural responses associated with Parkinson's disease. *CNS Neurosci Ther.* 18(9):781-90.
19. Yeo S, Choe IH, van den Noort M, Bosch P, Jahng GH, Rosen B, Kim SH, Lim S. 2014. Acupuncture on GB34 activates the precentral gyrus and prefrontal cortex in Parkinson's disease. *BMC Complement Altern Med.* 14(1):336.
20. Wang F, Sun L, Zhang XZ, Jia J, Liu Z, Huang XY, Yu SY, Zuo LJ, Cao CJ, Wang XM, Zhang W. 2015. Effect and Potential Mechanism of Electroacupuncture Add-On Treatment in Patients with Parkinson's Disease. *Evid Based Complement Alternat Med.* 2015:69279.
21. Liu CH, Wang R, Jin YB, Sun ZL, Zhou X, He JY. 2015. Acupoint injection of kakkonein for early- or mid-stage Parkinson's disease: a multicenter randomized controlled clinical trial. *Zhen Ci Yan Jiu.* 40(1):56-60.
22. Chen FP, Chang CM, Shiu JH, Chiu JH, Wu TP, Yang JL, Kung YY, Chen FJ, Chern CM, Hwang SJ. 2015. A clinical study of integrating acupuncture and Western medicine in treating patients with Parkinson's disease. *Am J Chin Med.* 43(3):407-23.
23. Chae Y, Lee H, Kim H, Kim CH, Chang DI, Kim KM, Park HJ. 2009. Parsing brain activity associated with acupuncture treatment in Parkinson's diseases. *Mov Disord.* 24(12):1794-802.
24. Lam YC, Kum WF, Durairajan SS, Lu JH, Man SC, Xu M, Zhang XF, Huang XZ, Li M. 2008. Efficacy and safety of acupuncture for idiopathic Parkinson's disease: a systematic review. *J Altern Complement Med.* 14(6):663-71.
25. Lee HS, Park HL, Lee SJ, Shin BC, Choi JY, Lee MS. 2013. Scalp acupuncture for Parkinson's disease: a systematic review of randomized controlled trials. *Chin J Integr Med.* 19(4):297-306.
26. Kim HJ, Jeon BS. 2014. Is acupuncture efficacious therapy in Parkinson's disease? *J Neurol Sci.* 341(1-2):1-7.
27. Lee MS, Shin BC, Kong JC, Ernst E. 2008. Effectiveness of acupuncture for Parkinson's disease: a systematic review. *Mov Disord.* 23(11):1505-15.

28. Zhang G, Xiong N, Zhang Z, Liu L, Huang J, Yang J, Wu J, Lin Z, Wang T. 2015. Effectiveness of traditional Chinese medicine as an adjunct therapy for Parkinson's disease: a systematic review and meta-analysis. *PLoS One.* 10(3):e0118498.
29. Huang Y, Jiang XM, Li DJ. 2006. Effects on electro-scaip acupuncture on cerebral dopamine transporter in patients with Parkinson' s disease. *Zhongguo Zhong Xi Yi Jie He Za Zhi.* 26(4):303-7.
30. Jiang XM, Huang Y, Li DJ, Tang AW, Wang SX, Zhuo Y, Li QS, Chen J, Gao YP. 2006. Effect of electro-scalp acupuncture on cerebral dopamine transporter in the striatum area of the patient of Parkinson's disease by means of single photon emission computer tomography. *Zhongguo Zhen Jiu.* 26(6):427-30.
31. Jeon S, Kim YJ, Kim ST, Moon W, Chae Y, Kang M, Chung MY, Lee H, Hong MS, Chung JH, Joh TH, Lee H, Park HJ. 2008. Proteomic analysis of the neuroprotective mechanisms of acupuncture treatment in a Parkinson's disease mouse model. *Proteomics.* 8(22):4822-32.
32. Huang Y, Jiang X, Zhuo Y, Tang A, Wik G. 2009. Complementary acupuncture treatment increases cerebral metabolism in patients with Parkinson's disease. *Int J Neurosci.* 119(8):1190-7.
33. Kim SN, Doo AR, Park JY, Bae H, Chae Y, Shim I, Lee H, Moon W, Lee H, Park HJ. 2011. Acupuncture enhances the synaptic dopamine availability to improve motor function in a mouse model of Parkinson's disease. *PLoS One.* 6(11):e27566.
34. Wang YC, He F, Ma J, Zhou D, Liang Y, Gong YX. 2013. Impacts of electroacupuncture on ubiquitin-proteasome system in rats with Parkinson's disease *Zhongguo Zhen Jiu.* 33(8):725-9.
35. Wang S, Fang J, Ma J, Wang Y, Liang S, Zhou D, Sun G. 2013. Electroacupuncture-regulated neurotrophic factor mRNA expression in the substantia nigra of Parkinson's disease rats. *Neural Regen Res.* 8(6):540-9.
36. Ghaffari BD, Kluger B. 2014. Mechanisms for alternative treatments in Parkinson's disease: acupuncture, tai chi, and other treatments. *Curr Neurol Neurosci Rep.* 14(6):451.
37. Wang SJ, Ma J, Gong YX, Wang YC, Zeng XL, Liang Y, Sun GJ. 2014. Effect of electroacupuncture intervention on ERK 1/2 signaling and TNF-α and IL-1β protein levels in the substantia Nigra in rats with Parkinson's Disease. *Zhen Ci Yan Jiu.* 39(6):456-60.
38. Kim SN, Doo AR, Park JY, Choo HJ, Shim I, Park JJ, Chae Y, Lee B, Lee H, Park HJ. 2014. Combined treatment with acupuncture reduces effective dose and alleviates adverse effect of L-dopa by normalizing Parkinson's disease-induced neurochemical imbalance. *Brain Res.*

1544:33-44.
39. Wattanathorn J, Sutalangka C. 2014. Laser Acupuncture at HT7 Acupoint Improves Cognitive Deficit, Neuronal Loss, Oxidative Stress, and Functions of Cholinergic and Dopaminergic Systems in Animal Model of Parkinson's Disease. *Evid Based Complement Alternat Med.* 2014:937601.
40. Li J, Wang LN, Xiao HL, Li X, Yang JJ. 2014. Effect of electroacupuncture intervention on levels of SOD, GSH, GSH-Px, MDA, and apoptosis of dopaminergic neurons in substantia nigra in rats with Parkinson's disease. *Zhen Ci Yan Jiu*. 39(3):185-91.
41. Park JY, Choi H, Baek S, Jang J, Lee A, Jeon S, Kim J, Park HJ. 2015. p53 signalling mediates acupuncture-induced neuroprotection in Parkinson's disease. *Biochem Biophys Res Commun*. 460(3):772-9.
42. Tu Q, Liang Y, Ma J, Wang S, Shen F, Wang Y. 2015. Effects of electroacupuncture on proteasomes of substantia nigra in rats with Parkinson's disease. *Zhongguo Zhen Jiu.* 35(4):355-60.
43. Tu Q, Liang Y, Ma J, Wang SJ, Shen F, Wang YC. 2015. Effect of Electroacupuncture on 26 S Proteasome and Nuclear Factor kappa B in Substantia Nigra of Rats with Rotenone-induced Parkinson's Disease. *Zhen Ci Yan Jiu*. 40(4):259-64.
44. Wang S, Ma B, Ma J, Liu F, Wang Y, Sun G. 2015. Effects of electroacupuncture on the expression of related protein mRNA in the striatum in rats with Parkinson's disease. *Zhongguo Zhen Jiu*. 35(7):697-701.
45. Yeo S, An KS, Hong YM, Choi YG, Rosen B, Kim SH, Lim S. 2015. Neuroprotective changes in degeneration-related gene expression in the substantia nigra following acupuncture in an MPTP mouse model of Parkinsonism: Microarray analysis. *Genet Mol Biol*. 38(1):115-27.

Chapter Six

1. Chen YB and Deng LY. 1987. *Essentials of Contemporary Chinese Acupuncturists' Clinical Experience*. Tianjin: Tianjin Science and Technology Press.
2. Zhu B and Wang HC. 2009. *Case Studies from the Medical Records of Leading Chinese Acupuncture Experts*. Beijing: People's Military Medical Press.
3. Yuan Q. 2004. *Jin 3-Needle Technique*. Shanghai: Shanghai Science and Technology Literature Press.
4. Shi XM. 2005. Clinical Research on the Treatment of 9005 Cases of Apoplexy With the Acupuncture Method of Sharpening Mind and

Inducing Consciousness, *Guiding Journal of Traditional Chinese Medicine and Pharmacy (Zhong Yi Yao Dao Bao)*. 1: 5-7.
5. Alexander DN, Cen S, Sullivan KJ, Bhavnani G, Ma X, Azen SP. 2004. Effects of acupuncture treatment on poststroke motor recovery and physical function: a pilot study. *Neurorehabil Neural Repair*. 18(4):259-67.
6. Cheng XK, Wang ZM, Sun L, Li YH. 2011. Post-stroke hand dysfunction treated with acupuncture at SJ 3 (Zhongzhu) and SJ 5 (Waiguan). *China Acupuncture and Moxibustion (Zhong Guo Zhen Jiu)*. 31(2):117-20.
7. Seki T, Kurusu M, Tanji H, Arai H, Sasaki H. 2003. Acupuncture and swallowing reflex in poststroke patients. *Journal of the American Geriatrics Society*. 51:726-7.
8. Chou P., Chu H., Lin JG. 2009. Effects of Electro-acupuncture Treatment on Impaired Cognition and Quality of Life in Taiwanese Stroke Patients, *Journal of Alternative and Complementary Medicine*. 15(10):1067-1073.
9. Wong AM, Su TY, Tang FT, Cheng PT, Liaw MY. 1999. Clinical Trial of Electrical Acupuncture on Hemiplegic Stroke Patients. *American Journal of Physical Medicine & Rehabilitation*. 78(2) – pp 117-122.
10. Hu H-H, Chung C, Liu TJ, Chen RC, Chen C-H, Chou P, Huang W-S, Lin JCT, Tsuei JT. 1993. A Randomized Controlled Trial on the Treatment for Acute Partial Ischemic Stroke with Acupuncture, *Neuroepidemiology* 12:106–113.
11. Zhu HH. 2010. The Clinical Research on Treating Spastic Paralysis after Stroke with Different Methods of Acupuncture Therapy. *China's Outstanding Master's Theses,* Guangzhou University of Traditional Chinese Medicine, Guangzhou.
12. Chau AC, Fai Cheung RT, Jiang X, Au-Yeung PK, Li LS. 2010. An fMRI Study Showing the Effect of Acupuncture in Chronic Stage Stroke Patients with Aphasia. *Journal of Acupuncture and Meridian Studies.* 3(1): 53-7.
13. Hsiu H, Huang SM, Chen CT, Hsu CL, Hsu WC. 2011. Acupuncture Stimulation Causes Bilaterally Different Microcirculatory Effects in Stroke Patients. *Microvascular Research*. 81(3):289-94.
14. Li G, Yang ES. 2011. An fMRI Study of Acupuncture-Induced Brain Activation of Aphasia Stroke Patients. *Complement Ther Med*. 19 Suppl 1: S49-59.
15. Wu P, Mills E, Moher D, Seely D. 2010. Acupuncture in Poststroke Rehabilitation: A Systematic Review and Meta-Analysis of Randomized Trials. *Stroke*. 41(4):e171-9.

16. Zhang SH, Liu M, Asplund K, Li L. 2005. Acupuncture for Acute Stroke. *Cochrane Database Syst Rev*. Apr 18;(2):CD003317.
17. Wu HM, Tang JL, Lin XP, Lau J, Leung PC, Woo J, Li YP. 2006. Acupuncture for Stroke Rehabilitation. *Cochrane Database Syst Rev.* Jul 19;(3):CD004131.
18. Shiflett, S.C. 2007. Does Acupuncture Work for Stroke Rehabilitation: What Do Recent Clinical Trials Really Show? *Top Stroke Rehabil.* 14(4):40-58.
19. Editorial Staff. New Study Suggests Acupuncture Can Improve Recovery, Physical Functioning in Stroke Patients. *Acupuncture Today.* April 2005.

Chapter Seven

1. Uhrig S, Hummelsberger J, Brinkhaus B. 2003. Standardized acupuncture therapy in patients with ocular hypertension or glaucoma—results of a prospective observation study. *Forsch Komplementarmed Klass Naturheilkd.* 10(5):256-61.
2. Wu YH, Zhu GQ, Lin XY, Oyang L, Su H, Wu B. 2004. Effect of needling Quchi and Taichong points on blood levels of Endothelin and Angiotension Converting Enzyme in patients with hypertension. *Zhongguo Zhong Xi Yi Jie He Za Zhi.* 24(12):1080-3.
3. Gao XY, Zhu B. 2005. Analysis on blood-pressure-decreasing effect of electric pulse stimulation of auricular acupoint Jiangyagou in the patient of hypertension. *Zhongguo Zhen Jiu.* 25(7):474-6.
4. Zhou W, Longhurst JC. 2006. Review of trials examining the use of acupuncture to treat hypertension. *Future Cardiol.* 2(3):287-92.
5. Huang F, Yao GX, Huang XL, Liu YN. 2007. Clinical observation on acupuncture for treatment of hypertension of phlegm-stasis blocking collateral type. *Zhongguo Zhen Jiu.* 27(6):403-6.
6. Cao L, Hou GY, Fan WS. 2007. Analysis on the therapeutic effect of acupuncture of Jiaji (EX-B 2) for treatment of cervical hypertension. *Zhen Ci Yan Jiu.* 32(3):195-8.
7. Yin C, Seo B, Park HJ, Cho M, Jung W, Choue R, Kim C, Park HK, Lee H, Koh H. 2007. Acupuncture, a promising adjunctive therapy for essential hypertension: a double-blind, randomized, controlled trial. *Neurol Res.* 29 Suppl 1:S98-103.
8. Flachskampf FA, Gallasch J, Gefeller O, Gan J, Mao J, Pfahlberg AB, Wortmann A, Klinghammer L, Pflederer W, Daniel WG. 2007. Randomized trial of acupuncture to lower blood pressure. *Circulation.* 115(24):3121-9.

9. Song YH. 2007. Observation on therapeutic effects of combined acupuncture and medicine therapy and simple medication on renal hypertension of chronic kidney disease. *Zhongguo Zhen Jiu*. 27(9):641-4.
10. Wan WJ, Ma CY, Xiong XA, Wang L, Ding L, Zhang YX, Wang Y. 2009. Clinical observation on therapeutic effect of electroacupuncture at Quchi (LI 11) for treatment of essential hypertension. *Zhongguo Zhen Jiu*. 29(5):349-52.
11. Zhang J, Ng D, Sau A. 2009. Effects of electrical stimulation of acupuncture points on blood pressure. *J Chiropr Med*. 8(1):9-14.
12. Park SU, Ko CN, Bae HS, Jung WS, Moon SK, Cho KH, Kim YS, Park JM. 2009. Short-term reactions to acupuncture treatment and adverse events following acupuncture: a cross-sectional survey of patient reports in Korea. *J Altern Complement Med*. 15(12):1275-83.
13. Chen J, Li J, Wang ZR. 2010. Therapeutic effect on essential hypertension treated with combined therapy of acupuncture and medication. *Zhongguo Zhen Jiu*. 30(11):896-8.
14. Orekhova EM, Solodovnikova TS, Radzievskiĭ SA, Konchugova TV, Bobkova AS, Lebedeva OD, Lebedeva EV, Luk'ianova TV. 2010. The application of trans-auricular low-frequency electrical puncture for the treatment of arterial hypertension. *Vopr Kurortol Fizioter Lech Fiz Kult*. 6:16-8.
15. Yang DH. 2010. Effect of electroacupuncture on Quchi (LI11) and Taichong (LR3) on blood pressure variability in young patients with hypertension. *Zhongguo Zhen Jiu*. 30(7):547-50.
16. Chen NY, Zhou Y, Dong Q, Zhou CX. 2010. Observation on therapeutic effect of acupuncture in the treatment of German hypertension patients. *Zhen Ci Yan Jiu*. 35(6):462-6.
17. Park JM, Shin AS, Park SU, Sohn IS, Jung WS, Moon SK. 2010. The acute effect of acupuncture on endothelial dysfunction in patients with hypertension: a pilot, randomized, double-blind, placebo-controlled crossover trial. *J Altern Complement Med*. 16(8):883-8.
18. Xing XM, Wang RC, Sun QW, Li H. 2011. Effect on blood pressure and microcirculation of nail fold in primary hypertension patients treated with acupuncture according to syndrome differentiation. *Zhongguo Zhen Jiu*. 31(4):301-4.
19. Yin C, Du YZ. 2012. Observation of anti-hypertensive effect on primary hypertension treated with acupuncture at Renying (ST 9) mainly. *Zhongguo Zhen Jiu*. 32(9):776-8.
20. Dong YS, Xing SL. 2012. Effect of acupuncture needle-retention duration at Baihui (GV 20) and sishencong (EX-HN 1) on blood

pressure in hypertension patients. *Zhen Ci Yan Jiu.* 37(3):233-6.
21. Kim HM, Cho SY, Park SU, Sohn IS, Jung WS, Moon SK, Park JM, Ko CN, Cho KH. 2012. Can acupuncture affect the circadian rhythm of blood pressure? A randomized, double-blind, controlled trial. *J Altern Complement Med.* 18(10):918-23.
22. Severcan C, Cevik C, Acar HV, Sivri AB, Mit SS, Geçioğlu E, Paşaoğlu OT, Gündüztepe Y. 2012. The effects of acupuncture on the levels of blood pressure and nitric oxide in hypertensive patients. *Acupunct Electrother Res.* 37(4):263-75.
23. Chen H, Dai J, Zhang X, Wang K, Huang S, Cao Q, Wang H, Liang Y, Shi C, Li M, Ha T, Ai L, Li S, Ma J, Wei W, You Y, Liu Z, Tian J, Bai L. 2013. Hypothalamus-related resting brain network underlying short-term acupuncture treatment in primary hypertension. *Evid Based Complement Alternat Med.* 2013:808971.
24. Cevik C, Işeri SO. 2013. The effect of acupuncture on high blood pressure of patients using antihypertensive drugs. *Acupunct Electrother Res.* 38(1-2):1-15.
25. Litscher G, Cheng WP, Cheng GY, Wang L, Zhao J, Litscher D, Gaischek I, Sheng Z, Kuang H. 2014. Acupuncture Point Laterality: Investigation of Acute Effects of Quchi (LI11) in Patients with Hypertension Using Heart Rate Variability. *Evid Based Complement Alternat Med.* 2014:979067.
26. Xie B, Lin YP. 2014. Efficacy observation on acupuncture for essential hypertension of yin deficiency due to yang hyperactivity pattern. *Zhongguo Zhen Jiu.* 34(6):547-50.
27. Li YM. 2014. Efficacy on borderline hypertension treated with acupuncture combined with anti-hypertensive plaster intervention. *Zhongguo Zhen Jiu.* 34(11):1057-60.
28. Yang X, Liu W. 2015. Primary hypertension treated with acupuncture combined with auricular point sticking: a randomized controlled trial. *Zhongguo Zhen Jiu.* 35(3):227-31.
29. Liu Y, Park JE, Shin KM, Lee M, Jung HJ, Kim AR, Jung SY, Yoo HR, Sang KO, Choi SM. 2015. Acupuncture lowers blood pressure in mild hypertension patients: A randomized, controlled, assessor-blinded pilot trial. *Complement Ther Med.* 23(5):658-65.
30. Li P, Tjen-A-Looi SC, Cheng L, Liu D, Painovich J, Vinjamury S, Longhurst JC. 2015. Susan-Samueli Long-Lasting Reduction of Blood Pressure by Electroacupuncture in Patients with Hypertension: Randomized Controlled Trial. *Med Acupunct.* 27(4):253-266.
31. Lee H, Kim SY, Park J, Kim YJ, Lee H, Park HJ. 2009. Acupuncture for lowering blood pressure: systematic review and meta-analysis. *Am*

J Hypertens. 22(1):122-8.
32. Kim LW, Zhu J. 2010. Acupuncture for essential hypertension. *Altern Ther Health Med.* 16(2):18-29.
33. Wang J, Xiong X, Liu W. 2013. Acupuncture for essential hypertension. *Int J Cardiol.* 169(5):317-26.
34. Xiong X, Liu W, Yang X, Feng B, Wang J. 2014. Moxibustion for essential hypertension. *Complement Ther Med.* 22(1):187-95.
35. Li DZ, Zhou Y, Yang YN, Ma YT, Li XM, Yu J, Zhao Y, Zhai H, Lao L. 2014. Acupuncture for essential hypertension: a meta-analysis of randomized sham-controlled clinical trials. *Evid Based Complement Alternat Med.* 2014:279478.
36. Zhao XF, Hu HT, Li JS, Shang HC, Zheng HZ, Niu JF, Shi XM, Wang S. 2015. Is Acupuncture Effective for Hypertension? A Systematic Review and Meta-Analysis. *PLoS One.* 10(7):e0127019.
37. Kim DD, Pica AM, Durán RG, Durán WN. 2006. Acupuncture reduces experimental renovascular hypertension through mechanisms involving nitric oxide synthases. *Microcirculation.* 13(7):577-85.
38. Zhou W, Longhurst JC. 2012. Neuroendocrine mechanisms of acupuncture in the treatment of hypertension. *Evid Based Complement Alternat Med.* 2012:878673.
39. Li P, Longhurst JC. 2010. Neural mechanism of electroacupuncture's hypotensive effects. *Auton Neurosci.* 157(1-2):24-30.
40. Jin CN, Zhang TS, Ji LX, Tian YF. 2007. Survey of studies on mechanisms of acupuncture and moxibustion in decreasing blood pressure. *Zhongguo Zhen Jiu.* 27(6):467-70.
41. Guo YH, Zhao XF, Wang S. 2011. Discussion on clinical trial design of treatment of hypertension with acupuncture and moxibustion. *Zhongguo Zhen Jiu.* 31(2):177-80.
42. Longhurst J. 2013. Acupuncture's Cardiovascular Actions: A Mechanistic Perspective. *Med Acupunct.* 25(2):101-113.
43. Yu Z, Wu QF, Liang FR. 2014. Considerations about mechanisms of acupuncture therapy for improving hypertension by regulating immune system. *Zhen Ci Yan Jiu.* 39(4):333-6.

Chapter Eight

1. Andreasen NC, Liu D, Ziebell S, Vora A, Ho BC. 2013. Relapse duration, treatment intensity, and brain tissue loss in schizophrenia: a prospective longitudinal MRI study. *Am J Psychiatry.* 170(6):609-15.

2. Bosch P, de Rover P, Staudte H, Lim S, van den Noort M. 2015. Schizophrenia, depression, and sleep disorders: their traditional Oriental medicine equivalents. *J Acupunct Meridian Stud.* 8(1):17-22.
3. Tian DH. 2004. *Huang Di Nei Jing: Ling Shu (Yellow Emperor's Classic of Medicine: Spiritual Pivot)*. Beijing: People's Medical Publishing Press.
4. Sun SM, 2014. *Qian Jin Yao Fang (Essential Formulas Worth a Thousand Pieces of Gold*), Beijing: People's Medical Publishing Press.
5. Sun SM. 1992. Ode to Thirteen Ghost Acupoints for the Treatment of Mental Disorders, translated by Ralph Alan Dale and Yan Cheng, *American Journal of Acupuncture.* 20(3).
6. Tao Y, Hou W, Liang Y, Zong L. 2015. Clinical application and mechanism on the ghost points in the treatment of mental diseases. *Zhongguo Zhen Jiu.* 35(2):179-83.
7. Zhao J, She Y, Huang M. 2007. *Selected Readings from Famous Acupuncturists Case Studies*. Beijing: People's Military Medical Press.
8. Bosch P, Staudte H, van den Noort M, Lim S. 2014. A case study on acupuncture in the treatment of schizophrenia. *Acupunct Med.* 32(3):286-9.
9. Feng-Ju Y, Fu-Gen S, Zhi-Hua Z. 2006. Short-term curative effect of electroacupuncture as an adjunctive treatment on schizophrenia. *Zhongguo Zhong Xi Yi Jie He Za Zhi.* 26(3):253-5.
10. Zhang BR, Li S, Yuan PY, Zhang XB, Cheng LX, Zhou HH, Zhou CY, Liu XY, Wang XL, Tian GZ, Lin QG, Sha WW. 2006. Effects of injection of Huangqi injection into Zusanli (ST 36) on immune function in the patient of schizophrenia. *Zhongguo Zhen Jiu.* 26(9):625-8.
11. Xiong DZ, Yi Y, Zhu XG, Hu W. 2009. Controlled study on therapeutic effects of electroacupuncture and modified electric convulsive therapy on catatonic schizophrenia. *Zhongguo Zhen Jiu*. 29(10):804-6.
12. Jing Cheng, Gaohua Wang, Ling Xiao, Huiling Wang, Xiaoping Wang, Chengyan Li. 2009. Electro-acupuncture versus sham electro-acupuncture for auditory hallucinations in patients with schizophrenia: a randomized controlled trial. *Clin Rehabil.* 23(7):579-88.
13. Xiong DZ, Liu LL, Yi-Yan, Ye-Feng. 2010. Observation on the therapeutic effect of electroacupuncture combined with small dose of clozapine in clinical treatment of refractory schizophrenia. *Zhen Ci Yan Jiu*. 35(2):134-7.
14. Ronan P, Robinson N, Harbinson D, Macinnes D. 2011. A case study exploration of the value of acupuncture as an adjunct treatment for patients diagnosed with schizophrenia: results and future study design. *Zhong Xi Yi Jie He Xue Bao*. 9(5):503-14.

15. Bouhlel S, El-Hechmi S, Ghanmi L, Ghaouar M, Besbes C, Khaled M, Melki W, El-Hechmi Z. 2011. Effectiveness of acupuncture in treating schizophrenia: a clinical randomized trial of 31 patients. *Tunis Med.* 89(10):774-8.
16. Bosch P, van den Noort M, Yeo S, Lim S, Coenen A, van Luijtelaar G. 2015. The effect of acupuncture on mood and working memory in patients with depression and schizophrenia. *J Integr Med.* 13(6):380-90.
17. Lee MS, Shin BC, Ronan P, Ernst E. 2009. Acupuncture for schizophrenia: a systematic review and meta-analysis. *Int J Clin Pract.* 63(11):1622-33.
18. Shen X, Xia J, Adams CE. 2014. Acupuncture for schizophrenia. *Cochrane Database Syst Rev.* 10:CD005475.
19. Bosch P, van den Noort M, Staudte H, Lim S. 2015. Schizophrenia and Depression: A systematic Review of the Effectiveness and the Working Mechanisms Behind Acupuncture. *Explore (NY).* 11(4):281-91.

Chapter Nine

1. Coco A. 1999. Primary Dysmenorrhea, *Am Fam Physician.* 60(2):489-496.
2. Grandi G, Ferrari S, Xholli A, Cannoletta M, Palma F, Romani C, Volpe A, Cagnacci A. 2012. Prevalence of menstrual pain in young women: what is dysmenorrhea? *J Pain Res.* 5:169-74.
3. Zhou HG, Yang ZW. 2010. Students Group, Prevalence of dysmenorrhea in female students in a Chinese university: a prospective study, *Health.* 2(4):311-314.
4. Chia CF, Lai JH, Cheung PK, Kwong LT, Lau FP, Leung KH, Leung MT, Wong FC, Ngu SF. 2013. Dysmenorrhoea among Hong Kong university students: prevalence, impact, and management. *Hong Kong Med J.* 19(3):222-8.)
5. Bazarganipour F, Lamyian M, Heshmat R, Abadi MA, Taghavi A. 2010. A randomized clinical trial of the efficacy of applying a simple acupressure protocol to the Taichong point in relieving dysmenorrhea. *Int J Gynaecol Obstet.* 111(2):105-9.
6. Wu LL, Su CH, Liu CF. 2012. Effects of noninvasive electroacupuncture at Hegu (LI4) and Sanyinjiao (SP6) acupoints on dysmenorrhea: a randomized controlled trial. *J Altern Complement Med.* 18(2):137-42.
7. Xiong J, Liu F, Zhang MM, Wang W, Huang GY. 2012. De-qi, not psychological factors, determines the therapeutic efficacy of acupuncture treatment for primary dysmenorrhea. *Chin J Integr Med.*

18(1):7-15.

8. Ma YX, Ye XN, Liu CZ, Cai PY, Li ZF, Du DQ, Guo G, Chen SZ, Zhao JP, Liu JJ, Yi HQ, Gao SZ. 2013. A clinical trial of acupuncture about time-varying treatment and points selection in primary dysmenorrhea. *J Ethnopharmacol.* 148(2):498-504.
9. Liu YQ, Ma LX, Xing JM, Cao HJ, Wang YX, Tang L, Li M, Wang Y, Liang Y, Pu LY, Yu XM, Guo LZ, Jin JL, Wang Z, Ju HM, Jiang YM, Liu JJ, Yuan HW, Li CH, Zhang P, She YF, Liu JP, Zhu J. 2013. Does Traditional Chinese Medicine pattern affect acupoint specific effect? Analysis of data from a multicenter, randomized, controlled trial for primary dysmenorrhea. *J Altern Complement Med.* 19(1):43-9.
10. Kiran G, Gumusalan Y, Ekerbicer HC, Kiran H, Coskun A, Arikan DC. 2013. A randomized pilot study of acupuncture treatment for primary dysmenorrhea. *Eur J Obstet Gynecol Reprod Biol.* 169(2):292-5.
11. Liu CZ, Xie JP, Wang LP, Liu YQ, Song JS, Chen YY, Shi GX, Zhou W, Gao SZ, Li SL, Xing JM, Ma LX, Wang YX, Zhu J, Liu JP. 2014. A randomized controlled trial of single point acupuncture in primary dysmenorrhea. *Pain Med.* 15(6):910-20.
12. Zhao MY, Zhang P, Li J, Wang LP, Zhou W, Wang YX, She YF, Ma LX, Wang P, Hu NJ, Lin C, Hu SQ, Wu GW, Wang YF, Sun JJ, Jiang SZ, Zhu J. 2017. Influence of *de qi* on the immediate analgesic effect of SP6 acupuncture in patients with primary dysmenorrhoea and *cold and dampness stagnation*: a multicentre randomised controlled trial. *Acupunct Med.* 35(5):332-338.
13. Gao J, Wang Q, Xian S, Feng YM, Cao WX, Ye JY, Zhang QQ, Zou CL, Wu QG, Liu SJ. 2015. The effect of moxibustion on alleviating menstrual pain in a population of young nursing students: A prospective randomized cross-over pilot study. *Complement Ther Med.* 23(6):773-81.
14. Wade C, Wang L, Zhao WJ, Cardini F, Kronenberg F, Gui SQ, Ying Z, Zhao NQ, Chao MT, Yu J. 2016. Acupuncture point injection treatment of primary dysmenorrhoea: a randomised, double blind, controlled study. *BMJ Open.* 6(1):e008166.
15. Armour M, Dahlen HG, Smith CA. More Than Needles: 2016. The Importance of Explanations and Self-Care Advice in Treating Primary Dysmenorrhea with Acupuncture. *Evid Based Complement Alternat Med.* 2016:3467067.
16. Yang M, Chen X, Bo L, Lao L, Chen J, Yu S, Yu Z, Tang H, Yi L, Wu X, Yang J, Liang F. 2017. Moxibustion for pain relief in patients with primary dysmenorrhea: A randomized controlled trial. *PLoS One.* 12(2):e0170952.

17. Cha NH, Sok SR. 2016. Effects of Auricular Acupressure Therapy on Primary Dysmenorrhea for Female High School Students in South Korea. *J Nurs Scholarsh*. 48(5):508-16.
18. Armour M, Dahlen HG, Zhu X, Farquhar C, Smith CA. 2017. The role of treatment timing and mode of stimulation in the treatment of primary dysmenorrhea with acupuncture: An exploratory randomised controlled trial. *PLoS One*. 12(7):e0180177.
19. Bazarganipour F, Taghavi SA, Allan H, Hosseini N, Khosravi A, Asadi R, Salari S, Dehghani R, Jamshidi Z, Rezaei M, Saberian M, Javedan F, Salari Z, Miri F. 2017. A randomized controlled clinical trial evaluating quality of life when using a simple acupressure protocol in women with primary dysmenorrhea. *Complement Ther Med.* 34:10-15.
20. Gaubeca-Gilarranz A, Fernández-de-Las-Peñas C, Medina-Torres JR, Seoane-Ruiz JM, Company-Palonés A, Cleland JA, Arias-Buría JL. 2018. Effectiveness of dry needling of rectus abdominis trigger points for the treatment of primary dysmenorrhoea: a randomised parallel-group trial. *Acupunct Med.* 36(5):302-310.
21. Proctor ML, Smith CA, Farquhar CM, Stones RW. 2002. Transcutaneous electrical nerve stimulation and acupuncture for primary dysmenorrhoea. *Cochrane Database Syst Rev.* 1: CD002123.
22. Yang H, Liu CZ, Chen X, Ma LX, Xie JP, Guo NN, Ma ZB, Zheng YY, Zhu J, Liu JP. 2008. Systematic review of clinical trials of acupuncture-related therapies for primary dysmenorrhea. *Acta Obstet Gynecol Scand*. 87(11):1114-22.
23. Cho SH, Hwang EW. 2010. Acupuncture for primary dysmenorrhoea: a systematic review. *BJOG.* 117(5):509-21.
24. Smith CA, Zhu X, He L, Song J. 2011. Acupuncture for primary dysmenorrhoea. *Cochrane Database Syst Rev.* 1:CD007854.
25. Chung YC, Chen HH, Yeh ML.2012. Acupoint stimulation intervention for people with primary dysmenorrhea: Systematic review and meta-analysis of randomized trials. *Complement Ther Med.* 20(5):353-63.
26. Chen MN, Chien LW, Liu CF. 2013. Acupuncture or Acupressure at the Sanyinjiao (SP6) Acupoint for the Treatment of Primary Dysmenorrhea: A Meta-Analysis. *Evid Based Complement Alternat Med*. 2013:493038.
27. Xu T, Hui L, Juan YL, Min SG, Hua WT. 2014. Effects of moxibustion or acupoint therapy for the treatment of primary dysmenorrhea: a meta-analysis. Altern Ther Health Med. 20(4):33-42.
28. Smith CA, Armour M, Zhu X, Li X, Lu ZY, Song J. 2016. Acupuncture for dysmenorrhoea. *Cochrane Database Syst Rev.* 4:CD007854.

29. Abaraogu UO, Igwe SE, Tabansi-Ochiogu CS. 2016. Effectiveness of SP6 (Sanyinjiao) acupressure for relief of primary dysmenorrhea symptoms: A systematic review with meta- and sensitivity analyses. *Complement Ther Clin Pract*. 25:92-105.
30. Armour M, Smith CA. 2016. Treating primary dysmenorrhoea with acupuncture: a narrative review of the relationship between acupuncture 'dose' and menstrual pain outcomes. *Acupunct Med.* 34(6):416-424.
31. Xu Y, Zhao W, Li T, Bu H, Zhao Z, Zhao Y, Song S. 2017. Effects of acupoint-stimulation for the treatment of primary dysmenorrhoea compared with NSAIDs: a systematic review and meta-analysis of 19 RCTs. *BMC Complement Altern Med.* 17(1):436.
32. Stux G, Berman B, Pomeranz B. 2003. *Basics of Acupuncture*. 5th Edition, Springer.

Chapter Ten

1. Hofmeyr GJ, Hannah ME. 2003. Planned caesarean section for term breech delivery. *Cochrane Database Syst Rev*. 3:CD000166.
2. Lee HC, El-Sayed YY, Gould JB; 2008. Population trends in cesarean delivery for breech presentation in the United States, 1997-2003. *Am J Obstet Gynecol*. 199(1):59.e1-8.
3. Pasupathy D, Wood AM, Pell JP, et al; 2009. Time trend in the risk of delivery-related perinatal and neonatal death associated with breech presentation at term. *Int J Epidemiol*. 38(2):490-8.
4. *The Management of Breech Presentation,* 2006. Royal College of Obstetricians and Gynecologists.
5. Guittier MJ, Pichon M, Dong H, Irion O, Boulvain M. 2009. Moxibustion for breech version: a randomized controlled trial. *Obstet Gynecol*. 114(5):1034-40.
6. Mitchell M, Allen K. 2008. An exploratory study of women's experiences and key stakeholders views of moxibustion for cephalic version in breech presentation. *Complement Ther Clin Pract*. 14(4):264-72.
7. Smith CA, Betts D. 2014. The practice of acupuncture and moxibustion to promote cephalic version for women with a breech presentation: implications for clinical practice and research. *Complement Ther Med*. 22(1):75-80.
8. Cardini F, Basevi V, Valentini A, Martellato A. 1991. Moxibustion and breech presentation: preliminary results. *Am J Chin Med*. 19(2):105-14.